Medical Office Management and Technology
An Applied Approach

Brandy G. Ziesemer, MA, RHIA, CCS

Health Information Management Program Manager
Lake–Sumter State College
Leesburg, Florida

Wolters Kluwer | Lippincott Williams & Wilkins
Health

Philadelphia · Baltimore · New York · London
Buenos Aires · Hong Kong · Sydney · Tokyo

Acquisitions Editor: Michael Nobel
Product Manager: Paula C. Williams
Marketing Manager: Shauna Kelley
Designer: Steve Druding
Compositor: SPi Global

351 West Camden Street   **Two Commerce Square**
Baltimore, MD 21201   **2001 Market Street**
                                Philadelphia, PA 19103

Printed in the United States of America

Library of Congress Cataloging-in-Publication Data
Ziesemer, Brandy G.
   Medical office management and technology : an applied approach / Brandy G. Ziesemer. — 1st ed.
       p. ; cm.
   Includes bibliographical references and index.
   ISBN 978-1-60831-742-4
   I. Title.
   [DNLM: 1. Practice Management, Medical—organization & administration. 2. Medical Informatics—organization & administration.   W 80]
   610.68—dc23
                                                                            2011032651

DISCLAIMER
Care has been taken to confirm the accuracy of the information present and to describe generally accepted practices. However, the authors, editors, and publisher are not responsible for errors or omissions or for any consequences from application of the information in this book and make no warranty, expressed or implied, with respect to the currency, completeness, or accuracy of the contents of the publication. Application of this information in a particular situation remains the professional responsibility of the practitioner; the clinical treatments described and recommended may not be considered absolute and universal recommendations.

The authors, editors, and publisher have exerted every effort to ensure that drug selection and dosage set forth in this text are in accordance with the current recommendations and practice at the time of publication. However, in view of ongoing research, changes in government regulations, and the constant flow of information relating to drug therapy and drug reactions, the reader is urged to check the package insert for each drug for any change in indications and dosage and for added warnings and precautions. This is particularly important when the recommended agent is a new or infrequently employed drug.

Some drugs and medical devices presented in this publication have Food and Drug Administration (FDA) clearance for limited use in restricted research settings. It is the responsibility of the health care provider to ascertain the FDA status of each drug or device planned for use in their clinical practice.

To purchase additional copies of this book, call our customer service department at (800) 638-3030 or fax orders to (301) 223-2320. International customers should call (301) 223-2300.

Visit Lippincott Williams & Wilkins on the Internet: http://www.lww.com. Lippincott Williams & Wilkins customer service representatives are available from 8:30 am to 6:00 pm, EST.

                                        9 8 7 6 5 4 3

practice both administrative and clinical application, using a robust and integrated practice management and electronic health record system (Optum).

Text Features

- **Learning Outcomes** at the beginning of each chapter guide both students and instructors to the material in the chapter and help to prepare you for the information provided.
- **Leadership Boxes** highlight leadership concepts and how they relate to medical office management.
- **Case Studies** provide real-world examples throughout the text to illustrate key concepts.
- **Video Clips** feature scenarios related to the case studies and are included on thePoint Web site.
- **Key Terms** appear at the beginning of each chapter and are highlighted throughout the text with definitions in the margin.
- **Tips** illustrate a best-practice approach for a management task.
- **Chapter Review Questions** appear at the end of each chapter and challenge students to use critical thinking to recall concepts and theories learned in each chapter.
- **Workbook Activities** are included at the end of each chapter to allow students to apply the management principles that they have learned.
- The **Glossary** lists terms and definitions at the end of the text.
- The **Appendix** includes forms frequently used by medical office managers.

It is exciting to present a comprehensive set of resources (text, workbook, and Web-based ancillaries) that help prepare future medical office managers and practice administrators as well as supplement the knowledge and skills of existing medical managers in the demands of today's medical practice.

The physician practice is a key component in the delivery of health care in the United States. As an aging population looks toward longer life expectancy, the fact remains that older people tend to have numerous chronic health conditions to manage. When these conditions are not in an acute phase, physicians of various specialties coordinate the care for these patients in addition to providing routine and nonroutine care to patients of all ages on a daily basis.

Over the past several years, the business side of medicine has grown more complex with increasing regulations and data collection needed to obtain proper reimbursement and to avoid penalties. Practices have more complicated coding requirements and these requirements change frequently. There is a national plan to increase the use of health information technology, such as electronic health records and health information exchange networks with penalties for practices that do not meet the requirements. These systems require ever-increasing vigilance on the part of health care professionals as well as policies and procedures to protect patient security. At the same time, new methods of protecting consumers from medical identity theft are being introduced.

All of these changes contribute to the need for very strong administration of medical practices. Physicians and other clinicians should be able to dedicate all of their time to practicing medicine. This ideal is only possible with strong leadership in practice management and administration.

Today's practice administrators and managers must be knowledgeable about competition, marketing, technology, reimbursement, confidentiality, privacy, security, and relationships between physicians and other health care entities. The successful leader will also be savvy at motivating a staff to work as a team to build patient loyalty and continually improve the performance of all aspects of the practice.

ADDITIONAL RESOURCES

Medical Office Management and Technology: An Applied Approach includes additional resources for both instructors and students that are available on the book's companion Web site at http://thePoint.lww.com/Ziesemer.

Instructor Resources

Approved adopting instructors will be given access to the following additional resources:

- PowerPoint Presentations
- Test Bank
- Answers to Chapter Review Questions and Workbook Suggestions and Answers
- Lesson Plans

Student Resources

Students who have purchased *Medical Office Management and Technology: An Applied Approach* have access to the following additional resources:

- Interactive Question Bank
- Video Clips
- Abbreviations
- EHR Activities: Real-world application exercises and Web-based practice management with electronic health record software transactions

In addition, purchasers of the text can access the searchable full text online by going to the *Medical Office Management and Technology: An Applied Approach* Web site at http://thePoint.lww.com/Ziesemer. See the inside front cover of this text for more details, including the passcode you will need to gain access to the Web site.

The author is delighted to have this opportunity to work closely with Lippincott Williams & Wilkins and their competent and dedicated staff in developing a textbook that is both relevant to the needs of the health professions and critical in meeting the ever-increasing expectations of a watchful and wary public.

Brandy G. Ziesemer, MA, RHIA, CCS
AHIMA Approved ICD-10-CM/PCS Trainer
Health Information Program Manager/Associate Professor
Lake–Sumter State College
Leesburg, Florida

CONTRIBUTORS

Robert E. Hoyt, MD, FACP
Director, Medical Informatics
University of West Florida
Pensacola, Florida
Assistant Professor of Medicine
Adjunct Assistant Professor of Family Medicine
Uniformed Services University of the Health Sciences
Bethesda, Maryland

Sandi L. Zeljko, PhD
Instructor, School of Business & Technology
Excelsior College
Albany, New York
Program Manager/Faculty, Bachelor of Applied Science
    in Organizational Management
Lake–Sumter State College
Leesburg, Florida

Thomas G. Ziesemer, JD, MS
Associate Professor, Criminal Justice
College of Central Florida
Ocala, Florida

ACKNOWLEDGMENTS

A special thank-you to the following individuals for their positive input on
improving the quality of this book and ancillaries:

Michael Baxter, MBA
Richard and Karen Blanchette (PAHCOM)
Rita E. Crews, MHSA, PA-C
Steve Verno, CMBS, CEMCS, CMSCS, CPM-MCS
Alexander Ziesemer, RN

REVIEWERS

Lori Andrews, ASN, BS, MSEd
Medical Assisting Program Chair
Department of Medical Assisting
Ivy Tech Community College
Indianapolis, Indiana

Katie Barton, LPN, BA
Director of Allied Health
Allied Health Department
Savannah River College
Augusta, Georgia

Brenda Edwards, LPN, CPC, CPC-I, CEMC
Medical Support Faculty
Clinical Documentation Specialist
Minnesota State Colleges & Winona Health
Winona, Minnesota

Cyndi Ferguson, AAS, RHIT
Instructor
Allied Health
Texas State Technical College
Sweetwater, Texas

Terri Fleming, BSN, MS
Health Sciences/Medical Assisting
Ivy Tech Community College
Indianapolis, Indiana

Cheri Goretti, MA, BS
Medical Assisting Professor and Program Director
Quinebaug Valley Community College
Danielson, Connecticut

Rosalie Jaenisch, MBC, BS, BA
Instructor
HIT and Medical Coding
Ridgewater College
Willmar, Minnesota

Wendyanne Jex, MPA-HS
Program Department Chair
Medical Office Management
School of Health Sciences
Kaplan University
Fort Lauderdale, Florida

Teresa Jolly, MA
Instructor
Business Department
South Georgia Technical College
Cordele, Georgia

JoAnn Jordan, MPH
Assistant Professor
Health Information Technologies
Springfield Technical Community College
Springfield, Massachusetts

Paul Lucas, AA
Medical Assisting Program Director
Medical Assisting and Health Care Administration
Brown Mackie College
Fort Wayne, Indiana

Jeanne McTeigue, CPC, CMA
Director of Allied Health Programs
Medical Assisting and Medical Billing
Branford Hall Career Institute
Albany, New York

Lane Miller, MBA/HCM
LMS Administrator
LMS and Continuing Education
Medical Careers Institute
Virginia Beach, Virginia

Kimberly Rash, AAS
Adjunct Instructor
Medical Information Technology
Gateway Community & Technical College
Edgewood, Kentucky

Georgina Sampson, BS
Program Director
Health Information Technology and Medical Coding
Anoka Technical College
Anoka, Minnesota

Tamera Schulze, AA
Medical Department Chair
Medical Administrative Assisting
Medical Coding and Billing and Medical Assisting
Antonelli College
Cincinnati, Ohio

Geri Kale-Smith, MS, CMA
Coordinator
Medical Office Administration Programs
Health Administration
Harper College
Palatine, Illinois

Kerri Yingst, BA
Adjunct Faculty
Health Information Management
Ivy Tech Community College
Bloomington, Indiana

CONTENTS

Chapter 7 Managing Quality and Performance Improvement 149

Chapter 8 Customer Service, Patient Loyalty, and Marketing 173

Chapter 9 Managing the Legal Aspects of Health Information 197

Chapter 10 Managing Health Information Technology   225

Chapter 11 Managing the Physicians and Keeping Up with Emerging Trends   259

1

The Basics of Today's Medical Offices

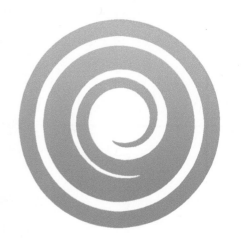

LEARNING OUTCOMES

Upon completion of this chapter, the student should...

- Describe strategic goals that guide most medical practices
- Document the flow of work in a modern medical office
- List the main tasks performed in each step of the workflow
- Define the revenue cycle
- List the most common positions on the medical office team
- Describe the most important aspects of the relationship between the managing physician and the practice manager or administrator
- Explain the major external forces influencing medical practices in the United States today

KEY TERMS

Ad Hoc
Adjudication
Allowed Amount
Center for Medicare & Medicaid Services (CMS)
Certified Coder Specialist, Physician Based (CCS-P)
Certified Professional Coder (CPC)
Chain of Command
Claim
Clearinghouse
Covered benefit
Current Procedural Terminology (CPT)®
Electronic Health Records
Encoder
Established Patient
Explanation of Benefits
Federal Register

Health Insurance Portability and Accountability Act (HIPAA)
International Classification of Diseases (ICD)
Medical Necessity
New Patient
Participating Physician
Physician Extender
Practice Management (PM) System
Registered Health Information Administrator (RHIA)
Registered Health Information Technician (RHIT)
Registration Form
Remittance Advice (RA)
Revenue Cycle
SOAP Order
Source Document
Superbill
Voice Recognition

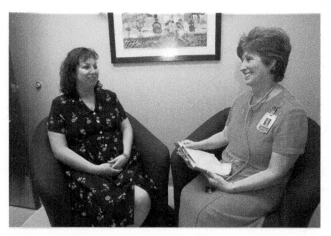

Figure 1.1 Teammember smiling at patient after communicating care instructions.

OVERVIEW

Although a career in any aspect of health care is an ever-changing, lifelong learning commitment, there are aspects of a successful health care practice that have endured through the decades and continue to be keys to success. These aspects provide a foundation of excellence in leadership and team building, based on the premise that the single most critical factor for an outstanding medical practice is a loyal patient base (Fig. 1.1). Patient loyalty is the hallmark of an outstanding medical practice and requires every single employee to consistently embrace the following principles outlined in Fred Lee's book "If Disney Ran Your Hospital: 9½ Things You Would Do Differently." These principles are

- Sense people's needs before they ask (initiative)
- Help each other out (teamwork)
- Acknowledge people's feelings (empathy)
- Respect the dignity and privacy of everyone (courtesy)
- Explain what's happening (communications)[1]

Case Study

JANE AND MRS. JONES

Jane, the billing supervisor, is meeting with Mrs. Jones, the widow of a recently deceased patient. Mrs. Jones is also a patient. Mr. Jones had not been ill. He had been rushed to the hospital where it was determined he had an aortic abdominal aneurysm. He was admitted through the ED for emergency surgery. He died during the operation. Jane works for the patient's primary care physician who had gone to the ED and stayed with the patient until the patient was sedated for surgery. Mrs. Jones is still somewhat shocked at having lost her husband so unexpectedly (he had been in his late 50s and otherwise healthy). She is trying to figure out all of the charges from this practice, what her husband's policy will pay and how to make arrangements to make small payments on the balances since she is losing her husband's income and is only getting enough for burial expenses from the small life insurance policy her husband carried.

What would you do?

One good approach for Jane is to use the SHARE principles as a guide in her meeting with Mrs. Jones. For example, in order to sense or anticipate needs, acknowledge feelings, and respect the patient's dignity, one has to listen first. Jane was so busy "doing her job" of collecting money due to the practice that she was missing the point altogether—Mrs. Jones wasn't trying to get out of paying, she was simply trying to verify that the amounts on the statements were correct and to see if there was a way to make payments instead of paying everything at once. Had Jane listened more carefully, she would have acknowledged Mrs. Jones's feelings not only about the sudden loss of her husband but also about the humiliation of not being able to pay her debt immediately after being accustomed to doing so. Therefore, Jane would have respected the dignity of the patient and explained the charges thoroughly. She then would have asked Mrs. Jones if she thought she'd be able to make payments with no interest of at least $75.00 per month until the debt was settled. The practice would have had a loyal patient and still be paid the full amount owed.

GOALS OF A MEDICAL PRACTICE

The overarching goal of any medical practice is to provide exceptional, accessible health care, as efficiently as possible, so that the practice can focus on its health care mission from a financially secure base of operations. This goal is achieved by a management philosophy that

- Focuses on the SHARE principles above
- Uses effective tools to measure the degree to which the practice achieves its desired outcomes on a regular basis—clinical and financial
- Promotes awareness of the internal and external environment to identify problematic areas, opportunities for improvement, and emerging changes that may impact the practice
- Facilitates a team approach to resolving issues, implementing changes efficiently, and continually improving performance (Fig. 1.2)

THE FLOW OF WORK IN A MODERN MEDICAL OFFICE

Several steps are common to almost any medical practice with regard to treating patients and getting reimbursed properly for the services provided. The steps are subdivided based on whether the patient has

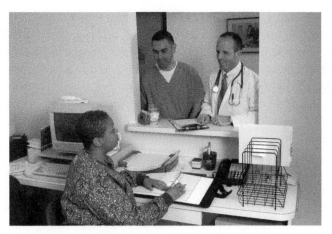

Figure 1.2 Teammembers working together.

been to this practice previously for any type of service. Either way, the first step is to get the patient registered. This can be accomplished via a practice Web site or by the patient calling the office to schedule an appointment. Figure 1.3 demonstrates a typical outpatient office workflow. Later in this book, the workflow is discussed in further detail from the perspective of the benefits available by using practice management software integrated with a robust electronic health record system.

Patient Registration

This step includes obtaining demographic information, including any health care plan or plans the patient has and establishing which member

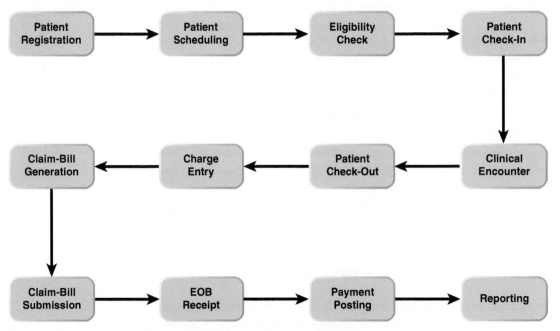

Figure 1.3 Typical outpatient office workflow (EOB, explanation of benefits).

of the patient's household is financially responsible for any amount that is not covered by insurance. Depending on the type of insurance, there may be an amount that is paid by the patient, to the practice, at the time of the office visit. In other cases, the patient may have a balance due to the practice after claims adjudication. Adjudication means that any health insurance company to which the practice submitted a bill on behalf of the patient has paid the full amount they are going to pay for those services.

Adjudication: The determination by a third party of its financial obligations after applying the patient's health insurance benefits to a claim.

Patient Scheduling

Once financial responsibility is determined, the patient is then scheduled for an appointment. If the patient is an established patient, meaning he or she has been seen by a physician in the same practice and of the same specialty within the past 3 years, or, if a physician from the practice has seen the patient previously in the hospital, the patient will be in the database. The receptionist simply has to update any changes to the patient information that is already on file.

Established Patient: A patient who has been seen by the same physician or another physician of the same specialty in the same practice within 3 years of a current appointment.

Eligibility Check

If the patient is a new patient to the practice, meaning he or she has not seen any physician of the same specialty in the practice during the previous 3 years, the insurance information given by the patient must be verified to ensure (A) the patient is a current member of the health plan, and (B) the planned services are a covered benefit. If the practice does not participate with that particular plan, the patient must be notified in advance of the visit so they can decide if they want to cancel the appointment and find a participating physician. A participating physician is one who agrees to accept the amount a health insurance plan allows for a service as payment in full. For example, if the physician bills the insurance company $110 for a service, and the insurance company only allows $100 for that service, a participating physician will write off the $10 difference while a nonparticipating physician is able to charge the patient for that extra $10. If a patient has an insurance plan that will pay regardless of whether the physician is a participating member, but the patient's share of cost is less when the services are conducted by a participating physician, the patient may agree to pay a greater share of cost because of the reputation of that physician for a specific type of treatment.

New Patient: A patient who has not been seen by the same physician or another physician of the same specialty in the same practice within 3 years of a current appointment.

Covered Benefit: A term referring to whether a specific third-party payer reimburses for certain services or procedures. For example, one plan may cover an annual physical exam for all of its participants and another may only pay for physicals for children of certain ages.

Participating Physician: A physician who is contractually bound to a particular program (e.g., one enrolled in the Medicare program) and agrees to accept compensation thereunder.

Patient Check-In

The patient arrives and signs in at the receptionist's desk at the time a visit has been scheduled. If the patient is new, and the data gathered to schedule an appointment was obtained via telephone, the patient is asked to complete a registration form which contains all pertinent contact information and financial information such as health insurance coverage and who is financially responsible for the services provided, and provide a copy of his or her insurance card(s). Any information not

Registration Form: Forms, checklists, and guidelines to meet the management needs of registration department in hospitals and health care providers.

Practice Management System (PM): A system (modernly software) that deals with the day-to-day operations of a medical practice allowing for the capture of patient demographics, scheduling of appointments, maintenance of lists of insurance payers, performance of billing tasks, and generation of reports and which is often connected to and overlapping with the electronic health records system.

Source Document: A document in which data collected for a clinical trial is first recorded.

Physician Extender: A health care provider who is not a physician but who performs medical activities typically performed by a physician, most commonly a nurse practitioner or physician assistant.

SOAP Order: A standardized method of documentation of patient symptoms, diagnosis, and care consisting of subjective component, objective component, application or assessment, and plan.

Voice Recognition: A combination of speaker recognition (recognizing who is speaking) and speech recognition (recognizing what is being said). It uses learned aspects of a speaker's voice to determine what is being said. Many electronic medical records (EMRs) applications can be more effective and may be performed more easily when deployed in conjunction with a speech–recognition engine.

Electronic Health Records (EHRs): An electronic record of health-related information on an individual that conforms to nationally recognized interoperability standards and that can be created, managed, and consulted by authorized clinicians and staff across more than on health care organization.

previously obtained is keyed into the computer system for use by the practice management (PM) system, which is a specialized software that provides the practice with computerized tools to manage the process of getting reimbursed for services rendered, and the source document (registration form in this example but any original document from which information is keyed into a computer system) is filed in the paper medical record, if applicable. Electronic registration is covered in a later chapter.

Clinical Encounter

The patient is seen by a physician extender, such as a nurse, to have vitals taken, blood and urine samples collected, if needed, and the patient's medical history, which is considered subjective because the patient is not a medical professional, updated. The patient is then examined by the physician who completes a physical exam, which is considered objective because the physician is using medical knowledge to perform the examination, including any test results (Fig. 1.4). The physician then makes an assessment of the patient's specific condition and any other conditions that need to be addressed. Finally, the physician determines a plan of treatment for this patient. The physician documents this clinical aspect of the patient encounter in what is called SOAP order because the order is Subjective (history), Objective (exam), Assessment, and Plan. In a paper system, the physician dictates either during the visit or as soon afterward as possible and a transcriptionist creates a paper copy of the notes. Alternatively, some physicians use voice recognition technology to dictate directly into a laptop or other device, and then print out the report generated by the software to file in the paper record. For a sample of a full range of voice recognition software that can be used as a stand-alone product for creating a paper document or that interfaces with electronic health records (EHRs), visit Nuance's corporate Web site.[2] Other options for inputting clinical information using an EHR are discussed in a later chapter.

Patient Checkout

The patient is discharged after a receptionist collects any money due and schedules any follow-up visits (Fig. 1.5). The patient is given paper

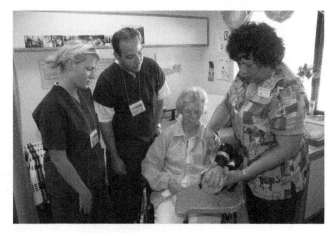

Figure 1.4 A patient's clinical encounter.

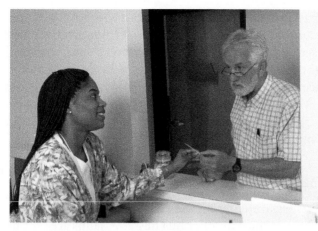

Figure 1.5 Patient receives appointment card during checkout.

Current Procedural Terminology (CPT): A copyrighted coding system by the American Medical Association that provides a listing of descriptive terms and identifying codes for reporting medical services and procedures performed by physicians and other qualified practitioners.

copies of any physician orders for tests or prescriptions for facilities not linked using either an EHR or any electronic prescribing or electronic patient referral systems.

Charge Entry

In a stand-alone PM system (not affiliated with an EHR), the charges are keyed into the system. The charges are linked to Current Procedural Terminology (CPT)® codes. CPT is a registered medical coding system consisting of five-digit codes, which provides standardized descriptions of surgeries, other procedures, and services performed by a physician or other qualified practitioner. CPT is a registered, proprietary system published and maintained annually by the American Medical Association (AMA). In order to select an appropriate CPT code, the medical necessity must be demonstrated by one or more codes from the International Classification of Diseases (ICD) codebook that describe the condition or conditions that required the services. Many practices have the clinicians complete a superbill. See Figure 1.6 for an

International Classification of Diseases (ICD): The official system used to code and classify health conditions, reasons for encounters with health professionals, inpatient hospital procedures for the use of the facility, and other health-related information.

Superbill: An itemized form utilized by health care providers for reflecting rendered services; the main data source for creation of a health care claim, which will be submitted to payers (insurances, funds, and programs) for reimbursement.

Patient Information (Name, Address, Account Number...)	Payment/Third Party Payer Information	Encounter Information (Date, Physician Name...)		
Diagnosis:		**Other, Not on Form:**		
_X_ **250.00** Diabetes Mellitus, Not Otherwise Specified		*2nd degree burn on wrist from a hot iron; New patient history and physical; patient is diabetic.*		
____ Diabetes Mellitus (see 250.00-250.93)				
____ **401.9** Hypertension, Not Otherwise Specified		*Code(s) 944.27,*		
____ Hypertensive Disease (401-405; note 4th/5th digits)		*E924.8* ____		

Procedures by Category:							
E&M – New	**Code**	**Charge**	**Modifier**	**Injuries**	**Code**	**Charge**	**Modifier**
X Level I (Lowest)	99201	$55.00	25	__Initial Burn	16000	____	
__Level II	99202	____	____	X Dress/debrid	16020	$90.00	____
__Level III	99203	____	____	__Eschar...		____	____

Figure 1.6 Excerpt from a superbill.

excerpt of a superbill that contains a list of the most common diagnostic and procedure codes for a given practice. Other practices have a medical coder, described later in this chapter, who reviews the medical record and selects the appropriate codes based on the documentation. Whether the practice uses a superbill or a professional coder, the codes are keyed into the PM system. All the other information required, such as patient name, address, and date of birth, is already in the PM system from the registration process.

Claim Generation and Submission

Claim: A standardized document—CMS 1500 in the case of health care practitioners containing all necessary information and submitted to a third-party payer in order for the practitioner to be reimbursed for eligible services provided to a patient who has health insurance.

Once the codes are entered, the PM system creates a claim, which is like a bill or an invoice in other businesses. Claims are sent to the payers electronically in all but rare cases, but they are sent in cycles so once the PM system is updated, the claim is in queue waiting for transmission to a claims' clearinghouse. A clearinghouse is a service that checks the claim data for accuracy (e.g., male having a female-only procedure, or a 50-year-old patient having a pediatric physical examination) and once it is free of errors, it routes the claims to the appropriate payer in batches. If a clearinghouse is not used, the claims are electronically sent directly to the payer such as Medicare.

Clearinghouse: Practices submit electronic claims to clearinghouses where the claims are scrubbed, formatted, and sent in real time to the appropriate insurance companies in a format acceptable by each insurance company regardless of the software used in the originating medical office.

Receipt of Remittance Advice (RA) and Explanation of Benefits (EOB)

Remittance Advice (RA): A notice of payments and adjustments sent to providers, billers, and suppliers after a claim has been received and processed.

After the claim is sent, the payer electronically (again, there are some exceptions in which the practice will actually get a paper check in the mail) sends a Remittance Advice (RA) to the physician containing the details for each charge paid or denied in that cycle. An RA can contain payment and denial details for multiple patients. The part of the RA that details any reasons for denied charges, reduced payments, patient responsibility, physician responsibility, or whether the balance was automatically transmitted to a secondary payer is the explanation of benefits (EOB) portion. An individual EOB is also mailed to each patient. Figure 1.7 shows an excerpt from an RA. A complete manual for reading a Medicare Remittance Advice is available free through the Medicare Learning Network at the following Web site: http://www.cms.gov/MLNProducts/downloads/RA_Guide_Full_03-22-06.pdf. The first half is the guide to institutional (e.g., hospital) RAs and the second half is the professional guide.

Explanation of Benefits (EOB): A statement from a third-party payer that explains to the patient the result of processing a claim and explains any amount that was not paid for that service.

Payment Posting

Allowed Amount: The amount a third-party payer determines is the full value of a specific service or procedure. Therefore, the total of a patient's responsibility plus the payer's responsibility will not exceed this amount.

The money generated for a given RA is electronically deposited into the practice's account. Billing team members also have to follow-up when a person has more than one payer, to determine that the claim was transmitted to the appropriate secondary payer. If there is still a balance after the biller has applied payments and written off any charges in excess of the allowed amount for a particular payer, which is the full amount that payer allows for that service regardless of what the physician normally charges, the system moves the balance into a queue to await patient

PERF PROV SRVC DATE POS NOS PROC MODS BILLED ALWD DED COINS GRP/RC AMT PROVPD											

NAME DOE JOE   HIC 9999999999 ACNNT DOEO1234566-01 ICN 010101010101 ASG Y, MOA MA01

11223344   0110 011020XX 11 1   99213   XX   66.00   49.83   0.34   9.97   PR-96   16.17   39.52

PT RESP 10.31   CLAIM TOTALS 66.00   49.83   0.34   9.97   16.17

　 NET 39.52

(Messages are in the online manual with MA01 simply stating the right to appeal if the provider doesn't agree with this determination of payment. Any other services for this patient on this RA would be below the first line with a different PROC. The top line and bottom line have their own headings but the headings for the middle line are on top of the first line in bold print. All other patients processed at this same time would be listed on the RA)

Figure 1.7 Excerpt from a paper remittance advice.

billing. The biller is also responsible for tracking claims and initiating the collections process if a balance due by the patient is not paid in a timely fashion.

Reporting

Daily reports are run and verified to ensure deposits match, all patients who were seen that day have charges in the system, etc. There are both routine reports (daily, weekly, monthly, quarterly, and end of year) and ad hoc or "as needed" reports used by the practice.

Ad Hoc: A committee or report that is not routine but formed or generated as needed for a specific purpose.

Telephone Calls in a Medical Office

Calls to the practice may be for various reasons from cancelling an appointment to asking if the doctor can see a patient who does not have an appointment. The calls should be prioritized into categories for emergency (in which the practice should advise the patient to hang up and dial 911 and then confirm the patient is capable of doing that before disconnecting), urgent, or nonurgent (Fig. 1.8). Strategies for optimizing efficiency in handling telephone calls are discussed in more detail

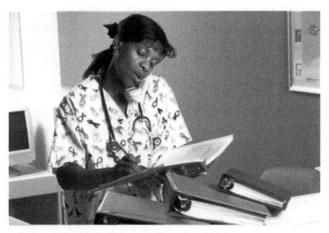

Figure 1.8 A member of the team takes a telephone call from a patient.

later in this book. It is important to realize that before any decisions are made about the various telephone technologies available, the manager needs to keep patient loyalty in the forefront and then develop a total telephone protocol which includes staff training and a solid plan for what to automate, what will be handled by a service, if applicable, and what to make available to the patient for speaking to a real person who works in that office.

THE MOST COMMON POSITIONS ON THE MEDICAL OFFICE TEAM

Several factors influence the level and diversity of positions in medical offices. The size of the practice with regard to both the number of physicians and the number of active patients typically help physicians determine the most appropriate level of the nonphysician administrator. Another factor is the degree to which one or more of the physicians choose to be involved in the day-to-day operations of the practice. The person at the highest level of nonclinical management is often called a practice administrator. Other titles include practice manager or office manager. Office managers may be the sole nonclinical member of management in a small practice or they may report to a practice manager or practice administrator in a larger office. Other titles found in larger offices to designate team members who report to an administrator include assistant managers or supervisors.

In a midsized practice, the most common positions and general qualifications usually include the following titles.

Practice Manager or Administrator

The practice manager or administrator must possess a unique combination of leadership ability, health-related business and technical knowledge, and the skills necessary to collaboratively manage routine and problematic processes. Collaboration is important so that all staff have an ownership stake in the solutions to problems or changes that are made to improve performance or to comply with new rules.

Registered Health Information Technician (RHIT): Individuals who have been trained and certified by examination to be licensed as a health information technician.

Registered Health Information Administrator (RHIA): Administrators who design and manage medical information systems, ensuring efficient record keeping while meeting state and federal requirements for medical confidentiality.

In a midsized practice, the practice manager or administrator typically has a college degree (associate or bachelor's) in health information management, business administration with a medical office specialization, health services administration, health care management, nursing, medical assisting, or another health-related field. For example, an experienced registered health information technician (RHIT), or registered health information administrator (RHIA), possess the knowledge and skills necessary to effectively manage a midsized or large practice. Another good candidate may be an experienced registered nurse (RN) with a bachelor's or master's degree in nursing or health administration. Ideally, any of these candidates should have experience either supervising in a large practice or managing a smaller one. A good career path for any allied health professional (e.g., medical assistant, registered nurse, coder specialist, or health information technician) interested in practice management is to obtain increasingly more challenging supervisory experience while taking college courses that focus on the business and technology aspects of health care and participating in professional development educational opportunities. The ideal candidate in a midsized practice will be a person who embraces lifelong learning, excels in all levels of communications and customer service, motivates people to stay on top of their game, and is savvy about optimizing the value of all investments in technology.

For more information on some of the more common professional organizations and certifications available specifically for medical practice management, visit the following Web sites: Professional Association of Health Care Office Management (PAHCOM) at www.pahcom.com, Practice Management Institute (PMI) at www.pmimd.com, Physician Office Managers Association of America (POMAA) at www.pomaa.net, and the Association of Registered Health Care Professionals (ARHCP) at www.iarhcp.org.

Assistant Manager, Supervisor, or Office Manager

In a midsized or large practice, the practice administrator may hire a health information technician or someone with equivalent knowledge to assist him or her with the management of health information and technology. This position is ideal for a recent graduate of a health information or informatics associate or bachelor's degree because it enables a person to develop the leadership aspect of a career under the coaching of a strong mentor. Meanwhile, these recent graduates already have a lot of knowledge and technical skills as a foundation to assist with the creation, maintenance, and communication of policies and procedures pertaining to any compliance requirements such as all aspects of the Health Insurance Portability and Accountability Act (HIPAA). An RHIT is also able to audit medical record documentation for compliance with rules and regulations. A health information technician is able to run reports from the PM system to help identify areas for performance improvement. A health information professional is also able to assist with workflow analysis and with the management of implementing and maintaining an electronic health record system. If neither the administrator nor the assistant manager are formally trained in health information management, then a health information technician with a degree from an accredited health informatics and/ or information management program should be hired to assist with all medical record compliance issues even if this person is also responsible for coding medical records.

Health Insurance Portability and Accountability Act (HIPAA): A law designed to define privacy standards in order to protect the privacy, confidentiality, and security of patient-specific health information.

Medical Coder, Biller, or Insurance Specialist

There are several options regarding coders and billers depending on whether the practice needs a professional to code from the medical record (paper or electronic) or if the clinicians use a superbill to select the appropriate diagnosis and procedure codes. If the practice does not use a superbill, an RHIT, a certified coder specialist, physician based (CCS-P), a certified professional coder (CPC), or other coding professional is able to code medical records without the use of a superbill.

Certified Coder Specialist, Physician Based (CCS-P): A credential offered through the American Health Information Management Association designating a professional coder specializing in the coding of physician-based documentation.

Certified Professional Coder (CPC): A credential offered through the American Association of Professional Coders designating a professional coder specializing in the coding of physician-based documentation.

Visit the following Web sites to learn about some of the professional organizations and certifications available for medical coder and billing specialists: The American Health Information Management Association (AHIMA) at www.ahima.org; The American Academy of Professional Coders (AAPC) at www.aapc.com; Medical Association of Billers (MAB) at www.e-medbill.com; Professional Association of Healthcare Coding Specialists (PAHCS) at www.pahcs.org; Professional Medical Billers Association (PMBA) at www.pmbausa.com; and National Certification Services—Med-Certification (NCS-MC) at www.med-certification.com.

If a superbill is used, a medical biller or an insurance specialist inputs the coded data into the practice management system. In some EHR systems that are interfaced or integrated with the PM software, a module that is called an encoder actually contains logic necessary to assess key terms from the data that is input into the EHR and to assign appropriate codes. In this instance, experienced insurance specialists double-check the codes to see if there are any inconsistencies. They are able to correct many inconsistencies by looking at information in the EHR.

In this case, as with the superbill, it is important to realize that sometimes physicians perform services that would legitimately increase the level of code and generate more reimbursement but they don't know what information the system needs to assign the best code. So, the auditor actually investigates a case by discussing it with the physician. For example, if the auditor notices a low-level code on a patient with severe systemic illness, the auditor asks the physician specific questions to see if the physician examined a body system more thoroughly than the documentation indicates. If yes, the auditor educates the physician regarding what to be sure is included in the documentation. On the other hand, if the diagnosis is something mild but the physician documents comprehensive history and physical exam which results in a higher code, the auditor has to explain that even if the physician performs these services at this level, the diagnosis does not justify the medical necessity of a comprehensive exam and the physician may have the reimbursement level dropped to that of a lower code or even be fined.

Remember from the workflow described earlier, the reimbursement process is initiated when a scheduled appointment is first entered into the system by a receptionist. Upon the patient's arrival for an appointment, the receptionist initiates the collection of encounter data in the PM system. The process of obtaining reimbursement, from initiation of that service through final payment, is called the revenue cycle.

Physician Assistant (PA), Nurse Practitioner (NP)

The degree to which a PA or an NP is licensed to perform certain procedures or services without the supervision of a physician may vary from state to state. In general, however, when a PA or an NP is employed by a medical practice, these professionals work under the supervision (the physician must be immediately available if needed) of a physician to perform procedures that are necessary as part of the patient's overall care, but the procedures or services are considered an incidental extension of the physician's services. For example, the physician may be in an examining room with one patient while a PA or an NP is in another

---

Encoder: Software that facilitates coding medical records by providing sophisticated search tools and logic. Encoders contain updates from coding resources for ICD, CPT, and HCPC codes.

Medical Necessity: A set of predetermined conditions for which a certain procedure or service is considered to be necessary for health purposes and therefore eligible for reimbursement by a third party. An example is urinalysis. Medicare may pay for this test under certain circumstances but not others.

Revenue Cycle: The process businesses use to describe the financial progression of their accounts receivables from the very beginning, when they first acquire product or deliver a service until they get paid and/or clear the balance owed.

examining room giving a different patient a steroid injection to treat an arthritic shoulder. Even if the patient doesn't physically see a physician during a specific encounter, the physician is the one who initially signed off on the plan of care for that patient's specific condition that included the administration of steroid injections.

Registered Nurse (RN), Licensed Practical Nurse (LPN), Certified Medical Assistant ([CMA] trained in both clinical and office administrative functions), Certified Nurse Assistant (CNA), and other clinical allied health professionals such as various technicians and therapists are involved in direct patient care at various levels. These professionals extend a physician's ability to care for more patients because, within the constraints of their licensure, they are able to provide direct patient care at the appropriate level while the physicians are seeing other patients. For example, a CMA who is also certified to draw blood (phlebotomy) may take all of the patient's vital signs, check blood pressure, weight, and height, collect a urine specimen, collect a blood specimen, check blood sugar, etc., before the patient sees the physician.

Receptionist

The receptionist is responsible for many steps in the office workflow: patient registration, scheduling, referrals, eligibility checks, patient check-in, and patient checkout. The receptionist is also responsible for answering the telephone and either taking a message or forwarding the call to the appropriate person. In addition to excellent technical skills, the receptionist is the first person many patients encounter and therefore, the crucial "first impression" by the patient must be very favorable. If it isn't, it's very hard to convince that patient that the practice is patient centric.

Medical Records, Clerical Support

Some degree of clerical support is needed in a medical practice regardless of the degree of automation (Fig. 1.9). In a practice with paper medical records, clerical support is needed to prepare new charts, file reports in the proper format in the medical record, file and retrieve the record itself, make copies, and to fax authorized reports from the medical

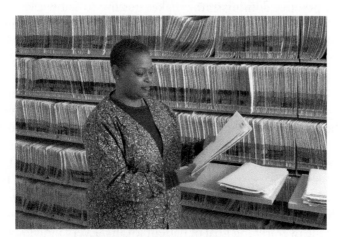

Figure 1.9 Medical records clerk team member.

record to other medical facilities. In an office that uses an EHR, clerical workers scan documents and shred original paper copies as appropriate.

THE RELATIONSHIP BETWEEN PHYSICIANS AND THE PRACTICE ADMINISTRATOR

Unlike many professionals, physicians are accustomed to being independent of supervision even when they work for another physician. This independence is important because every time a doctor cares for a patient, that patient's outcome is directly impacted by everything the physician says and does. Physicians don't typically obtain approval from a supervisor for what they plan to do, like many professionals do. The culture of being expected to work independently carries down through the staff in a practice with a well-coached team and in which anyone who is not dependable and self-directed creates a disruption in the otherwise busy but smooth workflow.

Chain of Command: A system of organization in which authority and decision making flows down from the top through a series of managers in which each manager is generally only accountable to one superior.

Nevertheless, there is a need for both large and small practices to have a defined chain of command. In smaller practices, a physician is usually a managing or lead physician. In these cases, an office manager is more of a liaison between the lead physician and the rest of the staff. The physician does the planning and major decision making while the manager is responsible primarily for day-to-day operations. A manager in a small office may be involved in staffing and supervisory decisions but generally requires the physician's approval on any major personnel matters. Even in this model, all of the same concepts apply to recruiting and retaining a team of workers who make it their number one priority to help the team develop and maintain a loyal patient base.

Midsized and large practices also have a lead physician, but the practice manager or administrator has more of a leadership role to accompany the management duties. Very large practices might have a lead physician for the clinical staff and another for the business side of the practice. In these large practices, a practice administrator needs to be autonomous, provide strong leadership, and possess the skills necessary to manage processes effectively. This level of administrator may participate in high-level, strategic planning meetings with the physicians.

A savvy practice administrator makes getting to know each physician a high priority. Some physicians prefer to solely practice medicine and leave the business aspect up to a good administrator. Some physicians want regular updates from an administrator regarding the business side of the practice. Some want to be involved in decisions about new technology—others just want the administrator to make recommendations. Some physicians are not open to any nonphysician discussing issues with him or her about documentation practices, so the administrator has to work with a physician to reach consensus on how the physician wants to be informed when they are not documenting properly.

Regardless of the way the physicians in a practice have chosen to organize themselves, the practice administrator must learn to work effectively with each physician—not just the managing or lead physician—in order to achieve the overarching goal of patient loyalty. Every individual must be cognizant of the team effort regardless of their own individual preferences.

Box 1.1

The Proactive Leader and External Forces Influencing the Practice

The most effective leaders stay tuned to the external environment so that they can start planning for changes and obtaining early input, and therefore acceptance, from the staff, before the practice is under the gun to implement a new mandate without adequate time to plan the most strategic approach and communicate the change effectively.

EXTERNAL FORCES INFLUENCING THE PRACTICE

All medical practices must comply with the licensure requirements that are applicable to medical practices in each state. Additionally, there are federal laws, rules, and regulations that require compliance—especially if a physician treats any Medicare or Medicaid Patients. The Center for Medicare & Medicaid Services (CMS) has several federal guidelines that dictate correct coding, quality measures, and other compliance laws, rules, and regulations that must be followed. For example, Figure 1.10 is a screen print of the introduction to the Physician Quality Reporting Initiative (PQRI) of 2006 and can be located at the following Web site: http://www.cms.gov/PQRI/. The PQRI is an example of a federal initiative with which all medical practices must comply.

As discussed earlier, compliance with HIPAA is mandatory for all health care providers and managers need to be aware that these rules are subject to change and new rules are published periodically. One recent example is what is called a "Red Flags Rule," which mandates certain procedures take place in every medical office (and other businesses) to protect patients from identity theft. It turns out that this rule was successfully challenged in December 2010 after 2 years of postponements for medical practices; however, had the challenge not been successful, any office that didn't have a plan in place ready to implement by a final deadline may

Center for Medicare and Medicaid Services (CMS): A division of the Federal Department of Health and Human Services concerned with administering the Medicare and federal portion of Medicaid programs.

Physician Quality Reporting Initiative (PQRI)

Click on the **"Spotlight"** link to the left to view

"What's New" (recently posted items) for PQRI

Background. The 2006 Tax Relief and Health Care Act (TRHCA) (P.L. 109-432) required the establishment of a physician quality reporting system, including an incentive payment for eligible professionals (EPs) who satisfactorily report data on quality measures for covered professional services furnished to Medicare beneficiaries during the second half of 2007 (the 2007 reporting period). CMS named this program the Physician Quality Reporting Initiative (PQRI). The PQRI was further modified as a result of the Medicare, Medicaid, and SCHIP Extension Act of 2007 (MMSEA) (Pub. L. 110-275) and the Medicare Improvements for Patients and Providers Act of 2008 (MIPPA) (Pub. L. 110-275).

Figure 1.10 Excerpt from the Physician Quality Reporting Initiative (PQRI) overview found at www. cms.gov/PQRI/

have incurred fines and have had to suspend business until they were in compliance. Additionally, the rules are still worthwhile for those practices desiring to reduce risks above and beyond what the law requires. Medicare sometimes changes its coverage rules. For example, in January 2010, Medicare quit paying for consultations as consultations but did allow for the services at the lower paying regular evaluation and management service rate based on the location in which the services were rendered. Another example is the complex conversion of the entire diagnostic coding system from the 9th edition to the 10th edition. The implementation date was originally finalized in 2009 for October 1, 2013. However, in the spring of 2012, a proposal to delay the date by one full year was made. The American Recovery and Reinvestment Act of 2009 (ARRA) contained many provisions that impact the way physicians conduct business.

Administrators must monitor changes from the state, the federal government, payers with managed care agreements under which the practice participates, and any hospitals or other facilities where the physicians may have privileges. For example, regulatory changes initiated by the federal government are actually posted in the daily Federal Register for public comment before any decision is made to finalize the proposed change. Any federal regulation ever finalized as well as the status of any pending regulations can be researched using the Federal Register search engine. Figure 1.11 is a copy of the home page from the Federal Register Web site at http://www.gpoaccess.gov/fr/.

Federal Register: The daily publication of rules, proposed rules, and notices of the federal government.

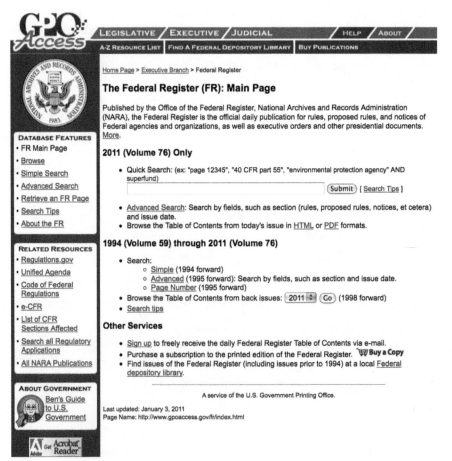

Figure 1.11 Home page for the Federal Register at www. http://www.gpoaccess.gov/fr/

A good leader analyzes the proposed change, determines if it is something that will require significant change or only minor changes and, depending on the results, writes a counterproposal during the public comment period, gleans support from colleagues for his or her alternative, and motivates these people to make a statement. At the same time, the leader is already formulating a plan for how to implement the proposed change with the least amount of cost and disruption to the practice possible.

SUMMARY

Regardless of the size of a medical practice, the savvy administrator of today will lead the building and retention of a patient-centric team, optimize the use of technology, anticipate and proactively prepare for changes in the health care delivery system, and draw upon the power of teamwork to effectively manage and continually improve the processes that are essential in any medical practice.

CHAPTER REVIEW QUESTIONS

1. List one word that summarizes each principle represented by the acronym SHARE.

_____

_____

_____

2. In your own words, describe the primary goal of a typical medical practice.

_____

_____

_____

3. Which steps in the workflow are usually performed by a receptionist?

_____

_____

_____

4. What is one task a clerk performs in an office that uses an EHR that is not done in an office that uses a paper medical record.

_____

_____

_____

5. What is the last step of the revenue cycle for any given patient?

_____

_____

_____

6. List three titles of clinical staff that are considered physician extenders.

_____

_____

_____

7. What is the name of the source that managers can monitor regularly to find out what federal changes are being considered and are open for public comment?

_____

_____

_____

8. What is the ultimate outcome of a patient-centric management philosophy?

_____

_____

_____

REFERENCES

1. Lee F. *If Disney Ran Your Hospital: 9½ Things You Would Do Differently*. Bozeman, MT: Second River Healthcare Press; 2004.
2. Nuance Communications, Inc. 2010. Available at: http://nuance.com. Accessed February 24, 2010.

Workbook for
Chapter 1

Workbook:
Chapter 1 The Basics of Today's Medical Offices

1.A: ILLUSTRATION: FLOW OF WORK

Using Figure 1-1 from your textbook as a template, list the title(s) of the team member or team members primarily responsible for each step of the work flow. Choices are: Physician, Physician Extender, Receptionist, Coder/Biller, Manager/Administrator, Medical Records Technician, Clerical Staff. Note any major tasks that are completed under each step other than the obvious. For example, under patient checkout, scheduling the next appointment is one of the functions.

1.B: WORKSHEET: COMPLETE A TABLE ON PATIENT SATISFACTION VERSUS PATIENT LOYALTY

The first one is done for you. Starting with number 2, apply the SHARE principles to the loyalty column.

Actions that result in patient satisfaction include…	Actions that result in patient loyalty include…
1. Waiting room time not to exceed the average for practices in the region.	1. Waiting room time rarely exceeds 10 minutes and when it does, the receptionist will go out to the lobby and let the patient know the reason for the delay and the anticipated remaining wait time if known.
2. Respond to each patient when he or she has a request.	
3. Each employee does his or her job very well.	

Actions that result in patient satisfaction include...	Actions that result in patient loyalty include...
4. When a patient is in the waiting room and starts to cry, the receptionist asks the patient if he or she would like to go to a private room to await the nurse or doctor.	
5. When a patient asks the receptionist if the patient will need to provide a urine sample and explains if he or she doesn't, the patient would like to go to the bathroom now, the receptionist says, "I'll find out as soon as possible, so please just take a seat and I'll let you know as soon as I find out."	
6. A nurse explains to the patient that they are going to draw blood and proceeds to do so.	

1.C: ASSIGNMENT: INTERVIEW ANY MEDICAL OFFICE EMPLOYEE

Call a physician's practice that you are familiar with and ask to speak to the practice manager regarding a school assignment. Identify yourself by name and by stating, "I am a student in the (insert program name) at (insert college or technical school name)." Ask if there is a convenient time in the next few days for you to come by and interview either the manager or an employee of your choice. Explain that you won't take more than 10 minutes of their time because you know how busy they are and that patients must take priority. You should have your questions ready and, if you don't take efficient notes, ask if you can bring a recorder. Dress professionally and treat the employee you interview with respect and appreciation of their time. Follow up with a nice thank-you note within a few days of the interview. Be sure to ask the employee what his or her primary job responsibilities are and what education, other training and experience were needed for the employee to have that position. Ask about the employee's approach to patients with regard to the SHARE principles (and explain what these are). Finally, ask any question you want to know, and be prepared to share your typed response with the instructor and your classmates.

1.D: VIDEO ACTIVITY (HOW NOT TO APPLY SHARE PRINCIPLES IN DEALING WITH A PATIENT ABOUT A SENSITIVE ISSUE)

 (See video clip on thePoint Web site to complete this activity.)

1. The video clip is based on the following case scenario presented in the chapter: *Jane, the billing supervisor, is meeting with Mrs. Jones, the*

widow of a recently deceased patient. Mrs. Jones is also a patient. Mr. Jones had not been ill. He had been rushed to the hospital where it was determined he had an aortic abdominal aneurysm. He was admitted through the ED for emergency surgery. He died during the operation. Jane works for the patient's primary care physician who had gone to the ED and stayed with the patient until the patient was sedated for surgery. Mrs. Jones is still somewhat shocked at having lost her husband so unexpectedly (he had been in his late 50s). She is trying to figure out all of the charges from this practice, what her husband's policy will pay, and how to make arrangements to make small payments on the balances since she is losing her husband's income and is only getting enough for burial expenses from the small life insurance policy her husband carried.

_____

_____

_____

2. Identify any mistakes you think were made by Jane.

_____

_____

_____

3. Jot down ideas for how Jane could have handled this situation more effectively at the same time as she used the SHARE principles to help build Mrs. Jones's loyalty without having to write off the balance due.

_____

_____

_____

4. Now, using the same scenario, write how you would have handled that situation had you been Jane. Include any dialogue from both parties—especially how Mrs. Jones may have responded had Jane employed the SHARE principles effectively. Remember, the goal in this exercise is to demonstrate the effectiveness of the SHARE principles in satisfactorily achieving the business objective of the practice while simultaneously building patient loyalty. Be prepared to either submit your findings and solution or to role-play your solution with a classmate.

_____

_____

_____

1.E: INTERNET SCAVENGER HUNT (STATE, FEDERAL AND ACCREDITATION AGENCIES)

Go to the following Web sites (since Web sites sometimes change, if you don't find what you are looking for, use your favorite search engine to find the new Web site) and answer the questions.

1. http://www.gpoaccess.gov/fr. What is the description of the Federal Register at the top of the page? What is the mailing address of the Government Printing Office (GPO)?

_____

_____

_____

2. http://www.aaahc.org/eweb/StartPage.aspx. What is AAAHC? Do they offer accreditation to both single-specialty and multispecialty medical practices?

_____

_____

_____

3. http://www.fdhc.state.fl.us/index.shtml. This Web site is for Florida's Agency for Health Care Administration (AHCA). Try searching for the equivalent AHCA in your state. For Florida, what is the definition of a health care advance directive?

_____

_____

_____

4. http://www.cms.gov. What does the acronym NCCI represent? Briefly describe what it is.

_____

_____

_____

2

The Application of Classic Management Principles in a Modern Medical Office

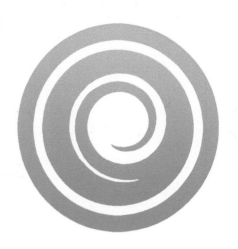

LEARNING OUTCOMES

Upon completion of this chapter, the student should...

- Describe the planning function of management and differentiate between long-term and short-term plans
- Identify the most common tools and resources for planning
- Demonstrate the use of a balanced scorecard for strategic planning and management
- Describe the organizing function of management
- Revise an organizational chart to accommodate growth
- Describe the leading or coaching function of management
- Describe the controlling function of management
- Explain how a budget is both a planning and a controlling tool

KEY TERMS

Authoritarian Leadership
Authority
Autocratic Leadership
Balanced Scorecard (BSC)
Bottom-up Budgeting
Bureaucratic Leadership
Capital Budget
Centralization
Chain of Command
Coercive Power

Controlling
Decentralization
Departmentalization
Depreciation
Ergonomics
Expert-Based Power
Fiscal Year
Formal Authority
Goals
Incremental Budgets

Informal Authority
Legitimate Power
Line Authority
Long-Term or Strategic Planning
Objectives
Operations Budget
Organization Chart
Participative Leadership
Policies
Power
Procedures
Reengineering

Representative Power
Referent Power
Reward-Based Power
Rules
Short-Term Planning
Span of Control
Staff Authority
Standards
SWOT Analysis
Top-Down Budgeting
Unity of Command

OVERVIEW

Practice managers and administrators support the mission of their practice using the four traditional functions of management:

- Planning
- Organizing
- Leading or coaching
- Controlling

Practice managers or administrators plan by starting with the overall mission of the practice and then developing various types of plans and strategies, discussed in the next section, to formally document the details of how the practice team will accomplish the mission based on a common understanding.

The organization function is comprised of grouping various types of work into logical units and determining any team members who will have supervisory authority. The next step is to determine how to design or redesign the office layout to ensure an efficient workflow—including how to place furniture, equipment, and team members to most effectively utilize the available space, technology, and workflow.

Practice administrators lead or coach by hiring, training, motivating, and retaining exceptional team members.

Finally, managers control by evaluating the effectiveness of the department as a whole, based on the projections in the various plans. Controlling is the function of continually assessing all aspects of practice performance and comparing these actual results with the planned outcomes for the current cycle. Based on the results, the practice team can work together to evaluate whether it is the plan or the performance that is causing a discrepancy. Then, adjustments can be made to either the plan or to the performance. This process provides feedback to improve the next planning cycle. Therefore, the classic principles of management are carried out in a circular manner that begins and ends with planning.

THE PLANNING FUNCTION OF MANAGEMENT

There are three categories of planning. The first category is long-term or strategic planning, the second is midterm operational planning, and the third is short-term planning. Strategic planning is almost always

Long-Term or Strategic Planning: Long-term planning is a function of senior or executive management as to how the practice is going to achieve its mission over a period of time—often 5 years with annual updates.

Short-Term Planning Management Strategy: A strategy that takes into account goals and objectives in the near future.

Planning

Planning is arguably the single most important function of any management team or manager but it is often the most neglected. It requires problem analysis and decision making to make predictions and to determine how to achieve goals. It is initiated at the highest level in an organization and flows to the lowest level.

conducted at the executive level. In large practices, they may have a board of directors in addition to one or more physician executives to whom the practice administrator reports. Regardless of size, executives identify the mission, which is the overall reason the practice exists, and plan how to achieve the mission over the next 5 to 10 years. Generally, the executive management team involves the practice administrator in this planning process. The key role of the administrator is to provide information based on research, generation and analysis of reports from the clinical and administrative data collected by the practice, and identification of any patterns or trends that are pertinent to the overall success of the practice. Even in small to midsized practices, the manager or administrator is generally responsible for analyzing data and presenting the information to the physicians. At times, this role includes making any recommendations they may have but it always involves providing useful information.

Strategic planning begins with what is known as a SWOT analysis, which is a process of analyzing

- Strengths
- Weaknesses
- Opportunities
- Threats

A SWOT analysis is done on both the internal environment of the practice and on any known external environmental influences. Internal analysis looks at what the practice already does well, what it could do better, what opportunities exist within the control of the practice to seize, and what internal factors may threaten the practice's plans for success. An example of an internal strength is a physician on the team who has been internationally recognized for developing a noninvasive, highly successful procedure to treat certain types of tumors. An example that involves the practice as an entity is a reputation for being patient centric in every aspect of the practice. An example of the "opportunities" part of a SWOT analysis is the practice manager learning that a regional health information exchange is planning to award incentives for physicians to join the exchange in sharing appropriate health information with its members. External analysis, on the other hand, is identifying the competition, determining what they do well and what they don't do well, how to be proactive in identifying potential threats from external forces in time to minimize disruptions, and to be competitive using all assets and strategies within the control of the practice.

SWOT Analysis: A strategic planning method used to evaluate the strengths, weaknesses, opportunities, and threats involved in a project or in a business venture by specifying the objective of the business venture or project and identifying the internal and external factors that are favorable and unfavorable to achieve that objective.

In addition to the SWOT analysis, the purpose of long-term planning is to establish the goals and strategies that will help the practice move forward toward achieving the vision and mission it has for existing in the first place. Certain assumptions must be made and then, as circumstances change, the assumptions are updated. For example, the strategic plan may be partially dependent on the premise that key people in the practice will be able to achieve certain goals that support the accomplishment of other goals. A tragedy may occur in which two key physicians are killed in a crash. Obviously, a tragedy of this nature would require adjustment of the strategic plan. Another important aspect of strategic planning is to develop one or more alternative approaches to achieving key goals. First, pick the best of these as the primary strategy but have one or more strategies to fall back on so that a major shift does not necessarily mean a major setback in progress.

Once the long-term plan is documented and communicated throughout the practice, a midrange plan generally breaks the strategic plan into what needs to be accomplished and by whom over the next 3 to 5 years in order to achieve the long-term goals.

Finally, the short-term plan is generally annual and it drives day-to-day operations of the practice. This plan is almost always the responsibility of the manager or administrator and the managing physician(s) and includes the annual budget. At the end of each year, the next annual plan is made based on an analysis of the current year but the planning process also looks at the mid- and long-range plans to identify any changes (positive or negative) as the result of current experience. Of course, if you have a 5–10-year plan and a 3–5-year plan, each year new goals and actions must be added because a year of each plan has expired. The idea is for all plans to act as working documents (meaning subject to adjustments) that use new experience to project forward one more year for every year that passes.

There are many documents and tools that are considered plans or parts of plans. Managers are primarily responsible for the creation, implementation, communication, and monitoring of these plans as well as any training that may be required for new or existing team members. In addition to the overall mission, these plans and planning tools include

Policies: Definitive courses or methods of action selected from alternatives and in light of given conditions to guide and determine present and future decisions.

- **Policies,** which are broad statements that guide management decisions. For example, when possible, internal candidates will be considered for promotion before an open position is announced outside of the practice. The manager has the discretion of determining if an internal candidate is qualified but is not required by this policy to select an internal candidate if no existing employee has the combination of skills and experience required for that job. A policy is a plan because it helps guide the direction the practice follows in certain circumstances on the way to accomplishing short- and long-term goals.

Procedures: In health care, a course of action intended to achieve a result in the care of persons with health problems.

- **Procedures,** which are plans of action that provide step-by step instructions on how to accomplish routine tasks. Procedures are also plans because without them, a practice does not have a way to determine how certain tasks are to be achieved which could result in planning based on incomplete information. An example of the first part of a procedure is shown in Figure 2.1. Notice how procedures refer back to the policy that is supported by the procedure.

Sunshine Health Systems
Anywhere, USA
Policy and Procedures Manual
Section I – Security, Privacy and Confidentiality of Patient Health Information

Policy 1.10
Procedure 1.10.1
Effective Date 6/1/20XX

Policy Statement 1.10:
Patient Protection Against Medical Identity Theft – Sunshine Health Systems will take every known precaution to protect every patient against being victimized by medical identity theft as part of its overall policy to aggressively protect the security, privacy and confidentiality of all patient health and financial information.

Procedure 1.10.1
Step I: Identify Red Flags and ensure all team members understand these alerts and how to detect any of these. The following are currently identified red flags:
    A. Suspicious documents
    B. Suspicious personal demographic information (e.g. unusual physical address)
    C. Alerts from other authorized persons such as the patient or law enforcement

Step II: Detecting Red Flags
    A. Sunshine Health Systems detects potential identity theft by:
    A.1. Creating thorough patient accounts for all new patients. Ensure all patient accounts contain, at a minimum – full legal name, date of birth….
    A.2 Verifying and maintaining thorough patient account for all established patients.

Figure 2.1 Procedure header and the policy it supports.

- **Rules,** which are black and white—no interpretation or decision making required. They are "must do" or "must not do" statements. For example, no smoking allowed. Rules are plans because they help provide a framework for achieving the goals in the strategic plan that have to do with the way team members are expected to behave in order to maintain a team of champions who work together to achieve success.

  Rules: Laws, bylaws, or regulations adopted to provide guidance for procedure, conduct, or action.

- **Standards,** which are measures established to determine acceptable job performance and are plans because if one doesn't know the average time it takes to perform a task, one can't project staffing needs to meet the demands. A standard is directed at individual performance expectations: Code seven surgery records per hour, for example.

  Standards: Models or examples; rules for the measure of quantity, value, extent, or quality.

- Strategies, which help achieve the goals and are also plans.

- **Goals,** which flow from the mission of the practice. The mission is the purpose of its existence and incorporates the philosophies of how the practice sees itself as distinguished from other medical practices. The goals are statements of long-range departmental and organizational intent.

  Goals: A goal is a desired outcome or end result of a planned course of action by an individual or a company–usually within a specific frame of time.

- **Objectives,** which define specific, attainable, clear, concise, and measurable expectations needed to accomplish goals. Objectives should include quality factors, time frames, and performance standards. For example, if the goal of the front office is to achieve excellence in health care information processing (flowing from the mission of the organization to provide excellent patient care), then an objective may

  Objectives: A desired result a person or a system envisions, plans, and commits to achieve—a personal or organizational desired end point in some sort of assumed development.

be to transcribe all history and physical examination records with 99% accuracy, within 24 hours of dictation.

As mentioned earlier, the budget, which is a plan, is also a powerful tool for the control function. The results of this control process of comparing actual performance against projected performance for productivity, quality, and cost-effectiveness feed into the planning process for the next cycle.

⊗ UTILIZING A BALANCED SCORECARD FOR STRATEGIC PLANNING

A balanced scorecard approach to strategic planning and management provides one high-level approach to the planning process. The details of how to design and implement a balanced scorecard that will meet the needs for a given practice are beyond the scope of this book. It is important, however, to be aware of this powerful process and to know where to learn more about customizing this tool for use in a specific medical practice. According to the Advanced Performance Institute, "The Balanced Scorecard (BSC) is a strategic performance management framework that allows organizations to identify, manage and measure its strategic objectives....

Balanced Scorecard (BSC): A strategic performance management framework that allows companies to identify, manage, and measure its strategic objectives from various perspectives.

Kaplan and Norton (original creators) identified four generic perspectives that cover the main strategic focus areas of a company. The idea was to use this model as a template for designing objectives and measures in each of the following perspectives:

- The Financial Perspective covers the financial objectives of an organization and allows managers to track financial success and shareholder value.
- The Customer (Patient) Perspective covers the customer objectives such as customer satisfaction (loyalty, in this case), market share goals as well as product and service attributes.
- The Internal Process Perspective covers internal operational goals and outlines the key processes necessary to deliver the customer objectives.
- The Learning and Growth Perspective covers the intangible drivers of future success such as human capital, organizational capital and information capital including skills, training, organizational culture, leadership, systems, and databases."[1]

As evidenced in Figure 2.2, this planning process is a map to outlining overall goals for the practice as a whole by looking at how the various perspectives are dependent upon one another for success. It is acceptable to place the financial perspective at the bottom instead of the top which is common in nonprofit or government service organizations but also emphasizes that in a private medical practice the patient perspective will drive the other perspectives if it is moved to the top. Organizational capital under learning and growth perspective is where

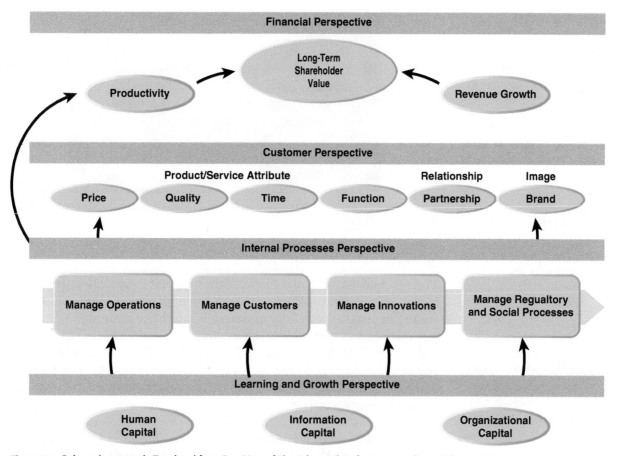

Figure 2.2 Balanced scorecard. (Reprinted from Ben Marr of The Advanced Performance Institute, with permission.)

the culture, leadership, teamwork, and management of knowledge in a practice falls as far as the goals for achieving the desired customer perspective of building patient loyalty which, in turn, increases revenue under financial perspective.

THE ORGANIZING FUNCTION OF MANAGEMENT

The classic principle of management that deals with organizing requires decisions regarding each of the following:

- Specialization of workers—do one thing and do it well
- Unity of command, which means reporting to only one supervisor
- Span of control, meaning the number of employees that report to a manager and that a manager can effectively supervise
- Departmentalization (e.g., billing and coding department and lab department)
- Centralization versus decentralization with regard to where the decisions are made in a company
- Authority, which is the right to act based on level or title of position
- Power or the ability to influence others regardless of official position

Unity of Command: Each employee has only one boss. One of the 14 principles of management.

Span of Control: In business management, refers to the number of subordinates a supervisor has.

Departmentalizing: A form of organization in which like tasks are grouped together into departments. For example, in a large medical office, laboratory staff may form one department while radiology staff forms another.

Centralization: An organizational theory in which decision making is centralized with top administration based on set policies and communicated down through the organizational structure to the bottom tier.

Decentralization: An organizational structure in which authority to make decisions is delegated downward in an organization rather than centralized with executive management.

Authority: The formal or legitimate authority or power to act on behalf of an organization including the authority to require other employees to act within the limits of the authority figure's scope and within the scope of the employee's job description.

Power: The ability to get things done regardless of the source of one's power.

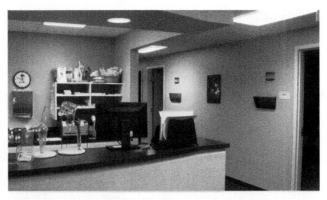

Figure 2.3 Layout of a modern, medium-size medical practice.

Specialization of Workers

For the modern, patient-centric, team-oriented medical practice, these classic cornerstones of management are important to understand but should be handled carefully in determining the organization of a practice initially and periodically reevaluating the initial plan as the practice grows (Fig. 2.3). As far as specialization, most allied health workers are specialized based on licensing and accreditation (Fig. 2.4). The practice administrator, however, has to make decisions about degree of specialization for functions like

- Receptionist—will this position be responsible for all of the clerical support or will there be a separate pure clerical position and how much of the billing process will be initiated by the receptionist including knowledge of which plans require prior approval of certain services
- Coding and billing—will there be a professional coder who codes from the medical record and an insurance specialist or will one position do both and does the office need a professional coder or do they use a superbill?

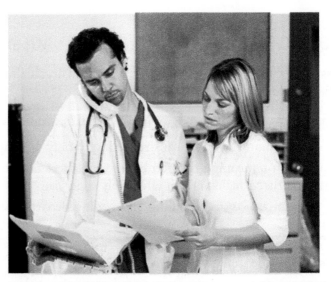

Figure 2.4 A Certified Medical Assistant and a Nurse Practitioner are both specialized team members.

- How will the data be input into an Electronic Health Record—a medical transcriptionist, a medical scribe, clinician direct input, voice recognition software, etc.?
- What level(s) of physician extenders will the office use and how specialized?

Unity of Command and Span of Control

Unity of command and span of control are very important. The practice needs to determine how much of the clinical supervision is done by the office administrator and how many, if any, supervisors are necessary. Much of this will be dictated by the number and type of employees but in order to be patient centric and have a champion team, it is crucial to ensure anyone with formal authority uses that authority to facilitate and coach, not to wield power.

Departmentalization

Departmentalization is another principle that is based, to a degree, on the size of the practice, and the variety of services offered. If it is a large practice, it will probably have both a lab department and a radiology department in addition to the physicians and the physician extenders. On the nonclinical side, there may be a coding and billing department with its own supervisor if the practice is large. Keep in mind that for the overarching goal of patient loyalty, regardless of what decisions are made about organization, all people who work in the practice must be consistent in working toward this goal as a whole team—not a team for every location. This may require extra work on the part of the administrator to visit all locations frequently enough to motivate each employee to remember the role they have on the team and the fact that in order to win, the team must work together to put the patient first with the secure knowledge that management is taking care of their individual needs.

Centralization versus Decentralization

Decentralization is based on having more than one location in which one has to determine if the central office is going to make all of the decisions or if the other locations have some autonomy and supervisors who report the administrator but can make certain decisions regarding day-to-day operations in the location in which they are the supervisor. This principle also pertains to whether or not certain functions like coding and billing will be centralized in a main location or if there will be a coder and/or biller at each location.

Authority and Power

Authority is the power to act for someone else. Line authority positions are responsible for direct supervision of employees, while staff authority positions are more advisory or consultative in nature such as a human resources specialist in an office that only has one human resources person. The specialist does not directly supervise anyone but

Line Authority: A position of authority in which at least one person reports to that supervisor. It differs from staff authority because staff authority is a person who has authority to make decisions that affect others but they are not the direct supervisors of those employees.

Staff Authority: Authority to advise, but not to direct, other managers.

Chain of Command: A system of organization in which authority and decision making flows down from the top through a series of managers in which each manager is generally only accountable to one superior.

Formal Authority: Formal authority is the power to influence or get things done by position—supervisory authority, for example.

Informal Authority: A source of power (the ability to get things done) derived based on employees looking to a coworker for leadership due to charisma or perceived expertise or some other non–company-sanctioned trait.

Organization Chart: A diagram that shows the structure of an organization and the relationships and relative ranks of its parts and positions/jobs.

Reengineering: The analysis and design of workflows and processes within an organization to help rethink or redesign for efficiency.

Ergonomics: The consideration of the human factors in the design of office equipment and furniture to optimize safety, minimize repetitive stress disorders, and facilitate efficiency.

they do have the authority to advise the office administrator of how to handle certain situations with other employees or how to fairly administer merit pay.

Traditionally, the chain of command was the most common model of authority in which the authority flows downward from the top. Another principle that is important to know before customizing these principals to meet the needs of a specific medical practice is that there is both formal and informal types of authority. Formal authority is by position—supervisory authority, for example. Informal authority, on the other hand, is employees accepting a person who is not in a formal position of authority as an influence on their decisions and behavior. Informal organizational structure is not under the control of management but must be recognized by management. A savvy leader respects the authority of a natural leader and works toward a collaboration in which the informal leader is actually a positive force in building a strong team.

It is very important not to misuse or abuse either authority or power and to be sure that every single person who has any authority also understands that they must use this authority and power to achieve the practice goals by optimizing the team effort.

The organization chart delineates the hierarchy of relationships within the practice and designates solid lines for "line authority" and dotted lines for "staff authority." See Figure 2.5 for an example of an organization chart for a midsized medical practice. The organization needs to illustrate the flow of formal communication.

Another concept that falls under the principle of organization of resources is reengineering. It is the process of looking at an established practice (or any business) from the perspective of designing the business from scratch in an effort to identify and redesign any inefficiencies in workflow or functions. This process always results in some degree of change.

Another function of organizing is the design of the office. It is important for a practice manager to understand and consider ergonomics, which is the design of furniture, equipment, and work processes to safely meet the requirements of those who work with them. A successful administrator is one who is aware of all rules, regulations, and laws pertaining to employee safety but who implements these practices because it is the right thing to do for the team, and not because it is dictated by law. The side benefits include reducing the risk of worker's compensation claims in addition to sending a message to all team players that management has their best interests in mind so they can focus on the patients.

THE LEADING OR COACHING FUNCTION OF MANAGEMENT

Leading or coaching involves effectively leading people to achieve their own and the organization's goals and objectives efficiently. To this end, the leader must not only do things right, the leader must identify and do the right things right so he or she can effectively coach the team into moving in the most effective direction toward building and maintaining a loyal customer base.

Orientation to the practice and to the specific job for all new members of the team is the first opportunity the administrator has to get the team

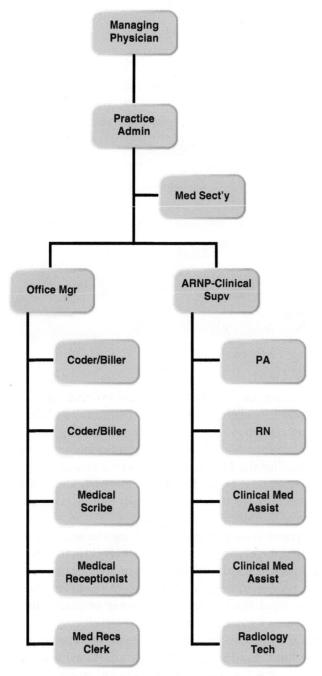

Figure 2.5 Sample organization chart for a midsized medical practice.

member off to a strong start. This is a unique opportunity to introduce the new member to the practice's patient-centric, team-oriented culture and to introduce him or her to the rest of the team and what positions each of them hold. Orientation is discussed in more detail in Chapter 3.

One of the classic motivation theories is Abraham Maslow's "Hierarchy of Needs." Although Maslow's original model has been modified in various ways over the years, his original work is central to the understanding basic principles of motivating humans. See Figure 2.6 for an illustration of Maslow's model of human needs. The Web site www.businessballs.com contains excellent information on Abraham

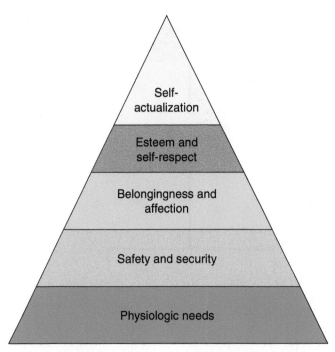

Figure 2.6 Maslow's hierarchy.

Maslow including the explanation: "Maslow developed the Hierarchy of Needs model in 1940 to 1950s United States, and the Hierarchy of Needs theory remains valid today for understanding human motivation, management training, and personal development. Indeed, Maslow's ideas surrounding the Hierarchy of Needs concerning the responsibility of employers to provide a workplace environment that encourages and enables employees to fulfill their own unique potential (self-actualization) are today more relevant than ever."[2]

The significance of Maslow's model for the medical practice leader is that any employee, regardless of skill level, is not going to be able to focus on patient loyalty when he's worried about whether or not he has enough money to keep his house from being repossessed. As each level of need is adequately met, employees are naturally motivated to work on the next higher level of needs. Therefore, the practice administrator has to be aware of individual team member needs (which can change), without invading the team member's privacy. Once the needs are identified, the leader coaches each individual toward achieving whatever level of needs they have, on an ongoing basis, so that the team member is able to progress toward self-actualization. This might mean that the coach locates free financial counseling for one employee and a support group for another to help deal with an alcoholic spouse or a parent who has Alzheimer disease. The goal is to help create a team environment where everyone helps themselves and each other achieve the overall goals of the practice while meeting each team member's personal needs. Meeting the lower needs, such as fair pay and a safe working environment, helps prevent dissatisfaction, while meeting the higher needs exponentially increases job satisfaction and loyalty. A loyal team player will do everything in his or her power to ensure patient loyalty.

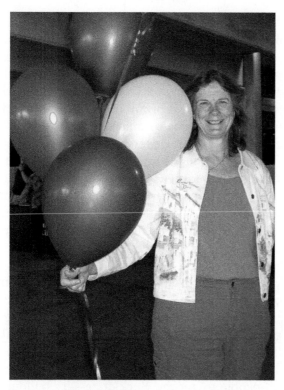

Figure 2.7 Office celebration.

Another pioneer of applying human psychological principles to a model of leadership, B. F. Skinner, believed behavior that is positively reinforced is repeated. This means that in order to shape the behavior of the team members and ultimately the team itself, a good coach is able to sincerely recognize and celebrate behavior that models the vision of a patient-centric practice. The practice manager should acknowledge all good behavior and celebrate behavior that goes beyond expectations (Fig. 2.7).

Yet another psychologist who influenced leadership styles is Douglas McGregor. McGregor's X-Y theory illustrates that if a manager is authoritarian or autocratic which is the "X" type of manager, then he or she believes people basically don't want to work, are only motivated to do their job by the threat of punishment for not doing it, and that people need to be directed in a dictatorial fashion to do what needs to be done. The source of power in an authoritarian style comes from the perception that the manager has the ability to punish and from the formal position the manager holds. These sources of power are known as coercive, which is the perception that the leader has the ability to punish, and legitimate source of power which is the perception that the manager has the right to supervise people based on official or legitimate or formal position held by the supervisor. This X style, authoritarian or autocratic type of manager, also believes that his or her approach to management is the only way to get the job done. As one might imagine, a theory X manager is not typically successful in achieving a motivated team of employees. Yet another style of leadership that won't work well in a medical practice is the bureaucratic style which uses an inflexible, literal interpretation of rules and regulations to gain the power needed to manage people.

Authoritarian Leadership: Also known as autocratic leadership, authoritarian leaders provide clear expectations of how, what, and when tasks need to be completed without input from subordinates and within a well-defined position of authority within the company.

Autocratic Leadership: See authoritarian leadership.

Coercive Power: One of five recognized forms of power (coercive, reward, legitimate, referent, and expert), coercive power is the power to force someone to do something against their will. It is often physical but may also be psychological or emotional and often uses demonstrations of harm to illustrate what will happen if compliance is not gained.

Legitimate Power: A source of power (the ability to get things done) which is the perception that the manager has the right to supervise people based on official or legitimate or formal position held by the supervisor.

Bureaucratic Leadership: Bureaucratic leaders are concerned with ensuring workers follow rules and procedures accurately and consistently.

Participative Leadership: A democratic leadership style that involves and engages team members.

Reward-Based Power: One of five recognized forms of power (coercive, reward, legitimate, referent, and expert), reward-based power is the ability to give other people what they want, and hence ask them to do things for you in exchange. Rewards can also be used to punish, such as when they are withheld.

Referent Power: One of five recognized forms of power (coercive, reward, legitimate, referent, and expert), referent-based power is the power derived from another person liking you or wanting to be like you. It is the power of charisma and fame.

Expert-Based Power: A source of power (the ability to get things done) that is derived from the supervisor having more knowledge than the workers about the work that needs to be accomplished and is therefore an expert in that area gleaning respect from subordinates.

Representative Power: Power democratically delegated by followers to a leader for the purpose of representing followers interests.

Controlling: One of the traditional functions of management in which the supervisor monitors actual performance against projected performance and determines when corrections need to be made during a certain period of time.

A theory Y manager, on the other hand, is a participative type of leader in which an assumption that people want to work, desire progressively more challenging responsibilities, respond to achieving goals from the perspective of feeling rewarded, and prefer to utilize their creativity and other talents at a higher level. Another aspect of the participative leadership style is that it promotes team input and feedback and values the democratic approach to achieving goals.

The sources of power for leadership, include those already mentioned plus reward based, in which the perception is that the leader has the ability to reward employees; referent power, in which the power to influence is derived from a charismatic person whom employees perceive can meet their needs; expert based, in which the leader has special knowledge that will benefit the team; and representative, in which followers democratically delegate power to a leader for purpose of representing followers interests.

The leading/coaching aspect of classic management principles involves, in collaboration with human resources staff when applicable, recruitment, selection, training, appraising, compensating, motivating, coaching, retaining, counseling, disciplining, and terminating employees as necessary to provide and maintain adequate staffing in any business. In medical practice, the goal of leadership is much more than having enough people to get the work done—it's building a powerful, efficient, patient-centric team composed of a mixture of clerical, technical, and professional members who are all treated like what they each contribute is equally vital to what any other member contributes.

THE CONTROLLING FUNCTION OF MANAGEMENT

The management principle of controlling, in its simplest form, is the leader's responsibility to assure that all aspects of what is done in a busy medical practice conform to the short-range plan, which in turn keeps the practice on target with longer-range plans. The trickiest part isn't so much monitoring as it is correcting variances. For example, production standards are plans because if you don't know the average amount of work that can be done in a typical day, whether it is coding medical records or how many patients a physician can treat, then you can't plan for how many coders to hire or how many patients to schedule. The control process for the plan involving production standards consists of monitoring individual team member actual productivity against the established standards for each function.

Controlling should work like a thermostat. Like a thermostat, slight variances up or down are acceptable. However, slight variances that stay over or under the plan for a period of time need to be audited more aggressively as do any significant variances. Upon closer scrutiny, the manager, often with input from the team, determines the reason for the variance and how to correct that variance. For example, if lab results are backlogged for some reason, it means that patients start to call because they've been told they should have results within five business days of the test. On the sixth business day, the phone calls will significantly increase causing yet another area to be backlogged. All this backlog directly impacts patient loyalty, so it must be analyzed and resolved immediately. The manager will first try to see if the team member who handles this function has a problem and, if so, how they can work together to resolve it. If it isn't an obvious change with the team member and that person doesn't know why they are backlogged, then the rest of the team should be brought together to help identify and then resolve the issue. For example, it could be that the main lab changed systems and is now electronically sending results but those results are getting held up from being accepted by the practice's system.

Work standards help the manager plan and need to be monitored as part of the control process. Standards can be set and audited using various techniques beyond the scope of this text but the important thing to know is that standards should be set with team member participation, be clear, specific and challenging, and be linked to positive reinforcement when met or exceeded.

> **T I P**
>
> Standards should have a method by which team members and the manager have input regarding the standard and also ability to provide feedback on the results of an audit in which the standard is not being met by one or more team members.

⊚ THE BUDGET, BOTH A CONTROLLING AND A PLANNING TOOL

As mentioned previously, the budget is a powerful tool for both planning and controlling functions of management. Basically, a budget is a projection of the amount of money that the practice anticipates earning (revenue), and then—the amount of that revenue it will take to accomplish all of the goals set by the practice for that year—expenses.

As a control tool, the administrator monitors the budget regularly to identify variances. Some variances are acceptable and some are not. An example of an acceptable variance is an increase in revenue over projected because the practice is operating at full capacity while the budget projected a continuance of the previous year's 85% of capacity. The correction, in this case, is a pleasant one to make. The manager may propose hiring an additional physician because the practice has grown to the extent that potential new patients are being turned away and existing patients often have to wait several weeks to see their physician for a nonemergency visit. For this scenario, the manager determines that if a physician (as an employee who is paid by the practice, not as a partner) is added, the practice can also afford a marketing campaign to make patients and potential patients aware of the new physician. The manager may decide that there is enough existing space for the new physician, without major expense, because they've recently converted from paper records to an electronic health record system thereby freeing up an extra exam room that had been being used to store older paper records. The manager may also decide that existing staff (clinical and nonclinical) can handle the increased workload until the new physician starts seeing enough patients to increase revenue as well as the patient-driven work the support staff does. With the physician's approval, the manager not only puts the proposal into effect but also adjusts the projected budget for the rest of the current year.

An unacceptable budget variance is a little less pleasant to deal with but very necessary. To get a better idea of how to control for a negative variance, read the following case study.

TROUBLESHOOTING AN UNACCEPTABLE BUDGET VARIANCE IDENTIFIED THROUGH THE CONTROL PROCESS

Fiscal Year: A 1-year financial cycle that may begin on any day of any month but the first date marks the new financial or budget year for a given practice.

Jean is the practice administrator. She has worked with the same team for going on 2 years. The practice starts each annual budget period on January 1 so that means the fiscal year is the same for the practice as the calendar year. A fiscal year can begin in any month.

Jean has many control tools to help her detect unacceptable variances in any aspect of performance. For example, she has several methods of surveying patients in an attempt to measure their ongoing degree of loyalty to the practice. But from the financial performance perspective, she generally checks daily and weekly reports that she has customized to graphically display any trends of categories that are either over or under budget. In June of this particular year, she notices 6 months into the fiscal year, the practice has already spent approximately 70% of its budget for staffing of nonclinical functions. She realizes that due to various reasons, she hasn't been checking the weekly variance reports. She panics because she realizes that the managing physician may take this out on her if she doesn't do something immediately to correct the problem. She notices that it is a few minutes before the practice closes for lunch so she walks into the front office and announces that all of the front-office staff must go to the conference room before they take their lunch break. Once the nonclinical workers gather in the conference room, Jean states the budget for their functions is way out of line and that everyone has been slacking off since the first of the year. She directly places the blame on the whole staff and threatens them with termination if each and every one of them doesn't start producing extra within regular work hours to make up for not being up to speed the past 6 months. She also says that if anyone is tardy or absent between now and the time they get the budget back in line, they better have a documented, life-threatening reason or else she will replace them with someone who wants to work. She then asks if everyone understands and if anyone has any questions.

What do you think Jean should do differently?

Jean should start by analyzing the details of expenses versus projections to determine whether the problem is the projections from which the budget was created (mostly driven by the projected number of patients and services provided for that year) or the actual performance of the team members. Jean needs to investigate this aspect before she seeks input from the team. For example, she may find that most of the overspending to date is in the category of temporary help and overtime related to coding and billing.

If this is the case, she would then look at the amount of revenue (money received to date in payment of services rendered) to see if coding and billing is up due to a corresponding spike in patient volume over what was projected, which would be evident in the revenue areas and actually a very positive explanation of the increased expenses. Assuming, however, that there is not an increase over projected revenue, what should Jean do next?

Jean needs to do one more analysis before bringing the team together to brainstorm the cause of the decrease in coding and billing productivity. She needs to check attendance to see if there has been an increase in absenteeism over normal during the past 6 months and then check productivity reports to see if there has been an individual drop in productivity. In either of these cases, the solution is an individual corrective action that is discussed in the next chapter. If neither of these individual issues is evident, then Jean needs to bring the team together to brainstorm. She will describe the issue and then have each person take turns calling out suggestions, without any judgment while Jean jots the list of suggestions on a dry erase board or large flip pad. Once everyone has run out of ideas, the group looks at the list and rules out anything that is highly unlikely. Then, the remaining ideas are grouped together. Finally, the group decides the most likely cause. For example, there may have been a change in procedures by a major payer or a change in workflow causing delays.

Once the potential cause is identified, the team will then brainstorm possible solutions. The best solution will be put into place on a trial basis and, if successful, adopted permanently with the team working together and embracing the solution. This approach results in the whole team having ownership in the solution. Another advantage is that the synthesis of ideas generated by a group often results in a solution that would have taken the manager a lot longer to discover without input. Once the problem and a solution are agreed upon, the manager monitors the results to ensure it actually does correct the problem.

During any given annual cycle, all the findings from using the budget as a control tool result in applying the lessons learned and also incorporating changes to the planning cycle for the following year with the budget at the short-range planning center.

In general, budgets can be zero based, which means the administrator starts from scratch rather than using past budgets as a starting place. This method may sound like it doesn't take advantage of the budget's role in planning but, in reality, it requires information learned from the previous year in order to make good decisions. The difference is that it enables the team to think creatively about improving various aspects of the practice instead of just assuming that everything will be done the way it has been done with the exception of whatever adjustments were made during the previous year to resolve budget variance issues. Bottom-up budgeting is when the practice team share in the ideas and planning process with the executives, while top-down budgeting is when the physicians dictate budget planning to the practice manager.

Incremental budgets adjust previous budgets to accommodate known variances such as the cost of health insurance is going to be raised by 5% for all employees. This method is perfectly adequate once a practice is performing exceptionally well but it's a good strategy to try zero-based budgeting periodically in an attempt to invigorate the practice.

Practices have an operations budget that includes the projected cost of labor, supplies, other routine expenses, and the

Bottom-Up Budgeting: A participative approach to budgeting in which each unit has input into the budgeting process up through senior management and then the final budget is approved.

Top-Down Budgeting: A budgeting process in which the costs of higher-level tasks are estimated and then those estimates constrain the estimates for costs of lower-level tasks; for example, the entire process of coming up with a budget begins with upper-level management and an overall estimate of the entire project which is then divided among the first level of tasks, and then the budget is divided among lower-level tasks and then lower-level tasks. This continues until funding has been given to all of the tasks necessary for a project.

Incremental Budgets: A form of budgeting in which an adjustment is made to the previous budget to accommodate known variances such as the cost of health insurance being raised by 5% for all employees.

Operations Budget: This is the annual budget of an activity and typically contains estimates of the total value of resources required for the performance of the operation as well as estimates of workload in terms of total work units identified by cost accounts.

Capital Budget: The amount of money projected in addition to the annual operational budget for long-term assets such as large equipment or facilities.

Depreciation: The gradual (usually over several years) converting of a capital expense, such as the amount of money spent at one time to purchase a $10,000.00 piece of equipment, into an operational expense (for the annual budget) over the useful life of the asset.

projected revenue. A capital budget, on the other hand, includes only major, nonroutine expenditures and sources of funding. For example, purchasing a new practice management computer system is a capital expense and the practice physicians getting paid to give lectures is a capital source of revenue, that is, it is other than minor amounts and it is nonroutine. Depreciation is a formal allocation of cost of a capital asset over a specific time.

It is evident from the process described above that the controlling function of the budget, as part of daily operations, is a valuable tool for both midyear adjustments with justification and for more accurate planning going into the next management cycle.

The full revenue cycle which, simply stated, is the steps involved from first contact with a patient through the process of getting fully reimbursed for the services provided to that patient, and the management of other financial aspects of the practice, beyond the budget, are discussed in Chapters 5 and 6.

SUMMARY

Although medicine and health care in the United States often lag behind optimizing the use of proven business management concepts, the classic principles of management are applicable in any medical practice and will promote the achievement of a patient-centric team of clinical and nonclinical people, an efficient and profitable medical practice, and the coveted loyal patient base.

These principles are applied in a cyclical or circular manner and include planning, organizing, coaching or leading, and controlling all aspects of the highly successful medical practice. Controlling provides feedback to improve the next planning cycle.

CHAPTER REVIEW QUESTIONS

1. What are the four traditional functions of management?

_____

_____

_____

2. Which function provides information for the next management cycle?

_____

_____

_____

3. List five types of planning tools.

_____

_____

_____

4. What is the key role of the office administrator in the strategic planning process?

_____

_____

_____

5. What does the acronym SWOT represent?

_____

_____

_____

6. What is a typical period for a short-term plan?

_____

_____

_____

7. What is the difference between a policy and a rule?

_____

_____

_____

8. Discuss the perspectives used in a balanced scorecard.

_____

_____

_____

REFERENCES

1. Marr B. What is a Balanced Scorecard? Management White Paper. The Advanced Performance Institute. 2008.
2. Maslow's Hierarchy of Needs. http://www.businessballs.com/maslow.htm. Accessed May 15, 2010.

Workbook for
Chapter 2

Workbook:
Chapter 2 The Application of Classic Management Principles in a Modern Medical Office

2.A: WORKSHEET: MATCH THE FOLLOWING TOOLS AND TASKS WITH MANAGEMENT PRINCIPLES

For each of the following tools or tasks, indicate which classic management function it falls under:

(A) Planning, (B) Organizing, (C) Leading or coaching, (D) Controlling, (E) Both planning and controlling

__A__ Mission		__C__ Motivation
__E__ Budget		__B__ Floor Plan
__B__ Power		__A__ Objectives
__C__ Bureaucratic		__B__ Ergonomics
__D__ Monitoring performance		__A__ Rules

2.B: VIDEO ACTIVITY (HOW NOT TO APPROACH SOLVING A NEGATIVE BUDGET VARIANCE ISSUE)

 See video clip on the Point Web site to complete this activity.

1. The video clip is based on the following case scenario presented in the chapter:

_____

_____

_____

2. *Jean is the practice administrator. She has worked with the same team for going on 2 years. From a financial performance perspective, she generally checks daily and weekly reports that she has customized to graphically display any trends of categories that are either over or under budget. In June of this particular year, she notices 6 months into the fiscal year, the practice has already spent approximately 70% of its budget for staffing of nonclinical functions. She realizes that due to various reasons, she hasn't been checking the weekly variance reports. She panics because she realizes that the managing physician may take this out on her if she doesn't do something immediately to correct the problem. She notices that it is a few minutes before the practice closes for lunch so she walks into the front office and announces that all of the front-office staff must go to the conference room before they take their lunch break. Once the nonclinical workers gather in the conference room, Jean states the budget for their functions is way out of line and that everyone has been slacking off since the first of the year. She directly places the blame on the whole staff and threatens them with termination if each and every one of them doesn't start producing extra within regular work hours to make up for not being up to speed the past 6 months. She also says that if anyone is tardy or absent between now and the time they get the budget back in line, they better have a documented, life-threatening reason or else she will replace them with someone who wants to work. She then asks if everyone understands and if anyone has any questions.*

_____

_____

_____

3. View the video clip.

_____

_____

_____

4. Identify any mistakes you think were made by Jean.

_____

_____

_____

5. Jot down ideas for how Jean could have handled this situation more effectively at the same time as she used the principles of "controlling" to resolve the issue while maintaining high team morale.

_____

_____

_____

6. Now, using the same scenario, write how you would have handled that situation had you been Jean. Include any dialogue from the team meeting. Be prepared to either submit your findings and solution or to role-play your solution with a classmate.

_____

_____

_____

2.C: ILLUSTRATION: UPDATE ORGANIZATION CHART IN FIGURE 2.5 TO REFLECT AN EXPANSION IN THE PRACTICE

Look at Figure 2.5 in the textbook. Redo the organization chart to accommodate a new wing housing a full-service laboratory staffed by a lab technologist and three lab technicians and a new imaging center requiring a new radiologist (physician) and three more radiology techs. (Hint: Remember to move existing radiology tech under the new radiologist.)

2.D: YOUR TURN: DEVELOP A MISSION STATEMENT FOR A MEDICAL PRACTICE

Using the concepts presented in the chapter, draft a concise mission statement for a new practice you have been hired to manage. Keep in mind that a mission statement tells others what your purpose is for existing but also what distinguishes you from other practices.

2.E: EXPERT PANEL

Read the following real-life scenario. Your instructor may have you break into teams or respond as an individual expert. Each team or individual needs to write down how they would solve this problem if they were the practice administrator. Once each team or individual response is prepared, the instructor may ask students to choose the top three solutions and describe why they are the best.

Jean is the practice administrator. Dr. Jones is the managing physician. The practice is a year old and is mostly on target working toward the long-term plan by aggressively monitoring the short-term plan. An area that is not up to planned performance, however, is the lab department. Jean doesn't think it is any particular individual but she does think that the lab workers are all loners who haven't bought into the teamwork or the patient-centric philosophy upon which the mission is based. The lab consists of a supervisor and four lab technicians. While all of them are competent and productive, none of them have responded to Jean's subtle efforts to interact well with other team members or even, when contact is necessary, the patients.

What should Jean and Dr. Jones do?

3

Leading the Medical Office Team

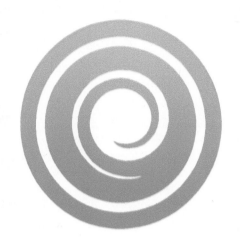

Upon completion of this chapter, the student should...

- Describe how to plan for replacing an employee or adding to staff
- Develop a recruitment plan to recruit and hire the best person for each job opening
- Design a training plan and provide in-service training to employees
- Evaluate strategies for retaining and motivating excellent employees
- Demonstrate team building skills
- Document a four-step process to handle misconduct and performance problems

KEY TERMS

Delegate
Discrimination
Insurance or Billing Specialist
Job Analysis

Job Description
Professional Journal
Soft Skills
Telephone Interview

> **Box 3.1**
>
> **Patient Loyalty, Not Just Satisfaction**
>
> The most important guiding principle in a highly successful medical practice is to be ever mindful of building and maintaining patient loyalty to the practice.

OVERVIEW

There are many aspects to leading a medical practice toward the goal of serving a strong, loyal patient base in which the patients become the practice's most effective marketing ally. A practice manager or administrator must not only model patient-focused behavior but also build a team that is patient centric. To accomplish and maintain a winning team, the administrator must have a plan that includes selecting the best person for each open position, motivating individuals to be responsible for their own performance and behavior, and coaching them to form a cohesive team in which all members are strong and in which strength increases with teamwork. The outcome is a team of medical practice professionals who are champions at winning patient loyalty.

THE GAME PLAN

Imagine a baseball coach with a reputation for building winning teams. The best coach would be unsuccessful if he or she recruited players based only on selecting applicants who had experience playing baseball. The coach would need to know what positions are needed and what the ideal qualifications are for each position. Likewise, the most successful medical office manager or administrator has to have a plan before hiring anyone, regardless if he or she is starting a new practice from scratch or hiring a single employee to fill a vacancy.

Keeping in mind patient loyalty, an element of which is how the patient perceives the quality of each interaction between the patient and any member of the practice's team, the game plan is to take the necessary steps that result in recruiting, hiring, retaining, and motivating the best employee for each job every single time a hiring decision is made. There are several planning tools that help the manager or administrator consistently accomplish this goal.

The first tool is a job analysis template that forms the basis for writing a job description that is most reflective of the work the person will be doing. This is important because you shouldn't hire an overqualified candidate anymore than you would hire a person who doesn't meet the minimum requirements for the position. For example, an extraordinary professional coder with billing experience shouldn't be hired to fill a billing or insurance specialist position in an office that uses a superbill (listing of the most common diagnosis and procedure codes

Job Analysis: A template that provides a tool for defining the work that is expected to be done by anyone in a specific job title. It forms the basis of the job description.

Job Description: A document that describes each job, by job title, as to what work is performed, the qualifications necessary, the pay grade, and whether or not it is an exempt or nonexempt position, reporting structure, etc.

encountered by that practice). The coder may be able to do the job, but may not be satisfied long term because the challenges of coding are different than the challenges of an insurance or billing specialist. Additionally, without more training, the coder may not be as effective at dealing with insurance companies as a billing specialist may be. The coder is motivated most by the specific challenges of abstracting information from a variety of medical records and assigning the appropriate codes in the proper sequence, while a billing specialist is more geared toward the revenue cycle of processing claims, resolving edits, and dealing with insurance companies to collect proper reimbursement for each service. An employee who is not challenged according to his or her main strengths may not stay with the practice any longer than it takes to find a more challenging position no matter how much the job pays or how well the team works together.

The format of a job analysis is not important, but the contents should include the following:

- Job title (the title should be a direct reflection on the type of responsibilities the job requires)
- Job overview (a short description that defines the overall function of the specific job)
- Job qualifications (both required and preferred education, experience, and applicable credentials or licensure including any applicable specialized training)
- Job duties and responsibilities (details of the major duties performed by the employee)
- Job interactions (list of the most frequent communications this person encounters daily with other internal employees, staff from other offices, diagnostics centers, or hospitals, vendors, insurance representatives, auditors, patients, etc.)
- Job relationships (list the title of the person this person will report to and any subordinates by job title)

Once the job analysis is completed for each position, the next step is to write a job description that provides a meaningful tool for both the manager and the employees. A good job description, as shown in Figure 3.1, defines how that employee interacts with all other positions in the practice as well as delineates formal lines of communication. The job description also ties to the organization chart mentioned previously to define the lines of authority, including any positions supervised and who supervises the person in each job.

The job description is helpful in other ways, too. Once general new employee orientation is completed, the job description is a guide to any job-specific training necessary. Also, on an ongoing basis, the job description is a good reference for both the manager and the employee either when there are any questions regarding work assignments or when it's time to formally evaluate the employee's performance.

Finally, the job description provides the highlights that will be used in advertising for an open position.

Insurance or Billing Specialist: A person who is responsible for all of the steps in the revenue cycle that occur from the time a patient is seen by a practitioner until there is a zero balance for that particular encounter.

SUNSHINE SURGERY CENTER
Anywhere, FL
Job Description

JobTitle: Certified Medical Coder

Reports to: Practice Administrator

Job Type: Full Time, Hourly

Salary Range: $12-$16/hr

Location: 123 Oak St., Anywhere, FL

Description:

This position is primarily responsible for the coding of all practice encounters for consultations and surgeries. Coders are also responsible for part of the billing process and must work closely with the insurance specialists to ensure accurate coding and billing. The practice is extremely patient-focused and the staff works as a team to ensure all of every patient's needs are met or exceeded. The practice is a large, busy, well-respected surgical center specializing in a wide-range of outpatient surgical procedures.

Primary duties and responsibilities:

- Code and sequence all relevant diagnoses and procedures from medical records.
- Utilize coding software (encoder) and manual resources as needed
- Apply current ICD-CM conventions, guidelines and coding clinic publications
- Apply CPT-4 conventions, guidelines and CPT Assistant publications
- Follow National Correct Coding Initiatives
- Obtain and follow any payer-specific guidelines including when to use HCPCs Level II Codes.
- Utilize database reports and spreadsheet software to analyze trends
- Assist patients with any questions and answer questions from hospital coders who call for physician documentation clarification.

Qualifications:

This position requires...

- Excellent verbal and written communication skills
- The ability to both work independently and as an integral part of a team
- National certification as a CCS, CCS-P, CPC or CPC-H
- Strong computer skills in all applications of M/S Office, especially Word, Excel and Access
- Experience with practice management software and encoding software
- A minimum of 2 years of experience or graduation within the past 6 months from an approved college coding certificate or health information technology degree program.

Figure 3.1 Job description.

RECRUITING AND HIRING THE RIGHT PLAYERS

The first thing to keep in mind is that hiring the best employee for each job every time means you must attract a good pool of qualified candidates. The actual advertisement that is placed and where it is placed can be crucial to success. The ad must succinctly but accurately reflect the most important aspects of the job based on the highlights from the job description. Managers should realize that the hiring process is a two-way street. On the one hand, the manager is looking for the best person for the job. On the other hand, an experienced applicant who is looking for a better opportunity often has options. Therefore, the applicant carefully checks out the initial ad and, if interested, submits an application with an eye as to whether or not the job is the right one for him or her. So you want to look at the recruitment process from your perspective and from the perspective of a strong potential candidate.

Once you have a pool of applicants for a specific job opening, you should look at each application carefully using the job description as a guide. Remember to be objective in matching the candidate to the key requirements, duties, and responsibilities of the position. Once you look through all of the applications and eliminate those that do not meet the minimum requirements (or are overqualified), you'll be able to focus on what's left. There is no magic number, but if there are over five promising applicants, it may be a good strategy to choose the top five to seven candidates based on the applications and resumes, and then conduct a quick telephone interview.

Upon completion of the phone interview, the pool can be narrowed to the top three candidates. Next, do reference checks on these finalists before inviting them to a seated interview. The reference checks, at a minimum, will confirm the candidates haven't exaggerated their work experience. Ideally, you will be able to speak directly with a previous supervisor instead of a human resource representative. If this is the case, they still may only be able to verify job dates, title, and salary, but often an astute manager can either solicit a little extra information or hear reservations in the person's voice. You should have already discussed with the managing physician(s) if you are willing to pay the expenses for a strong candidate to come to an interview from greater than 50 miles away and also if you are willing to help with relocation expenses if the successful candidate does have to move closer to the job.

The purpose of the phone interview is to ascertain whether the candidates have the soft skills (conscientious, self-motivated, customer-focused, etc.) you are seeking to complement the technical skills and experience documented on their applications and resumes. You aren't trying to verify facts at this point but to determine if they know how to respond to some specific questions appropriately and to get a feeling about their work ethic and ability to work with others. From a legal perspective, it is important to ask each candidate the same set of questions so you can't later be accused of discrimination on any grounds (age, sex, race, creed, etc.). A few ideas that may be good to ask during the phone interview are:

1. Why are you leaving your current position?
2. What do you like best about working in this field?
3. What do you like the least?
4. Give an example of a situation in which you worked with others to solve a problem or accomplish a task.
5. Give an example of a situation in which you did something in your job that was above and beyond the requirements. How did you feel about doing this?
6. What are some of the words or phrases you think your supervisors, coworkers, and patients would say about you if they were asked to briefly describe you?

TIP

Try looking online or in a **professional journal** or field-specific magazine at ads for some positions such as Medical Coder, Billing or Insurance Specialist, Medical Office Manager or Administrator, etc. A professional journal is one that relates to the health information management or medical office management field, in this case, and is produced by a related professional organization, while a field-specific magazine typically contains fewer articles that have been reviewed by the author's peers but contains very useful suggestions, articles, and advertisements. Get ideas of what is appealing to you and what doesn't work well. Use these ideas to design your own ad as part of a recruitment plan at the end of this chapter. Note that you can capitalize on your practice's location if there is anything special about the area such as a beach, national park, or other appealing characteristics.

Telephone Interview: A meeting or consultation between a provider and a patient over the telephone to solicit information regarding treatment, payment, or health care operations.

Soft Skills: A term relating to a cluster of personality traits, social graces, communication, language, personal habits, friendliness, and optimism (sometimes called an "EQ" or emotional intelligence quotient) that characterize relationships with other people. Soft skills complement hard skills which are the occupational requirements of a job.

Professional Journal: Publication intended for target marketing to a specific industry or type of trade; examples range from professional magazines to peer-reviewed journals.

Discrimination: Employment discrimination occurs when an individual receives unequal treatment in an employment situation. In other words, promoting one person over the other based on age discrimination.

The personal interview is an extension of what you've learned thus far about each of the candidates remaining in your pool (Fig. 3.2). The best interviews place the candidates in as comfortable of a situation as possible so they can relax enough to feel they can respond to questions openly. Some managers reserve some time at the end of the interview to enable the employees who will work the most closely with the prospective candidate a chance to ask the candidate a few questions or just to introduce themselves and interact casually with the candidate. Other managers invite one or two employees in for the full interview. It's a good team building strategy to involve existing coworkers in the selection process to some degree.

Employment-related laws are discussed in the next chapter but it is important to mention that neither the application form nor the interviewer is legally able to solicit information directly or indirectly about age, race/ethnicity, religion, sexual orientation, health or disabilities, marital status, credit history, or whether or not the candidate has children living at home. Although the sex of the applicant will be obvious at some point, don't ask any questions of a woman that you wouldn't also ask a man. To avoid any gray areas, don't ask any questions you don't need answered to help you make a decision about the candidate's qualifications. For example, if the position doesn't require the employee to drive a company car or to drive his or her own car on company business, there is no reason to ask if he or she has a valid state license.

The most important goal of the personal interview is to get a better understanding of the candidate's technical skills and experience than is evident on the application and to get a good feeling for his or her work ethic and how well he or she interacts with others at all levels—from supervisors, to coworkers, to subordinates if applicable, to patients and other customers. The interview should be conversational. The candidate should be asked questions that reveal how flexible the candidate is about the work schedule, working in more

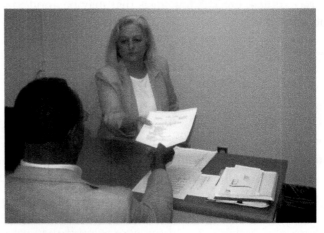

Figure 3.2 The job interview.

than one location if applicable, working overtime when necessary, or helping out coworkers even if the tasks are not directly related to the position in question. Other characteristics to explore include how well the candidate collaborates/cooperates with others, enthusiasm, and so forth.

The actual questions should require more than a simple yes or no response. The questions about the technical skills are dependent on the position. For example, for a receptionist, you might ask the candidate to describe a typical encounter with a patient in the office and how he or she handled multitasking if the phone rang and if the face-to-face patient required something involving the computer. For a medical coder, you might ask the candidate to describe the steps used to code a typical operative report and what the candidate did if he or she had a question about the correct code. The questions regarding interaction with people and work ethic can be the same for any candidate. Some examples are:

1. Can you give an example of a situation in which you helped get others excited about a project or task?
2. How do you handle a situation in which more than one issue must be addressed immediately to avert a possible crisis?
3. Do you consider yourself to be a person others look to when they need reassurance or advice?
4. How do you deal with an irate patient?

NEW TEAM MEMBER ORIENTATION AND HANDBOOK

Once the hiring decision has been made, all newly recruited team members need to have a clear orientation to the office including a tour of the full office with an explanation of who does what functions and how each function interacts with other functions (Fig. 3.3). Always remember to continually reinforce the concept of a patient-centric focus in everything the practice does.

Another part of orientation is to review the *Employee Handbook* with each new member of the team and to provide a copy of the handbook to the employee. The team member should sign a statement within 3 business days of employment that he or she has received and read the manual and agrees to comply with the policies and procedures contained therein. This manual, at a minimum, should contain policies and procedures regarding

- General information about the office including physical address and phone numbers
- A listing of all office job descriptions
- Pay schedule including any policy regarding cost of living increases and or merit increases/bonuses
- Orientation and training period

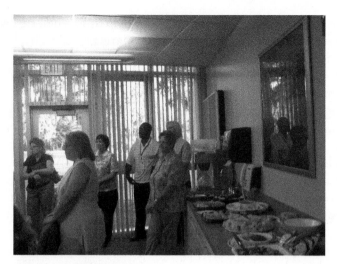

Figure 3.3 Group orientation.

- Employee evaluations
- Disciplinary policies including any appeals process
- Employee resignation notice
- Meals and other breaks (length, frequency, and whether or not the meal break is paid time)
- Benefits including any paid or unpaid time off, vacation, holidays, insurance, retirement, and any benefits for continuing education required for maintenance of licenses or credentials
- General policies such as confidentiality of patient and employee information, smoking, personal use of any employer or employee communications device, dress code, parking, and the expectations of each employee regarding keeping work areas neat and break areas clean.

TRAINING, RETAINING, AND MOTIVATING A TEAM OF CHAMPIONS

Once a new team member is thoroughly oriented to the office and the general policies and procedures, job-specific training is crucial for new employees and as an ongoing part of the culture for existing employees.

In addition to the orientation, the new employee needs to be trained in his or her job. Regardless of the amount of experience an employee has, each office has its own way to accomplish the tasks. Some of the differences that impact all employees include

- Practice management system
- Content and format of medical records and where paper records (if applicable) are stored
- The features of any electronic health records and degree of integration with other computer applications or interface with other facilities

- Protocols with regards to taking telephone calls or assisting a patient face to face
- Interacting with external customers or associates

Finally, the employee's individual job responsibilities require some degree of on-the-job training. Additionally, each major task should have a written procedure indicating how that task is carried out in that office.

For the ongoing training of all employees, the office manager should be aware of and consider the following training opportunities:

- Appropriate training any time an employee's job duties change due to promotion, lateral moves, or just a shift in procedures
- Training any time any of the office technology is upgraded or changed
- Training any time the office adopts new technology
- Training when rules, regulations, initiatives, or external requirements change or are officially clarified
- Free or inexpensive Web-based seminars for the employees affected by coding, reimbursement, or other third-party payer information
- Arranging for employees to take advantage of high-quality, economically reasonable continuing education offers
- Refresher training when it's been awhile since an employee did a task that now has to be done again
- Share information you find with your staff that should be of interest to all health care workers like a new medical device that's being tested or an emerging trend in any aspect of health care

The teamwork aspect of medical office management is a very rewarding aspect for the leader and for the employees. Simply stated, teams are comprised of two or more individuals working together to achieve specified outcomes or goals. Team members must communicate effectively, listen well to each other, and collaborate with the idea that each individual member can only succeed if the whole team succeeds. Teamwork consistently results in better service to the patients and other customers, continuous assessment and improvement of performance, increased morale and job satisfaction, and a less stressful work environment.

Sometimes teams are formed for a specific objective but a good manager is able to facilitate a team environment, office-wide, on an ongoing basis to help achieve continuous improvement of services and functions. Cross-training employees, when feasible (you can't cross-train a physical therapist assistant with a coding specialist, for example), increases the appreciation each team player has for the other players and the team as a whole.

The office culture should be one of courtesy and respect for everyone—internally and externally.

The office manager can help motivate individuals to become better teammates and more dedicated to their jobs in many ways. Managers

TIP

A recent graduate of a college or other reputable educational program, especially one that results in certification (e.g., a coding program that leads to the graduate becoming a certified procedural coder [CPC] or a certified coding specialist–physician based [CCS-P]), will require more training than an experienced coder who learned on the job but may make a better employee long term for several reasons. The inexperienced graduate takes longer to reach full productivity, but then there tends to be a period in which the experienced employee levels off, while the formal education of the recent graduate kicks in on issues such as researching the most current regulations or interpretations of policy, problem solving, improving procedures to increase efficiency and quality, and working toward continuous assessment and improvement of all related processes. Also, the person will feel loyal to the employer for providing the employee an opportunity to prove himself or herself.

should brainstorm occasionally with employees to determine what they think might make them more satisfied or increase morale—even if job satisfaction and morale are already relatively good.

People like to be recognized by others no matter how self-motivated they are. Managers should make a point of complimenting employees—especially in meetings or other gatherings. For example, when someone handled a particularly delicate situation extremely well or a group of employees pulled together to complete a backlog of work that accumulated during someone's absence. In a good team environment, each employee will be happy for the others when someone achieves special recognition, and it is even more rewarding when the office is recognized by the manager or physician(s) for achieving a goal that required good teamwork.

Employees often appreciate an office that acknowledges personal milestones too. Employees should be asked for suggestions regarding celebrating birthdays and work anniversaries. Be cautious, however, because celebrating something like an employee's wedding anniversary may not be a good idea since many employees have experienced divorce or death of a spouse or just regret that they never married.

Good communications are very important to motivating team players. Active listening is a crucial element of communicating effectively. Regular staff meetings, when well organized, facilitate team-wide communications in all directions—to and from physicians, the manager, and employees. The meetings should be kept on track as far as time, scheduled at a time that isn't likely to be interrupted, and conducted in a manner that encourages everyone to participate as appropriate.

Other motivational strategies include maintaining an environment in which employees feel respected and appreciated. Some examples of demonstrating that you trust your employees are

Delegate: To ask a subordinate to perform a task for which he or she has the authority to act on the superior's behalf but the superior is still ultimately responsible for the work getting done in a timely and accurate manner.

- Delegate thoughtfully—don't just dump on the employees. When you delegate effectively, you give the employee a chance to shine. Always remember that you delegate the authority the employee needs to get the job done, and you need to make sure that anyone the employee needs to deal with knows the employee has that authority. You don't, however, delegate responsibility, so if something does go wrong, you need to explain how the employee could have been more successful, and then you must do whatever is necessary to resolve the issue by taking the responsibility for it not getting done right the first time. Most of the time, a problem arises due to the manager overestimating an employee's abilities or not giving clear direction. Be sure the employee understands what is expected by when and what the consequences will be if the employee is not successful so that the employee understands there is a sense of urgency to let you know immediately if he or she runs into a snag. By the same token, don't hover and micromanage because that defeats the whole purpose of delegation.

- Whenever possible, ask the employees for ideas and let them participate in making decisions. Employees who were involved in a decision are the most likely to treat it as their own decision.

- Set goals with the staff and then work together to ensure the objectives are on track
- Be fair and consistent in dealing with all employees.

COACHING, CORRECTIVE ACTION, AND DISCIPLINE

Even under the best of circumstances, occasions arise in which an employee needs to do something differently. There are basically two types of issues that require management intervention to correct an employee issue. These are (1) problems with the performance of the employee's job or (2) problems with the employee's behavior/conduct.

Problems related to job performance are often correctable through coaching and mentoring. On the other hand, behavioral actions can be extreme enough to result in immediate termination or suspension pending further investigation (violence or direct threat of violence, theft, severe insubordination, breach of confidentiality of protected health information, etc.). Other behavioral issues may be resolved using corrective action. Examples include inappropriate dress, tardiness, excessive absenteeism, rudeness in dealing with patients, excessive personal calls during work hours, etc.

Performance issues relate to quality or productivity, while behavioral issues deal with violation of office rules or policies. Rules are black and white statements that leave no room for interpretation. For example, "NO SMOKING INSIDE THE FACILITY." Policies are guidelines that a manager uses to make decisions. An example of a policy addressing behavior or conduct is "EMPLOYEES ARE EXPECTED TO DRESS PROFESSIONALLY AND APPEAR NEAT AND WELL GROOMED."

With the exception of the category of behavior that needs to be dealt with by suspension or termination, an effective 4-step process to effectively address almost every other type of problem is delineated below.

Step 1: Always meet with the employee privately in your office. It is ineffective to talk with the employee about an issue in front of any other employees or in a public place where someone can interrupt your discussion.

Step 2: Focus on the behavior or performance issue, not the employee personally. For example, "Joe, I need your help. Why can't you get to work on time every day?"

Step 3: Get the employee to commit to what they are going to do to correct the problem. This makes the employee feel like he or she is in control of the situation, and it forces him or her to take responsibility for his or her action. Be sure both you and the employee are clear about the steps necessary and the time frame in which the steps must be carried out. Always document any discussions you have with an employee about performance or behavioral issues. The documentation should be dated and contain a summary of the steps to be taken, the time frames, and what will happen if the employee does not meet the agreed-upon outcomes. The employee should sign and date the documentation indicating that he or she understands and agrees with the steps necessary to prevent further disciplinary action.

Step 4: Before the employee leaves your office, make him or her feel like you are the employee's advocate. You want the employee to succeed, and you are there if he or she needs more guidance.

Let's look at two case studies. The first addresses a performance issue and the second a behavioral issue.

Case Study

PERFORMANCE ISSUE

The production standard for completing a claim form online is 20 per hour. Joe, a billing specialist who has been with the office about 9 months, had been meeting the standard most days, but over the past few weeks, has been averaging closer to 15 per hour. Sue, the office administrator, has noticed the drop in productivity but hasn't said anything to Joe yet. At the time Sue was analyzing month-end reports, she noticed that the days between services rendered and claim form submission for billing had increased that month from 2 days to 3 days. She knew this fact would cause the physician who owned the practice to grill her on the cause. Assuming it was due entirely to Joe's recent productivity drop and wanting to be able to tell her boss she has taken action, she went out to the billing area. She noticed Joe was at his desk and nobody else was within earshot, so she stood over Joe and said, "Joe, your production has been off lately, and it has caused us to lose a full day in the revenue cycle. What's the problem?" Joe immediately became defensive and replied, "How should I know? I just do my job." This really angered Sue who responded, "You're obviously not doing it very well." Joe responded, "If you think you can do it better, then knock yourself out because I quit!

OK, so how could this situation have been handled in a way that would have resulted in a win-win solution to the problem rather than a lose-lose case?

If you apply the 4-step process, Sue would have asked Joe to come to her office. Once Joe got there, Sue should have said, "Joe, we have a problem, and I need your help to solve it. Your productivity level has dropped significantly over the past few weeks. What do you think you can do to bring it back to an acceptable level?" This approach would make Joe feel like he wasn't being attacked and like Sue valued his input. He might say something like, "I've been trying to meet the standard every day, but lately it seems like I'm getting almost double the phone calls I was getting. Lisa (the new receptionist) doesn't seem to be able to handle more than one call at a time, and I back her up if the phone rings more than three times."

At this point, Sue needs to thank Joe and let him know that she will try to figure out how to minimize the number of calls he has to take on backup. Therefore, the last two steps aren't necessary. However, if Joe had said something about his productivity being slower because he hadn't been getting much sleep and was finding it difficult to concentrate, then the third step would be for Sue to tell him that she appreciates his honesty but that he needs to outline for her what he plans to do to correct the problem immediately and on a sustained basis. Finally, Sue would remind him that she is there for him if he has any obstacles in carrying out his commitment.

Case Study

BEHAVIORAL ISSUE

The office policy is for an employee to have no more than three absences in any 3-month period and that every third incident of being 5 minutes or more tardy counts as an absence. Sally has been with the office for 2 years as a professional coder. She has consistently managed to be absent the maximum number of times allowable under the policy. The office manager, Stan, notices a pattern—Sally's absences always occur on a Friday one time and a Monday the next time. Stan finally gets his chance to initiate corrective action when Sally gets to work late one morning after having already been tardy two other times recently, putting her over the allowable absences for that time frame. He calls her into his office and asks her if she thinks he's stupid enough to not notice that she is manipulating the attendance policy. She asks if he's calling her a liar. He says, "Nobody gets sick at the end of the week one month and the beginning of the week the next month for a whole year." She tells him she can get doctor's excuses. He says she probably is friends with a doctor who will write excuses for her. She finally yells, "I'm going to call my lawyer to file a workers' comp case against you since you are causing the stress that causes me to be sick so much."

This scenario could actually result in litigation, so managers must be cautious to not accuse employees of misconduct such as lying. How could Stan have turned this into a win–win scenario?

Using the 4-step process, Stan could have called Sally into his office. He should have told her that her absences had exceeded the allowable amount for the previous 90-day period. He should explain that she has not only exceeded the absences this time but that she consistently maxes out on the allowable absences in any 90-day period. He should further explain that he values her productivity but that her productivity is zero every day she is absent from work and that results in everyone in the office having to work harder to compensate. He should ask her what she can do to decrease the frequency of her absences—especially on Mondays, the highest volume day and Fridays, the day the office strives to catch up for the week with any work that has fallen behind. Depending on Sally's response, Stan can require her to bring a doctor's note for any future absences. If she commits to immediate and sustained improvement, Stan doesn't need to say anything further, but if he thinks she doesn't realize the severity of this situation, he can have her sign a note that she understands her responsibility and is aware that further absences will result in progressive disciplinary action up to and including termination of employment.

SUMMARY

Starting with the desired outcome of a loyal patient base, the successful medical practice administrator will create a staffing plan that includes recruiting, training, motivating, and retaining the best possible individuals. The effective leader will integrate individual employee development with coaching all employees to work as a team. There are many steps and tools that, when designed and implemented correctly, will assist the administrator in achieving the goal of building a patient-centric, championship team.

CHAPTER REVIEW QUESTIONS

1. List the minimum data that should be included on a job analysis.

_____

_____

_____

2. Describe how a job description assists in the hiring process.

_____

_____

_____

3. Describe how a job description assists in training a new employee.

_____

_____

_____

4. Describe how a job description assists with formal performance appraisals.

_____

_____

_____

5. What is the purpose of asking a candidate for a job in a medical office interview questions that aren't directly related to the technical aspects of the job for which he or she is being interviewed?

_____

_____

_____

6. Why is it important to have a policies and procedures manual instead of just verbally telling employees what the office policies are?

_____

_____

_____

7. List some instances in which it may be necessary for the manager to provide training.

_____

_____

_____

8. What are some things a manager can do to motivate employees?

_____

_____

_____

Workbook for
Chapter 3

Workbook:
Chapter 3 Leading the Medical Office Team

3.A: ILLUSTRATION: CREATE A RECRUITMENT AD

Using Figure 3.1 from your textbook as the description of a position that is open, create an advertisement to recruit certified candidates for this position. Highlight the aspects of your practice that make it a desirable place to work as well as any special draw your geographical region may have to offer. For example, collaborative or team environment, competitive pay with excellent benefits, pay for continuing education hours (CE) for credential maintenance, and located 10 miles away from a popular beach.

3.B: DESIGN AN IN-SERVICE TRAINING SESSION

Office administrators must be effective at writing up a training session and presenting it to the staff. Sometimes this is done for new employees or for employees who are promoted or cross-trained in other functions. Sometimes the training is for all staff to show them how to do a new procedure or use new technology.

In-Service Training: You have just hired a new receptionist. She learns quickly and is flexible, but she is inconsistent in the manner in which she answers the telephone. Sometimes she identifies herself and the name of the practice, sometimes she just says, "Hello, may I help you." She doesn't seem to have a consistent method of taking messages either. Design a short training session including a step-by-step procedure that addresses

- What to say upon answering the phone
- What to say if you need to place a caller on hold
- What information is needed for every telephone message

3.C: DEVELOP A RECRUITMENT PLAN

Recruitment Plan: See the sample job description in Figure 3.1 in your text, or find a job description online. Then, make a plan for recruiting a desirable candidate for that position. The plan should include a budget for the advertisement(s); whether the ad will be local, regional or national; whether the ad will be posted with college campuses, radio, tv, newspapers, websites, medical office management/health information management journals or some combination; and, whether or not some financial assistance will be offered to travel to an interview if more than 50 miles away and if there will be assistance for relocation.

3.D: VIDEO ACTIVITY (HOW *NOT* TO HANDLE A PERFORMANCE ISSUE)

 (See video clip on thePoint Web site to complete this activity.)

1. The video clip is based on the following case scenario presented in the chapter:

   The office policy is for an employee to have no more than three absences in any 3-month period and that every third incident of being 5 minutes or more tardy counts as an absence. Sally has been with the office for 2 years as a professional coder. She has consistently managed to be absent the maximum number of times allowable under the policy. The office manager, Sara, notices a pattern—Sally's absences always occur on a Friday one time and a Monday the next time. Sara finally gets the chance to initiate corrective action when Sally gets to work late one morning after having already been tardy two other times recently. Sara calls Sally into her office and asks Sally if Sally thinks Sara's stupid enough to not notice that Sally is manipulating the attendance policy. Sally asks if Sara's calling her a liar. Sara replies, "Nobody gets sick at the end of the week one month and the beginning of the week the next month for a whole year." Sally retorts that she can get doctor's excuses. Sara responds that she probably is friends with a doctor who will write excuses for her. Sally finally yells, "I'm going to call my lawyer to file a workers' comp case against you since you are causing the stress that causes me to be sick so much."

   _____

   _____

   _____

2. View the video clip.

   _____

   _____

   _____

3. Identify any mistakes you think were made by Sara.

_____

_____

_____

4. Jot down ideas for how Sara could have handled this situation more effectively at the same time as she used the 4-Step Corrective Action Process to give Sally an opportunity to correct her behavior and become a loyal member of the team.

_____

_____

_____

5. Now, using the same scenario, write how you would have handled that situation had you been Sara. Include any dialogue from Sara or Sally. Be prepared to either submit your findings and solution or to role play your solution with a classmate.

_____

_____

_____

3.E: EXPERT PANEL

Read the following real-life scenario. Your instructor may have you break into teams or respond as an individual expert. Each team or individual needs to create a dialogue depicting how a real-world conversation between Fran and Jenny may go in which Fran is attempting to resolve the issue without losing Jenny's enthusiasm or normally good work ethic. Once each team or individual response is prepared, the instructor may ask students to chose the top three solutions and describe why they are the best.

Jenny is an excellent receptionist who has been with the practice several years. She is usually fast, accurate, and good with the patients and other customers. Lately, however, she has been speaking with and texting her fiancé during work time. Fran, the office manager, notices that Jenny has started to make some careless errors when scheduling appointments and occasionally not getting all of her work done by the end of the day. One day, Fran asks Jenny a question and Jenny says, "Just a minute, I'll be right with you," and then finishes sending a text message.

4

Managing the Team Players

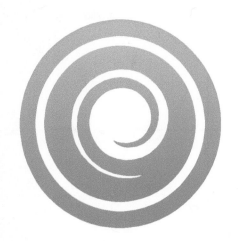

Upon completion of this chapter, the student should...

- Describe the basic function of human resource management
- Describe the basic employment laws pertaining to small practice management
- Describe and evaluate the various types of compensation and employee benefits available
- Evaluate employee incentive strategies
- Demonstrate the communication skills necessary for effective performance feedback
- Describe the basic options for managing payroll systems
- Design employee policies to address employee health and safety and emergency preparedness

KEY TERMS

Age Discrimination in Employment Act (ADEA)
Americans with Disabilities Act of 1990 (ADA)
Behaviorally Anchored Rating Scale
Civil Rights Act
Consolidated Omnibus Budget Reconciliation Act (COBRA)
Equal Pay Act (EPA)
External Equity
Fair Credit Reporting Act (FCRA)
Fair Labor Standards Act (FLSA)
Family and Medical Leave Act (FMLA)
Genetic Information Nondiscrimination Act (GINA)

Graphic Rating Scales
Immigration Reform and Control Act of 1986 (IRCA)
Incentive Plans
Internal Equity
Management by Objectives
Merit Pay
National Labor Relations Act (NLRA)
National Labor Relations Board (NLRB)
Occupational Safety and Health Act (OSHA)
Older Workers Benefit Protection Act (OWBPA)
Paired Comparison Method
Pay-for-Performance Plans

Personal Responsibility and Work Opportunity
    Reconciliation Act (PRWORA)
Pregnancy Discrimination Act (PDA)
Reasonable Accommodations
Scanlon Plan
SMART Goals

Society for Human Resource Management
    (SHRM)
Team-based Incentive Plans
Uniformed Services Employment and
    Reemployment Rights Act (USERRA)

OVERVIEW

A critical part of managing a medical practice is to understand and practice effective human resource (HR) management principles. The HR function is an essential part of any successful organization; however, the health care field has its own specific laws and policies with regard to employment law that must be recognized and communicated properly. Proper management of the medical practice's HRs will lead to higher levels of employee engagement and create a collaborative, patient-centric team environment where all stakeholders benefit. At the very least, attention to employment laws and regulations will save the practice time and money and avoid costly law suits and penalties.

HR management is a broad field that plays an important role in an organization's functioning, touching each part of the operation in specific ways. The first two roles of HR were discussed in the last chapter—find and hire the best people and train them to effectively work together to achieve the practice's goals. After these individuals have been hired, acclimated to the organization's culture, and trained, their performance needs to be appraised. Performance appraisals should be an interactive process that focuses on developing strengths rather than documenting failures. HR also includes compensation and benefits where managers decide which incentives will work best and how to manage payroll. Finally, HR oversees employee health and safety by ensuring policies and procedures are in place and communicated to employees on a regular basis.

EMPLOYMENT LAWS

One of the most important parts of managing employees is to know, understand, and communicate all laws and policies relevant to the medical practice. Mistakes in this area, even by managers who are trying to do the right thing, can cost your practice significant amounts of revenue and even result in criminal charges. Larger organizations have a legal department within HR that handles this area. While it is not practical for smaller organizations such as your practice to have a legal department, it is wise for the practice to have a lawyer it can consult who specializes in employment law. There are a considerable number of employment laws pertaining to medical practices; this section provides a brief overview of some of the more common and significant federal employment laws. While each state has their own regulations, this chapter does not touch on the wide variety of state laws that may impact your practice.

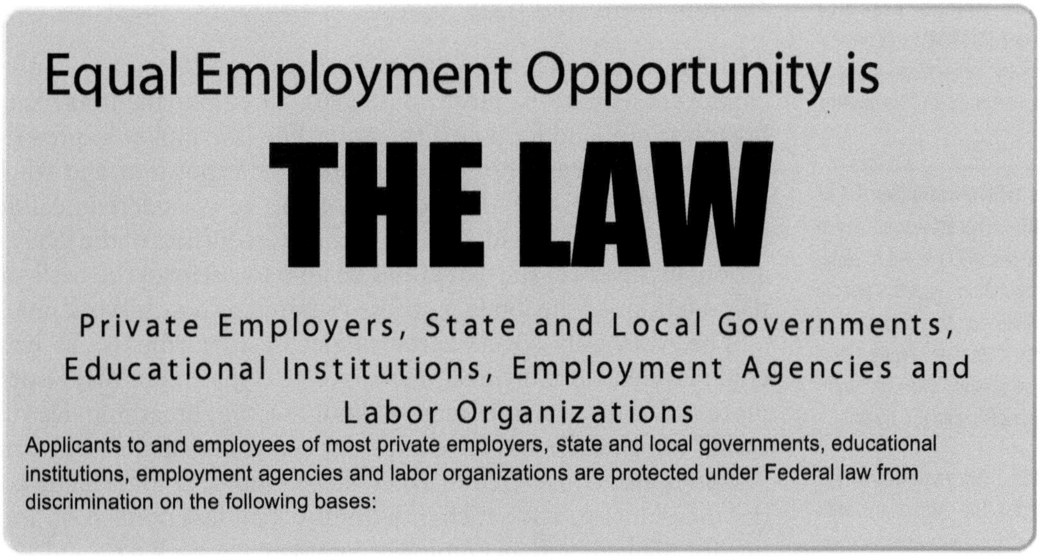

Equal Employment Opportunity is

THE LAW

Private Employers, State and Local Governments, Educational Institutions, Employment Agencies and Labor Organizations

Applicants to and employees of most private employers, state and local governments, educational institutions, employment agencies and labor organizations are protected under Federal law from discrimination on the following bases:

Figure 4.1 Header of poster from www.dol.gov/ofccp/regs/compliance/posters/pdf/eeopost.pdf

Federal employment law consists of statutes, regulations, and court decisions. The first set of federal laws that you should be aware of is meant to provide equal opportunity to all employees. These include the Age Discrimination in Employment Act (ADEA), the Americans with Disabilities Act of 1990 (ADA), the Equal Pay Act (EPA), the Pregnancy Discrimination Act (PDA), the Civil Rights Act of 1866 (Section 1981), Title VII of the Civil Rights Act of 1964 (Title VII), and the Uniformed Services Employment and Reemployment Rights Act (USERRA).

The Age Discrimination in Employment Act

The Age Discrimination in Employment Act (ADEA) applies to all employers with 20 or more employees. It prohibits discrimination against applicants and employees who are 40 years of age or older in all aspects of employment (e.g., hiring compensation, promotions, lay-offs, and time off). While there are no reporting requirements for this law, employers are required to post a notice regarding the ADEA. The Equal Employment Is the Law posters as seen in Figure 4.1 created and distributed by the Equal Employment Opportunity Commission fulfill this posting requirement.

Box 4.1

Motivation for Compliance with Employment Laws

The most effective managers or administrators, however, maintain a philosophy that policies and laws pertaining to equity and protection of the team members need to be communicated and enforced because it is the right way to build and maintain a team that makes establishing patient loyalty a high priority, due to knowing their own needs are being met by their "coach," and not because of fear of penalties.

TIP

The Society for Human Resource Management (SHRM) is a professional organization that specializes in the management of employees regardless of the business or service, and it provides a valuable tool for managers attempting to understand the myriad federal and state laws that pertain to their particular organization's situation. For example, some federal laws apply only to employers with 100 or more employees (e.g., Worker Adjustment and Notification Act [WARN]), while others apply to employers with 15 or more employees (e.g., Title VII of the Civil Rights Act of 1964). Still others apply to all private employers with one or more employees (e.g., Occupational Safety and Health Act [OSHA]).

Age Discrimination in Employment Act (ADEA): An act of Congress passed into federal law in the United States in 1967 making it illegal to discriminate against anyone over the age of 40 years.

Society for Human Resource Management (SHRM): A professional human resources association headquartered in Alexandria, Virginia.

Americans with Disabilities Act of 1990 (ADA): This act was amended in 2008. The law was passed to eliminate discrimination against people with disabilities for the purposes of employment including hiring, promoting, discharging, workers compensation benefits, and job training.

Reasonable Accommodations: Created under the Americans with Disabilities Act, reasonable accommodations are defined as any modification or adjustment to a job or the work environment that will enable a qualified applicant or employee with a disability to participate in the application process or to perform essential job functions. Reasonable accommodation also includes adjustments to assure that a qualified individual with a disability has rights and privileges in employment equal to those of employees without disabilities.

Equal Pay Act (EPA): Law passed in 1974 with the essential purpose of ensuring that women and men receive equal pay for equal work. However, the act protects both genders from wage discrimination based on sex.

The Americans with Disabilities Act of 1990

The **Americans with Disabilities Act of 1990 (ADA)** applies to all employers with 15 or more employees, all employment agencies, labor organizations, and local governments. The law applies to prospective or current employees who are qualified for the position and who have a disability that fits the ADA's definition. To be considered qualified for a particular job, an individual must fit the prerequisites of the job (e.g., education, experience, and skills) and be able to perform the basic or essential functions of the job (e.g., those required to do the work involved).

The ADA only covers certain types of impairments. To be considered disabled, an individual must have an impairment that limits one or more major life activities (e.g., walking, seeing, breathing, learning, and caring for oneself) and have a history of having such an impairment. A person is also considered disabled if the employer incorrectly considers the individual to have such a disability. The last point is an important one for managers. If an employee complains of back pain and a manager accommodates him by altering job tasks or moving his cubicle to a lower floor, the employee can then be classified as disabled because he was treated as if he had a disability.

The ADA requires employers to make **reasonable accommodations** for potential and current employees (Fig. 4.2). This means that accommodations that pose an unreasonable hardship on the organization do not have to be made (i.e., the cost of an accommodation would cause the practice financial hardship). While employers are prohibited from asking about a job applicant's disabilities, an employer may ask a job candidate how they will perform essential job functions. Finally, employers do not have to hire a qualified candidate with a disability if doing so would directly threaten the health and safety of the individual or other workers.

The Equal Pay Act

The **Equal Pay Act (EPA)** was passed in 1974 with the essential purpose of ensuring that women and men receive equal pay for equal work. However, the act protects both genders from wage discrimination based

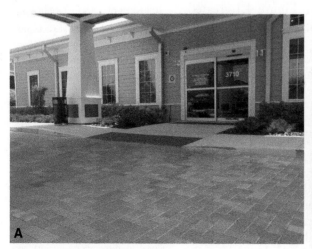
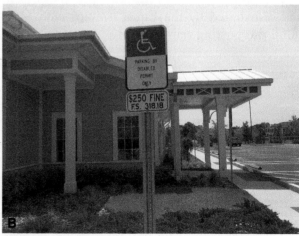

Figure 4.2 Reasonable accommodation.

on sex. Most businesses are covered by the act that requires workers performing equal work to be paid equal pay rates. This doesn't mean they are paid the same amount of money since pay can vary for a particular pay rate (e.g., pay grades). Along with equal pay is equal compensation in terms of fringe benefits and incentive pay. The only exceptions to the equal pay requirements are situations involving seniority, merit, the quantity or quality of production, and any other legitimate factor aside from sex (e.g., premiums for certain shifts).

The Pregnancy Discrimination Act

The Pregnancy Discrimination Act (PDA) essentially established that discrimination based on pregnancy, child birth, or related medical conditions in employment qualifies as illegal sex-based discrimination as outlined in Title VII of the Civil Rights Act of 1964. This means that employers are required to treat workers with pregnancy-related disabilities the same as workers with any other temporary disability (e.g., a broken leg).

Civil Rights Act of 1866 and Civil Rights of 1964 (Title VII)

While Title VII of the Civil Rights Act of 1964 is the most well known of EEO legislation, a lesser known law is Section 1981 of the Civil Rights Act of 1866. This earlier piece of legislation conferred a number of rights to African Americans, the most significant of which was the right to make and enforce contracts which the courts have interpreted as prohibiting racial discrimination in employment since this represents a contract between an employer and an employee. Section 1981 pertains only to intentional discrimination based on race or ethnicity.

Title VII (The Civil Rights Act of 1964) extends the protections first established in Section 1981 of the Civil Rights Act of 1866 to include discrimination and harassment based on sex, race, color, religion, and national origin in all aspects of employment. The law pertains to private employers with 15 or more employees.

Uniformed Services Employment and Reemployment Rights Act

Uniformed Services Employment and Reemployment Rights Act (USERRA) protects members of the uniformed services and covers all employers. Under this act, employers may not discriminate against members of the uniformed services; they must reinstate employees upon their return (from up to 5 years of leave for service); they must restore all benefits to the returning employee and treat time away as time worked (when determining eligibility for benefits, seniority and vesting); and finally, employers cannot fire returning employees for up to 1 year after they return from service (except for cause).

Other Important Federal Laws Related to Employment

Other federal laws that you should be aware of include the Consolidated Omnibus Budget Reconciliation Act (COBRA), the Fair Credit Reporting Act (FCRA), the Fair Labor Standards Act (FLSA), the Family and Medical Leave Act (FMLA), the Genetic Information

Pregnancy Discrimination Act (PDA): Make illegal discrimination on the basis of pregnancy, childbirth, or related medical conditions constitutes unlawful sex discrimination; women who are pregnant must be treated in the same manner as other applicants or employees with similar abilities or limitations.

Civil Rights Act: Originally passed in 1866 to outlaw certain discriminatory practices for African Americans after the Civil War, it was amended in 1964 to make any type of discrimination against blacks and women illegal. Amended again in 1968 to increase enforcement and include Fair Housing, this law continues to protect minorities from any form of employment discrimination.

Uniformed Services Employment and Reemployment Rights Act (USERRA): A law that establishes, with some exceptions, the cumulative length of time that an individual may be absent from work for military duty and retain reemployment rights to 5 years. USERRA clearly establishes that reemployment protection does not depend on the timing, frequency, duration, or nature of an individual's service as long as the basic eligibility criteria are met.

Nondiscrimination Act (GINA), the Immigration Reform and Control Act of 1986 (IRCA), the National Labor Relations Act (NLRA), the Older Workers Benefit Protection Act (OWBPA), the Personal Responsibility and Work Opportunity Reconciliation Act (PRWORA), and the Occupational Safety and Health Act (OSHA).

Consolidated Omnibus Budget Reconciliation Act

Consolidated Omnibus Budget Reconciliation Act (COBRA): An act established in 1985 to assist employees who find themselves involuntarily unemployed to continue health care benefits for themselves and their families at the employer's group rates. While the former employee pays the full amount, this option is typically less expensive than the individual or self-insured rate.

The Consolidated Omnibus Budget Reconciliation Act (COBRA) was established in 1985 to assist employees who find themselves involuntarily unemployed to continue health care benefits for themselves and their families at the employer's group rates. While the former employee pays the full amount, this option is typically less expensive than the individual or self-insured rate. Administration of COBRA can be complex given the notification requirements. For this reason, many organizations large and small outsource this duty to companies specializing in COBRA administration.

Fair Credit Reporting Act

Fair Credit Reporting Act (FCRA): A law that protects the privacy of individuals' consumer credit information, giving them the right to access their credit reports, know when someone has used this information in decision regarding credit, housing, employment, or other benefits, and dispute inaccurate information. With regard to employment, the FCRA places certain restrictions and obligations on employers who wish to access and use information in a potential employee's or current employee's credit report.

The Fair Credit Reporting Act (FCRA) covers all employers and essentially protects the privacy of individuals' consumer credit information, giving them the right to access to their credit reports, know when someone has used this information in decision regarding credit, housing, employment or other benefits, and dispute inaccurate information.

With regard to employment, the FCRA places certain restrictions and obligation on employers that wish to access and use information in a potential employee's or current employee's credit report. As a manager, you must first notify an employee or applicant in writing that you want their report and obtain written authorization from them before requesting the report. You must then verify with the credit reporting agency that you gave notice and received permission from the individual. The exception to this rule is when an employer uses an outside party to investigate alleged workplace misconduct. The FTC had previously interpreted third-party investigations as part of the FCRA's requirements which would mean that an individual could refuse to consent to an investigation, albeit fraud or sexual harassment.

If you receive notice of an address discrepancy from the credit reporting agency, it is your responsibility to ensure that the report received belongs to the person about whom you've requested a report. If you take an adverse action based on information in a report, you must provide the individual with specific information about the report and the consumer reporting agency it was received from. Finally, to guard the privacy of individuals, you must limit access to consumer reports that have been collected. Specific steps must be taken when destroying such information in order to prevent identify theft and other unauthorized uses of an individual's credit report data.

The Fair Labor Standards Act

Fair Labor Standards Act (FLSA): A federal law that regulates wages and hours. It determines how much workers must be paid, at a minimum, and how many hours they can be required to work.

The Fair Labor Standards Act (FLSA) is an important federal law for most employers since it regulates wages and hours. In particular, it determines how much workers must be paid and how many hours they can be required to work. It also contains rules with regard to younger workers. Those covered include any business with annual sales of at least $500,000 or that engage in interstate commerce—in today's market, this covers essentially all organizations. Medical practices are covered by the act's provision that employers whose employees use the mail, telephone, or other equipment (e.g., Internet) to communicate across state lines must comply.

This is the law that defines exempt and nonexempt categories and determines the rules for classifying employees in each group. Essentially, you can apply either the salary test or the job duties test to do so. As of 2008, the Department of Labor issued new guidelines on employee categories to help employers better understand the exempt and nonexempt classifications.

With regard to minimum wage, the FLSA sets the minimum and though state laws may set their own limits differently, if employers are covered under the FLSA provisions, they cannot go below the federal level. For example, since July 2009, the federal minimum wage has been $7.25 per hour for all covered nonexempt employees. Washington State's 2010 minimum wage is the nation's highest at $8.55 while Wyoming State has the lowest at $5.15. Employers in Wyoming that are covered under FLSA must pay a minimum wage of $7.25. Those that are not covered need only meet the state's minimum level.

Hours worked is another area regulated by the FLSA and the general rule is this: As an employer, you must pay employees for any of their time that benefits the organization and that you, the employer, control. For the typical medical practice, time that needs to be considered for pay includes on-call time, meals and breaks, and travel and commuting.

Overtime can be a complex calculation for some organizations, but basically, an employee should receive overtime pay (time and a half) for each additional hour worked above the 40 hours a week. Some states have daily overtime standards (i.e., employees who work more than 8 hours in a day are eligible for overtime pay), so it's important to be aware of your particular state's overtime regulations. The Department of Labor has created a fact sheet to assist you in calculating overtime pay. You can access this fact sheet at www.dol.gov/esa/whd/regs/compliance/whdfs23.pdf

The last area the FLSA deals with is child labor. While it is legal to employ teenagers as young as 14 or 15, they may only do certain types of tasks and may only work limited hours. Any employee 16 or younger may not perform work that has been deemed "hazardous" by the Secretary of Labor. Finally, child labor laws do not apply to certain younger employees such as children who work for their parents.

The Family and Medical Leave Act

The **Family and Medical Leave Act (FMLA)** applies to private employers with 50 or more employees in addition to the federal, state, and local governments and schools. Essentially, the law provides eligible employees with the right to take up to 12 weeks of unpaid leave per 12-month period for certain reasons. These include time to bond with a new child (whether by birth, adoption, or foster care), time to care for a family member with a health problem (you are allowed to ask for certification of the condition),

Family and Medical Leave Act (FMLA): A law that provides eligible employees with the right to take up to 12 weeks of unpaid leave per 12-month period for certain reasons such as to bond with a new child or care for a sick spouse.

time to deal with their own health problem, and time to deal with a qualifying exigency (i.e., all related to military service of a spouse, child, or parent). If your practice is covered by the FMLA, visit the DOL's FMLA page for complete information on the rights and responsibilities for both you and your employees: www.dol.gov/esa/whd/fmla/index.htm.

The Genetic Information Nondiscrimination Act

Genetic Information Nondiscrimination Act (GINA): The most recent new civil rights law–GINA prohibits health insurers from using genetic information in decisions about insurance coverage or premiums. With regard to employers, the act prohibits the use of genetic information in employment decisions such as hiring and promotion and requires employers to keep genetic information confidential.

The Genetic Information Nondiscrimination Act (GINA) is considered the most recent new civil rights law that was signed by President Bush in 2008. It is an extension of the protections afforded federal workers by President Clinton's Executive Order 13145 from 2000. The law covered private employers with 15 or more employees, federal and state governments, employment agencies, and labor organizations. GINA prohibits health insurers from using genetic information to decisions about insurance coverage or premiums. With regard to employers, the act prohibits the use of genetic information in employment decisions such as hiring and promotion and requires employers to keep genetic information confidential. Figure 4.3 is a genetic marker for breast cancer risk.

The Immigration Reform and Control Act of 1986

Immigration Reform and Control Act of 1986 (IRCA): A law containing three major provisions that require employers to verify that all employees are eligible to work in the United States; to keep records of employment verification; and to refrain from discrimination based on citizenship status or national origin.

The Immigration Reform and Control Act of 1986 (IRCA) of 1986 represented an overhaul of immigration policy as it applies to employment. Three major provisions of the act require employers to verify that all employees are eligible to work in the United States, to keep records of employment verification, and refrain from discrimination based on citizenship status or national origin. To assist you in verification of employee status, the USCIS allows employers to check Social Security Administration and Department of Homeland Security databases to verify the employment authorization of newly hired employees.

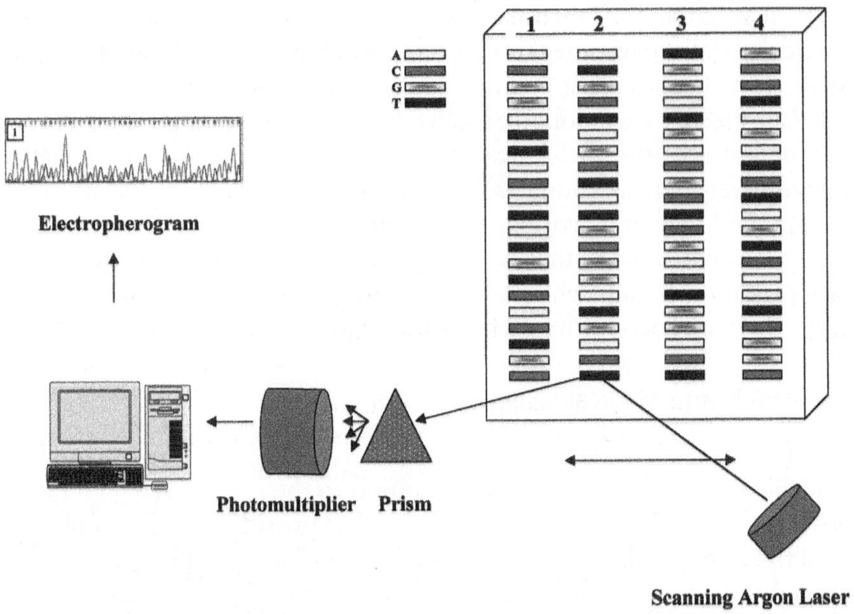

Figure 4.3 Genetic testing for disease markers.

Section 2. Employer Review and Verification (*to be completed and signed by employer. Examine one document for List A OR examine one document form List B and one from List C, as listed on the reverse of this form, and record the title, number, and expiration date, if any, of the document(s).*)

List A	**OR**	**List B**	**AND**	**List C**
Document title:_____		_____		_____
Issuing Authority:_____		_____		_____
Document#:_____		_____		_____
Expiration Date (if any):_____				

CERTIFICATION: I attest, under penalty of perjury, that I have examined the document(s) presented b the above-

Figure 4.4 Section of I-9 form.

This act has seen increased enforcement due to estimates that place the number of undocumented workers in the United States at between 6 and 8 million. The enforcement arm of the IRCA is the ICE (Immigration and Customs Enforcement). This agency reported more than 6,000 arrests between October 2008 and June 2009 that included business owners, office managers, supervisors, and HR professionals for knowingly hiring undocumented workers or failing to properly verify employment status. Figure 4.4 shows the middle section of an I-9 form in which the employer must verify they saw an original document from column 1 such as a passport, or an original document from column B and one from column C. After verifying that the authorized practice representative has seen the original document(s), a copy of those documents is attached to the I-9 form.

The National Labor Relations Act

The National Labor Relations Act (NLRA) applies to essentially all private employers and regulates what unions and management can and cannot do when interacting with one another and with employees. The National Labor Relations Board (NLRB) is the enforcement arm of the act and will only step in when certain jurisdictional standards are met. For medical practices, the standard is at least $100,000 in total business volume per year. When this limit is reached, the NLRB will enforce the provisions of the act in the event that employees exercise their right to organize.

The Older Workers Benefit Protection Act

The Older Workers Benefit Protection Act (OWBPA) helps protect older workers (those 40 years or older) from discrimination with respect to fringe benefits such as life insurance, health insurance, disability benefits, pensions, and retirement benefits. All employers are covered by the law which is actually an amendment to the ADEA. While an employer cannot discrimination against older workers with regard to these types of benefits, you are allowed to reduce the benefits of older workers when justified (e.g., cost), but only if offset with additional types of benefits (from you or the government). The rules associated with the act are detailed and can be confusing when attempting to calculate balanced benefits packages for older and younger workers. For explanations and examples of OWBPA's rules, see www.eeoc.gov/policy/docs/benefits.html

National Labor Relations Act (NLRA): A law that regulates what unions and management can and cannot do when interacting with one another and with employees.

National Labor Relations Board (NLRB): The enforcement arm of the NLRA. When a certain jurisdictional standard is reached, the NLRB will enforce the provisions of the act in the event that employees exercise their right to organize.

Older Workers' Benefit Protection Act (OWBPA): A law that forbids discrimination by employers based on age when providing employee benefits, such as severance, and also ensures that no employee is coerced or pressured into signing legal waivers of rights under the Age Discrimination in Employment Act (ADEA).

The Personal Responsibility and Work Opportunity Reconciliation Act

Personal Responsibility and Work Opportunity Reconciliation Act (PRWORA): A reform law that ended welfare as an entitlement program, required recipients to begin working after 2 years of receiving benefits, placed a lifetime limit of 5 years on benefits paid by federal funds, aimed to encourage two-parent families and discourage out-of-wedlock births, and enhanced enforcement of child support.

The **Personal Responsibility and Work Opportunity Reconciliation Act (PRWORA)** has been in effect since 1996 and was a major part of President Clinton's welfare reform initiatives. While the act is quite broad with respect to welfare law, this chapter centers on its employer-related provisions for the collection of child support. Employers are required to report all new hires to a state registry within 20 days of the hire date. The registry information is then used to track down parents who have failed to meet their child support responsibilities. You can fulfill this reporting requirement by supplying the registry with a copy of the new hire's IRS W-4 form. There is a $25 penalty for each new hire that is not reported to the state registry within the 20-day period.

THE OCCUPATIONAL SAFETY AND HEALTH ACT

Occupational Safety and Health Act (OSHA): The primary federal law that governs occupational health and safety in the private sector and federal government in the United States.

The **Occupational Safety and Health Act (OSHA)** was passed in 1970 to ensure safe working conditions for all U.S. workers. All private employers are covered under the act. Employers are required to know the specific standards that apply to their industry and business and maintain strict compliance with those standards. For a comprehensive list of employer responsibilities under OSHA, see www.osha.gov/as/opa/worker/employer-responsibility.html. As an employer, you have reporting requirements, post requirements, and record-keeping requirements to uphold. Penalties for violation of OSHA can be quite steep, costing an organization as much as $70,000 for each willful or repeated violation.

Case Study

NANCIE JONES AND EMPLOYMENT ISSUES AT HEALTHY YOU CLINIC

Nancie Jones has been hired as the practice administrator. Her predecessor left without notice due to a conflict with the managing physician. She has been oriented to the practice and is now accessing the e-mail that has been received since the previous administrator left. She notices several e-mail messages marked urgent and containing subjects such as morale, compliance, and legal issues. She opens the oldest message that is marked urgent and learns that her predecessor apparently denied a request for family leave from an employee whose husband had undergone bypass surgery and didn't have anyone else to care for him until he could regain his mobility. Other than the day of the surgery, the administrator had told the employee that the practice was short staffed and that they could not spare her. The employee had apparently sought legal advice because she had been forced to pay for a day-care provider for her husband that cost more than she earned on a daily basis. The attorney wants the new administrator to contact him as soon as possible.

What would you do?

One good approach for Nancie is to explain to the employee that she is going to contact the attorney immediately. Then, she should ask the attorney to fill her in on all the facts and what the attorney is requesting the practice do for this employee. She should be very careful not to comment or make any promises—just listen. If the attorney asks her what she plans to do, she should explain that she needs to gather the facts before she can determine any course of action. She should then refresh her knowledge of the family medical leave act and let the managing physician know she will contact the practice's attorney for advice before bringing a recommendation to the managing physician for approval. She should keep the employee fully informed so the employee has a chance to see that Nancie is going to make every effort to help the employee and, more importantly, that she is concerned for the mental, physical, and financial health of the employee.

PERFORMANCE APPRAISALS

Evaluating employee performance has not always been a manager's favorite task and in fact, when done incorrectly, the process can be a stressful experience for manager and employee alike. Appraising employee performance is now treated more as an integrated, collaborative process. In fact, HR professionals and managers refer to the evaluative process as performance management to capture the broader spectrum of activities that takes place.

This section addresses how the appraisal itself should be conducted, and the next sections discuss incentive options and compensation and benefits.

Employees will have difficulty performing well if they do not know what is expected of them in terms of goals and standards. Therefore, before you can evaluate their performance, it is important to make sure an employee knows what their job is, what goals they should meet, and how their success will be measured. As discussed earlier in the textbook,

Box 4.2

Collaborative approach to Performance Management

Performance appraisals should not start when you fill out the evaluation form. Instead performance management begins when you and your employees set goals for their performance together, you make sure they get the training they need to achieve those goals, and then appraise their performance. Based upon the results, you determine the type and amount of reward that makes sense.

job descriptions are a critical tool for communicating tasks to employees. These documents should be reviewed with employees and updated periodically based on input from those that actually perform the work. If there is agreement on the job description—that it is an accurate reflection of what the position requires—then you, as the manager, take the next step and meet with each employee to establish agreed-upon goals for a specific time period.

A useful guide to determining goals is the SMART goals system whereby good goals are ones that are

- Specific
- Measurable
- Achievable
- Results oriented
- Timetable specified (able to track time frames)

Goals set in collaboration with employees, rather than imposed on them by management, will result in higher levels of employee buy-in and commitment.

Once goals have been set, as the manager, you need to establish a timeline for when employee performance will be appraised and then communicate this to employees. Ideally, you should be observing employee behavior throughout the year and recording critical incidents—both positive and negative—that will assist you in making an overall assessment of an employee's performance for each 6-month appraisal period.

Collecting information on critical incidents throughout the year will assist you greatly in presenting employees with specific feedback about their performance that increases the credibility of the appraisal (Fig. 4.5). For example, John is an employee who has failed to meet performance standards with regard to his behavior with clients. You present John with a list of seven specific incidents that you observed in the last

SMART Goals: A mnemonic (specific, measureable, attainable, realistic, timely) used to set objectives in areas such as project management, employee performance management, or personal development.

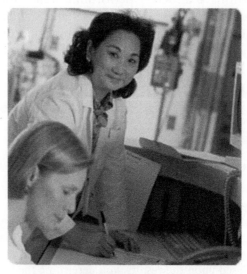

Figure 4.5 Manager reviewing documentation with employee.

3 weeks where he did not follow protocol when engaging a client, he was rude to clients by cutting them off, and failed to answer questions about basic information that all employees are expected to know. John is less likely to dispute your evaluation of his performance when faced with such facts.

Basic appraisal methods consist of the following: graphic rating scale, alternation ranking method, paired comparison method, forced distribution, behaviorally anchored rating scale, and the organization-wide management-by-objectives approach.

Graphic Rating Scale Approach to Performance Management

Graphic rating scales list a number of traits such as job knowledge, reliability, and quality, and ask you to rate each employee on a scale ranging from outstanding to unsatisfactory. The alternation ranking method identifies a relevant trait and asks you to alternate between identifying the highest ranking employee and the lowest ranking employee on that particular trait.

Paired Comparison Method of Performance Management

Paired comparison method is a form of ranking system that compares an employee to every other employee one by one on traits that are difficult to quantify. For example, on the trait of creativity, you would set up a chart as shown below that lists each of your five employees along the two axes. You would then make direct comparisons between each pair of employees on the chart as illustrated in Figure 4.6.

The Behaviorally Anchored Rating Scale Approach to Performance Management

The behaviorally anchored rating scale combines qualitative and quantitative measurement techniques to help managers more accurately evaluate employee performance. These scales take a skill, define it, and then present various levels of performance that are anchored by specific

Graphic Rating Scales: A method of performance management in which the supervisor lists a number of traits such as job knowledge, reliability, and quality and asks you to rate each employee on a scale ranging from outstanding to unsatisfactory.

Paired Comparison Method: A method of analysis where a range of options are compared and the results are tallied to find an overall winner.

Behaviorally Anchored Rating Scale: Combines qualitative and quantitative measurement techniques to help managers more accurately evaluate employee performance. These scales take a skill, define it, and then present various levels of performance that are anchored by specific types of behaviors.

As compared to	Simon	Terence	Emily	Yolanda	Sebastian
Simon		–	+	–	–
Terence	+		–	+	–
Emiliy	–	+		–	–
Yolanda	+	–	+		–
Sebastian	+	+	+	+	

Figure 4.6 Example of paired comparison method of performance management. Sebastian is the top performer on creativity, for example.

types of behaviors. For example, customer service is a skill defined as providing accurate information that addresses customer concerns in a timely, positive manner. At the bottom of the scale between a rating of 1 and 2 is the following behavior description: "the receptionist tells the patient that she does not know the answer to the question because the doctors keep changing policies." At the top of the scale at a rating of 9 is the following behavior description: "when the office is backed up and the waiting room is full, the receptionist continues to keep patients updated on the status and offers to rebook anyone whose schedules don't allow them to wait."

Management-by-Objectives Approach to Performance Management

Management by Objectives: An organization-wide goal-setting method that emphasizes collaboration and buy-in from one level to the next.

The last performance appraisal approach, management by objectives, is an organization-wide goal-setting method that emphasizes collaboration and buy-in from one level to the next. The first step is for top management, with input from organizational members, to set the organization's goals for the upcoming year. This then helps department heads to establish goals for their particular area with their subordinates. Once departmental goals are established, managers meet with each employee and ask them to develop their own goals that will help the department achieve department goals. With individual goals set and agreed-upon managers then conduct performance reviews that compare what employees have accomplished with the expected results and provide feedback to help employees adjust their course of action as necessary.

Effective Delivery of Performance Feedback

How appraisal feedback is delivered to an employee is an important consideration for you, as a manager. Although appraisal interviews should focus on remedying deficiencies and reinforcing strengths, few people like to give or receive negative feedback. To ensure the interview is done effectively, you should be sure to prepare adequately for the meeting. This includes the following preinterview activities: first, give the employee at least 1 week's notice that will allow you time to review their work, read over their job description, analyze issues, and put together a list of questions and comments; second, study the job description and compare their current performance with the job's standards as well as review past appraisals; and finally, choose a suitable place for the interview where you won't be interrupted, find a mutually agreeable time, and leave enough time.

A typical issue that managers must deal with in appraisal meetings is defensive behavior. It's important that the evaluation process is fair and the employee is given an opportunity to voice their opinion. Equally important, however, is that you maintain a professional demeanor and if necessary, allow an upset employee some time to calm down before continuing.

Another issue that managers content with in performance appraisals is bias. This can take the form of unclear measurements that lead to subjective ratings. Another source of bias is the halo effect where you take one trait and allow it to influence your overall assessment of an individual. For example, an employee who is generally unfriendly with her peers in the receptionist area could be rated as unsatisfactory for all traits even though in reality, she is pleasant to patients and works well with the medical staff. Central tendency is another bias that leads managers to rate all subordinates as average, avoiding high or low ratings.

Leniency or strictness is an opposite problem where you may tend to rate all subordinates positively or negatively. This can be linked to a manager's personality. Those who rate high on conscientiousness tend to be stricter in their evaluations, while those who score high on agreeableness are more positive in their evaluations.

Stereotyping is another source of bias and occurs whenever we use impressions about a group to influence our assessments of individuals who belong to that particular group. We have a wide range of stereotypes that can influence our perceptions of others that include bias due to an individual's sex, age, religion, or race.

Before an employee leaves an appraisal interview, you should get agreement from the employee on a plan of action to improve weak areas and continue to develop strong areas. The action plan should list specific activities with time frames so that you can check back with the employee on their progress.

As a final note on performance appraisals, it is critical for managers to take the necessary steps to ensure a legally defensible performance management system. Tips on making your performance management system legally defensible include the following:

- Make statements that never "attack" the person but provide constructive criticism related to a specific performance area that must be addressed.
- Keep appraisals objective and substantiated by documentation such as dates.
- Allow the team member to review the written appraisal before the interview.
- Address the employee's overall performance and not solely on a recent incident.
- Avoid biases such as those mentioned earlier in this chapter.
- Provide regular feedback throughout the cycle and make a note of the dates of an employee exceeding expectations as well as dates of any incident that required coaching or corrective action.
- Encourage the team member to discuss any concerns and listen well.

COMPENSATION, BENEFITS, AND PAYROLL

Compensation consists of two main components: direct financial payments (wages, salaries, bonuses, commissions, and incentives) and indirect payments (benefits). We'll take a look at both of these with a particular focus on incentive plans that are set up to improve employee motivation.

As discussed earlier in the chapter, there are several federal employment laws that deal directly with compensation. These include the Fair

Internal Equity: Determining that all employees within the same practice are paid within the same range as all other employees with similar job titles, responsibilities, and reporting structure.

External Equity: Determining an equitable amount to pay an employee compared to what other similar companies in the same geographic region pay for the equivalent of that employee's job title.

Incentive Plans: A method of rewarding either individual employees or groups of employees for meeting or exceeding goals, based on paying for performance by awarding extra money or other valuable incentives.

Pay-for-Performance Plans (Employee Incentive): Programs where employee compensation is generally given for specific performance results rather than simply for time worked.

Team-based Incentive Plans: Compensation plan offering a reward to the entire group for generating positive results.

Labor Standards Act, the Equal Pay Act, the Civil Rights Act of 1964, the Age Discrimination in Employment Act, the Americans with Disabilities Act, and the Family and Medical Leave Act.

A few issues to consider when discussing compensation at the organization level are its link to strategy and the role of equity. A practice's compensation strategy helps management determine how it will approach pay and benefits. A practice can adopt the philosophy that "you get what you pay for" and what they may wish to get is high quality. Therefore, they will strive to be a market leader when it comes to paying their employees and providing them with attractive benefits, hoping that this approach will lure and enable them to keep the best and the brightest. It is easy to see how this philosophy can work for an organization; pay is one way to let employees know how much they are valued. On the other hand, a practice might emphasize cost savings to such an extent that they decide to hire only part-time employees and keep hours below a certain amount per week to avoid paying for employee benefits. Either approach is a strategic decision and impacts the practice on every level.

Equity needs to be considered both internally and externally when determining pay levels. Internal equity essentially means that there is a perception among employees that pay differences are not unfair. External equity, on the other hand, requires employers to consider what the current market rate is for particular positions and match these to some extent in order to remain competitive with salaries and benefits. Balancing concern for internal and external equity can be difficult. For example, a practice that wishes to hire a new RN may need to offer the candidate a higher compensation package than its current RN's get if the current economy is especially competitive for this type of employee. While they've achieved external equity, they've done so at the expense of internal equity; bringing in someone new at a higher pay rate may cause problems in the practice and lead to lower levels of motivation.

Whether this happens or not depends on how the organization communicates its compensation strategy to its employees and finds other ways to motivate its members. Aside from salary, organizations can show employees they are valued through the use of incentive programs. A few common types of incentive plans are covered in the next section.

In the basic sense, incentive plans are pay-for-performance plans in that they provide employees with additional financial rewards based on how well they meet or exceed performance goals. These rewards can be determined on both the individual and group levels. Individual plans are typically referred to as piecework and represent one of the oldest types of incentives. Still used by many organizations, this technique ties pay directly to what an individual produces. A practice may reward a billing specialist for each claim, above a predetermined number, that is processed without error and paid within a particular time frame.

Group or team-based incentive plans are used when a practice wishes to reward teamwork and collaboration among its employees. For example, a practice implemented an initiative last year to measure and improve patient satisfaction. After a 6-month period, patient satisfaction increased 40% which has led to a 10% increase in new patients. The additional revenue from this success is shared among all employees to show appreciation and further encourage teamwork in improving the practice.

One such plan approach is the Scanlon Plan that has five distinct characteristics. Developed in 1937, the plan is still used in many organizations to encourage a collaborative culture and profit to share resulting from productivity-improving suggestions. The five elements of the plan include

1. A philosophy of cooperation
2. Shared identity
3. Employee competence across the board
4. Involvement system
5. The sharing of benefits formula that determines how extra profits will be distributed among employees

Another incentive approach is the stock ownership plan that allows employees to buy into the organization and share in its profits. This can be a lucrative approach for many organizations; when an employee or a manager shares ownership of an organization in the financial sense, they stand to gain or lose personally from the organization's performance. This can lead to higher levels of commitment and effort in being effective and finding ways to improve the practice's performance.

Merit pay is a form of individual incentive but differs from bonus payments in that merit pay becomes a part of an employee's base pay. It is a controversial topic given that while it can motivate an individual to increase their performance, it can also discourage collaboration among employees who are essentially competing for individual rewards. It is also tied directly to the performance appraisal system. This can present problems if employees perceive the appraisal system as unfair. A "rigged" evaluation system means decisions about who gets merit pay and who doesn't are also unfair and can cause conflict within the practice.

As stated earlier, compensation is more than just what an employee earns in take-home pay. It also includes an array of benefits defined as indirect monetary and nonmonetary payments received for continuing to work in the practice and represent a major expense for most employers. Some of these benefits are mandatory, such as unemployment insurance, while a host of others are voluntarily implemented by an employer to provide members with an incentive to stay with the organization and perform well. Overall, employee benefits account for approximately one-third of wages and salaries (28% of payroll). While it is a significant expense for employers, outside of the required benefits, elective benefits are a great way to show employees they are valued and increase motivation.

The first category of benefits is pay for time not worked and represents one of the most expense benefits for an employer. This includes unemployment insurance, vacation and holidays, sick leave, and severance pay.

The next category is insurance benefits and includes workers' compensation and insurance for hospitalization, medical, and disability. While workers' compensation is a required benefit, not all organizations elect to offer employees health benefits. Of those that do greater

Scanlon Plan: A gain-sharing program combining leadership, total workforce education, and widespread employee participation with a reward system linked to group and/or organization performance in which employees share in preestablished cost savings, based upon employee effort.

Merit Pay: A form of individual incentive that differs from bonus payments in that merit pay becomes a part of an employee's base pay. Merit pay is usually in addition to any across-the-board cost of living increases.

care is being taken to rein in the rising cost of employee health benefits by negotiating for group rates and outsourcing the administration of health plans that can become quite complex.

Retirement benefits are another category of employee benefits and include social security and pension plans. Social security benefits actually represent three types. The first is what is typically considered social security—income for those employees who retire at age 62 or later. The second are survivor or death benefits that represent income for dependents regardless of the age of an employee at the time of death. Finally, under certain conditions, social security provides income for an employee who becomes completely disabled. The second category for retirement benefits is the pension plan which only about half of all U.S. workers participate in. These consist of such plans as the 401 (k) which is one of the more common types.

In addition to indirect monetary benefits, employers can elect to offer a host of indirect nonmonetary benefits referred to as employee services. These include programs such as legal and personal counseling, child-care subsidies, education reimbursements, management perquisites, flex time, and subsidized physical fitness programs.

Taken together, salaries/wages and employee benefits make compensation an important tool for employers to show that they value their employees and motivate them to work together to achieve the practice's goals.

SUMMARY

Managing team players effectively requires managers to be familiar with the myriad employment laws affecting their practice. Major federal employment laws covered in the chapter include EEO-focused laws (ADEA, ADA, Civil Rights Acts, Equal Pay Act, and USERRA) as well as others (COBRA, IRCA, FLSA, and FMLA). Practice managers should know these and the various state laws that apply and keep up to date with changes that result from court cases and amendments. For this reason, it is wise to identify and consult with an employment law attorney on any employee-related legal issues. The chapter also discussed the importance of establishing an interactive performance management system that allows managers and employees to work together to determine performance-related goals. Appraisals should seek to develop weak areas while further developing employee strengths. This is done by using objective measures to evaluate performance, guarding against bias in evaluating behaviors and traits, and allowing employees to voice their own opinion with regard to the feedback interview. The last section of the chapter discussed what compensation is and described the two major ingredients in an employee's compensation package: direct financial payments (e.g., wages, salaries, and bonuses) and nondirect financial payments (benefits). Performance management and compensation systems that are seen as unbiased, fair, and developmental will increase employee motivation and help improve a practice's overall success—especially with regard to building a patient-centric team.

CHAPTER REVIEW QUESTIONS

1. List the three sources for federal employment laws.

_____

_____

_____

2. Briefly describe the basic requirements outlined by the ADA for a disability to be covered under the act.

_____

_____

_____

3. List three federal employment laws that would be considered under the broad umbrella of equal employment opportunity laws.

_____

_____

_____

4. Which federal law determines minimum wage and overtime?

_____

_____

_____

5. Describe the SMART system of establishing goals and how this helps create an effective performance management system.

_____

_____

_____

6. Which of the performance appraisal systems discussed in the chapter combines quantitative and qualitative measurements of performance?

_____

_____

_____

7. Define what the halo effect bias is and provide an example from your own experience.

_____

_____

_____

8. Define internal and external equity and discuss briefly why they need to be considered when making decisions about compensation and benefits.

_____

_____

_____

Workbook for
Chapter 4

Workbook:
Chapter 4 Managing the Team Players

4.A: YOUR TURN

Select any law discussed in this chapter and write an office policy and procedure to demonstrate the practice's compliance with the law selected.

4.B: TEAM PROJECT

Brainstorm with teammates on ideas for nonmonetary incentives and then develop a nonmonetary incentive plan. It is acceptable to use a small amount of money to purchase items for the incentive plan. For example, if there is an "employee of the month," money can be used to buy a plaque and, perhaps a cake.

4.C: ILLUSTRATION

Using Figure 4.6, complete a performance appraisal using the paired comparison method of performance management.

4.D: DESIGN A POSTER

Design a poster for a medical practice that will remind employees about the importance of safety and safe practices.

4.E: EXPERT PANEL

Recall the case scenario in this chapter (at the end of the Employment Laws Section).

Nancie Jones has been hired as the practice administrator. Her predecessor left without notice due to a conflict with the managing physician. She has been oriented to the practice and is now accessing the e-mail that has been received since the previous administrator left. She notices several e-mail mes-

sages marked urgent and containing subjects such as morale, compliance, and legal issues. She opens the oldest message that is marked urgent and learns that her predecessor apparently denied a request for family leave from an employee whose husband had undergone bypass surgery and didn't have anyone else to care for him until he could regain his mobility. Other than the day of the surgery, the administrator had told the employee that the practice was short staffed and that they could not spare her. The employee had apparently sought legal advice because she had been forced to pay for a day-care provider for her husband that cost more than she earned on a daily basis. The attorney wants the new administrator to contact him as soon as possible.

Nancie is now ready to address the other urgent e-mail messages. Chose one of the following additional e-mail messages pertaining to an urgent, legal issue, and document what steps the administrator should take to respond. You will most likely need to research your solution using one of the resources mentioned in this chapter. Your instructor may have you break into teams or respond as an individual expert. Each team or individual needs to create a step-by-step resolution to the issue including a response to the e-mail message.

1. Subject: Violation of ADA. From: Clinical Medical Assistant, John Jones. Message: I know that you are new but I have an urgent issue I need to discuss with you at your earliest convenience. I believe my rights under ADA have been violated by the previous administrator. About a year ago, I started experiencing severe back pain. I brought in a note from my chiropractor explaining that I had injured my back and that lifting should be restricted to no more than 35 lb, and that I shouldn't stand for more than 15 minutes without sitting for at least 15 minutes. There was no end date for this note. The previous administrator accommodated this disability until last month when she said that since my job description required that I am able to stand for long periods and lift up to 50 lb, and since I had not lost weight as recommended by my chiropractor, I had to go back to full duty immediately. My back is now worse than it was when the injury was first diagnosed. Please let me know how you intend to accommodate this disability.

---

2. Subject: Violation of Civil Rights. From: Attorney Smith. Message: It has been brought to my attention that your practice terminated my client's employment without cause. My client, a lab technician, believes he was terminated based exclusively on religious discrimination because of his Islamic faith. It is his contention that he was hired originally by the managing physician, and that the administrator constantly looked for fault with his performance. After 4 months of this treatment, she fired him for insubordination. My client maintains that she started asking him to do unreasonable tasks such as

take out the garbage and do clerical work for her. The first time he balked by telling her that she was not being reasonable, she fired him.

_____

_____

_____

3. Subject: Breach of confidentiality. From: Attorney Jones. Message: My client, Bill Smith, asserts that your practice mishandled his credit information resulting in his having his identity stolen. Mr. Smith gave his 2-week notice to your predecessor last month to take a higher-paying job. He maintains that his identity was stolen at approximately that time. He believes that the credit information was not maliciously mishandled but that when the administrator was processing his final paperwork, the security of the file was breached and somebody was able to steal his ID.

_____

_____

_____

5

Managing Third-Party Payers

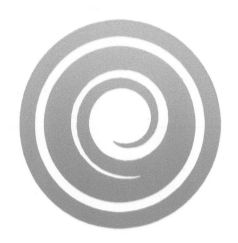

LEARNING OUTCOMES

Upon completion of this chapter, the student should...

- Describe how managing third-party payers impacts the success of the practice
- Develop a policy for all team members that governs the expectation that loyal patients rightfully expect information about the cost and quality of options available to them for additional tests, prescriptions, or procedures
- Distinguish between government and commercial third-party payers
- Distinguish between traditional and managed care plans
- Compare and contrast the types of managed care plans
- Differentiate Medicare, Medicaid, TRICARE, and the Civilian Health and Medical Program of Veteran Affairs (CHAMPVA) government health care plans
- Discuss the pros and cons from a practice perspective of current health care reform initiatives in the United States

KEY TERMS

Accountable Care Organizations (ACO)
Assignment of Benefits
Balance Bill
Capitation
Civilian Health and Medical Program of the
    Department of Veteran Affairs (CHAMPVA)
Coinsurance
Commercial Health Insurance
Coordination of Benefits (COB)
Deductible
Dual Eligibility

Evaluation and Management (E/M)
Fee Schedule
Formulary
Gatekeeper
Group Model
Health Maintenance Organization (HMO)
Indemnity Insurance
Individual Practice Association (IPA)
Managed Care Organization (MCO)
Medicaid
Medicare

Medicare Advantage
Medicare Part A
Medicare Part B
Medicare Part C
Medicare Part D
Medicare Secondary Payer (MSP)
Medigap
Network Model
Point-of-Service (POS) Plan
Preferred Provider Organization (PPO)

Premium
Primary Care Physician (PCP)
Resource-Based Relative Value Scale
    (RBRVS)
Staff Model
Sustainable Growth Rate (SGR)
TRICARE
Usual, Customary, and Reasonable
    (UCR)
Workers' Compensation

OVERVIEW

Regardless of the size of the medical practice or the expertise of its coding and billing staff, every team member from the physicians through to the clerical support staff should have a basic understanding of how the practice gets paid for the procedures and services it provides to its patients. The business of medicine is complicated but it is also the foundation that enables an exceptionally talented medical practice team to deliver outstanding health care to a loyal base of patients.

Although the practice will serve patients who do not have health insurance, the majority of patients will have some source of health care benefits through a third party such as one of several federal government health care programs or commercial insurance. This chapter discusses some of the basic concepts and the most common terminology associated with government and commercial third-party payers offering both traditional and managed care plans. The impact of health care reform on medical practice administration is also discussed.

BASIC CONCEPTS AND TERMINOLOGY REGARDING THIRD-PARTY PAYERS

There are two important reasons for a practice administrator to expertly manage third-party payers.

Box 5.1

Importance of Third-Party Payer Knowledge

First, as mentioned above, a practice cannot sustain itself without revenue and third-party payers generate the majority of revenue for all medical offices. The second reason is that today's patients expect to be active in managing their own health care—including cost. This means that the manager must know the differences between various benefit plans and ensure that physicians and other members of the practice team have the knowledge it takes to provide information to the patient about cost and quality of the various options available to that patient. For example, a patient should be informed of the pros and cons as well as the cost, based on what type of insurance they have, for options such as prescriptions (generic equivalents, mail order, cheaper to buy more, cut pills in half, etc.), diagnostic and therapeutic tests, consultations, or surgery.

In order to manage third-party payers and have the team provide the type of service that contributes to building and sustaining patient loyalty, the practice administrator must know the basics of the types of health care coverage, resources for learning more as specific questions arise, and how to communicate key information to the practice team so the team can consider options when making a decision and in communicating recommendations to a patient. For example, if a doctor only knows that drug A will help the patient resolve a health issue, and drug A doesn't have a generic equivalent, the patient will feel obligated to either pay a high amount or not take the recommended drug. However, if there is another drug, drug B, that is also effective in treating a certain condition and that drug has a generic equivalent, it could make the difference between whether the patient is able to afford the recommended prescription. The patient may know that their plan only covers generic drugs but they have no way of knowing that a drug without a generic version may not be the only drug that can successfully treat the patient's condition. Once a patient realizes that everyone on the team cares about the patient's ability to afford treatment and not just prescribing the most common treatment, that patient becomes a loyal patient.

There are several terms that are important to know as a foundation to understanding the concept of third-party payers. See Table 5.1 for a list of these terms and definitions.

Formulary: A prescription drug formulary is a list of prescription drugs that a given third-party payer will reimburse. Drugs not on that list are only reimbursed on an exception basis.

Table 5.1 Third-Party Payer Terminology	
Terms	Definitions
Centers for Medicare and Medicaid Services (CMS)	CMS is the agency under the U.S. Department of Health and Human Services charged with administering the federal Medicare program and the federal portion of Medicaid benefits. See www.cms.gov for detailed information about CMS and its programs. The third-party payer for Medicare and Medicaid is the federal government with state governments paying a portion of Medicaid expenses. Medicare and Medicaid are discussed in more detail later in this chapter.
TRICARE	TRICARE is another government program. It provides benefits to active duty military personnel and their dependents, and retired (officially retired from a military career, not just a person who served one or two enlistment periods) military personnel and their dependents, until age 65 when Medicare becomes primary and TRICARE becomes the secondary payer. There are traditional and managed care options under TRICARE. For more information on how physicians can become TRICARE providers, see http://www.humana-military.com/south/provider/tools-resources/new-tricare-provider.asp.
Civilian Health and Medical Program of the Department of Veteran Affairs (CHAMPVA)	CHAMPVA, another plan in which the government is the third-party payer, provides health benefits to veterans with service-related disabilities and their dependents.

(continued)

Table 5.1	**Third-Party Payer Terminology (*continued*)**
Workers' Compensation	Workers' compensation laws vary from state to state but the general premise is for employers to pay into a government fund so that when an employee gets injured on the job or is able to show an illness stems from the work environment, all treatment related to that injury or illness is paid for by the workers' compensation insurance plan. Practices must be careful not to submit claims for services rendered to a patient for other than the workers' compensation injury or illness. The release of information rules is different for employers when workers' compensation is involved, too, so be sure to keep the patient cases separate when the patient is treated for nonworkers' compensation and workers' compensation by the same physician or physicians in the same practice. For information state by state and for federal employees, see http://www.workerscompensation.com/workers_comp_by_state.php.
Indemnity Insurance	Indemnity insurance is also referred to as traditional or fee-for-service insurance and is considered a nonprovider network type of coverage. The covered patient (the policy holder or a dependent) is seen by a provider (e.g., physician or hospital). Either the patient or the provider submits a claim (bill) to the insurance company. The services that are listed as covered by the third-party payer in the plan summary of benefits are reimbursed based on the amount the health care plan allows called the allowed amount. The allowed amount for a physician is generally based on either **Resource-Based Relative Value Scale (RBRVS),** which is a formula that takes into account the cost of the physician's work, practice expenses, malpractice expenses, and the cost of professional liability insurance or **Usual, Customary, and Reasonable (UCR).** Usual is the amount a provider usually charges for that service or procedure; customary is a range of what most providers in that geographic area charge for the same service, and reasonable is either both usual and customary or justified as special circumstances. The patient is responsible for a **deductible,** which is a set amount per year and is collected at 100% of allowed amount of all covered services until it has been satisfied for that year; **coinsurance,** which is a percentage of the allowed amount (often 20% of allowed amount) after the annual deductible has been satisfied; and the difference between allowed amount and the amount charged by the physician unless the physician has agreed to accept the payer's allowed amount as payment in full. So, the deductible plus coinsurance plus amount paid by the third-party payer is equal to the allowed amount for each service rendered. (Note: Some indemnity plans incorporate concepts from managed care but are still indemnity plans overall. For example, requiring prior approval before the insurance company will pay for certain services, such as physical therapy, started with managed care plans but has been adopted by many indemnity plans.)
Managed Care	Managed care is a type of health care coverage that typically offers comprehensive health benefits to their members and relies on negotiating rates with providers who are then considered network or participating providers. Types of managed care plans are discussed in more detail later in this chapter.

MEDICARE AND MEDICAID

As mentioned earlier, the Center for Medicare and Medicaid Services (CMS) administers the federal Medicare program and the federal government portion of the Medicaid Program.

Medicare

Medicare is a federal government program administered by the CMS and provides health insurance benefits for people age 65 or older, people under age 65 with certain disabilities, and people of all ages with end-stage renal disease (permanent kidney failure requiring dialysis or a kidney transplant).

Medicare has four parts:

1. Part A is designed to provide insurance benefits to help pay for hospital, skilled nursing, and certain other facility charges. Most Medicare-eligible people don't have to pay for Part A coverage.

2. Part B is designed to provide medical insurance to help cover doctors' services and outpatient care. It also covers some other medical services that Part A doesn't cover, such as some of the services of physical and occupational therapists, and some home health care. Part B helps pay for these covered services and supplies when they are medically necessary. Most Medicare-eligible people have to pay a monthly amount, called a premium for Part B benefits.

3. Part C is called Medicare advantage, and it provides an option for Medicare-eligible people to choose a commercial, managed care option for their benefits under Part A, B, and D instead of traditional Medicare coverage. Medicare advantage plans may also cover benefits that aren't typically covered under traditional Medicare.

4. Part D coverage is coverage for prescription drugs.

Medigap

Medigap provides optional supplemental insurance to offset the patient's share of cost for those who have Medicare traditional coverage (not Medicare advantage), but no other health insurance, including Medicaid. Medigap is private insurance. Patients who choose to have a Medigap plan pay a monthly premium. Any company who offers this type of coverage must comply with standardization of packages and offer any or all of the standardized options ranging from A to N (in 2010, people who already had E, H, I, and J were able to keep these plans but no new plans under these standardized packages were sold; concurrently, new plans, M and N, have been added). For an outline of the standardized packages related to supplementing Medicare Part B, see Figure 5.1 and for a complete description of Medigap rules and other information, see the Medigap publication at http://www.medicare.gov/Publications/Pubs/pdf/02110.pdf. Note that Plan A must be available to all Medicare beneficiaries who purchase Medigap coverage, no matter where in the country they reside. Other options may or may

Medicare: A federal government program administered by the CMS that provides health insurance benefits for people age 65 or older, people under age 65 with certain disabilities, and people of all ages with end-stage renal disease.

Medicare Part A: Designed to provide insurance benefits to help pay for hospital, skilled nursing, and certain other facility charges.

Medicare Part B: Designed to provide medical insurance to help cover doctors' services and outpatient care. It also covers some other medical services that Part A doesn't cover.

Medicare Part C: Part C is also called Medicare Advantage and provides an option for Medicare-eligible people to choose a commercial managed care option for their benefits instead of traditional coverage.

Medicare Part D: Provides coverage for prescription drugs.

Premium: A payment paid by the insured to the insurer, in exchange for the insurer's promise to compensate (indemnify) the insured in the case of a loss to the insured.

Medicare Advantage: Provides an option for Medicare-eligible people to choose a commercial, managed care option for their benefits (Part A, B, and D) instead of traditional Medicare coverage.

Medigap: Provides optional supplemental insurance to offset the patient's share of cost for those who have Medicare traditional coverage (not Medicare Advantage), but no other health insurance, including Medicaid.

Medigap Benefits Related to Part B	A	B	C	D	F*	G	K	L	M	N
Medicare Part B Coinsurance or Copayment	X	X	X	X	X	X	50%	75%	X	X***
Medicare Part B Deductible			X		X					
Medicare Part B Excess Charges (billed versus allowed amount)					X	X				
Medicare Preventive Care Part B Coinsurance	X	X	X	X	X	X	X	X	X	X
Out of Pocket Limits**							$4,620	$2,320		

*Plan F also has a high-deductible option in exchange for it having low premiums. Patient must pay the Medicare Approved costs up to $2,000. before the Medigap high-deductible plan starts paying any benefits but then it covers coinsurance or copayments, deductible, excess charges and Preventive Care coinsurance.
**After the patient meets the specified out of pocket annual limit for coinsurance or copayments and the Part B deductible ($155 in 2010), these plans pay 100% of covered services for the rest of the year
***Plan N pays 100% of the Part B coinsurance except up to $20 copayment for office visits.

(This table abstracted from the publication at http://www.medicare.gov/Publications/Pubs/pdf/02110.pdf

Figure 5.1   Medigap standardized plans A to N as relevant to supplementing Part B Medicare (as of June 1, 2010)

Evaluation and Management: A service performed by a qualified practitioner (e.g., physician) whereby a patient's condition is evaluated by considering patient health history, results of a physical examination, and results of any tests to determine a diagnosis and a plan of managing the diagnosis.

Assignment of Benefits: The patient signs an agreement whereby the physician will receive any payment for services directly from the patient's insurance company including Medicare.

Balance Bill: The act of charging a patient (or person financially responsible for the patient) the difference between an insurer's allowed amount and the amount the practice charges for a service.

not be available, depending on where the Medicare beneficiary resides. The commercial insurance companies that offer these plans may choose to offer any combination of them. The patient does have to pay a premium for this coverage but it often saves the patient money in a typical year.

If a patient with Medicare Part B and Medigap coverage is seen by a physician for an office visit, which is also called an evaluation and management (E/M) service, the claim to get reimbursed for that service is sent to Medicare. Assuming the patient has satisfied the annual deductible, Medicare would pay 80% of the allowed amount. The 20% coinsurance balance would be submitted for payment by the Medigap plan.

At the point the Medigap plan pays the coinsurance balance to the physician, the physician will have been reimbursed for Medicare's full allowed amount. If the physician has accepted assignment of benefits for these services, it means that the practice must write off any difference between Medicare's allowed amount and the billed charges. If the physician has not accepted assignment, the practice may balance bill the patient for the difference between the allowed amount and the billed charges. Medigap plans do not pay the difference between Medicare's allowed amount and billed charges. See Figure 5.2 for an example.

While Medigap is standard regardless of which third-party payer offers these plans, many patients have a benefit plan as part of their retirement from an employer that offered group health insurance to its employees. In some cases, retirees (and sometimes spouses) who are eligible for Medicare benefits are able to retain their group benefits but the group plan becomes secondary to Medicare once the retiree is eligible for Medicare. In this case, the practice submits the claim to Medicare and then, once Medicare pays, the claim along with

Charges	Medicare Allowed Amount	Deductible	Coinsurance	Medicare Payment	$80.00
				Medigap Plan Payment	$20.00
				Physician Writes off (assigned) or bills the patient (not assigned)	
$125.00	$100.00	$0.00	$20.00		$25.00

Figure 5.2 **Medigap Part A example**

Medicare's payment information, is sent to the group plan to process whatever of the balance they will pay. Any balance at this point is billed to the patient. Secondary insurance is not standardized. Different plans pay different amounts without the governmental standards that must be followed for Medigap plans. The process of coordinating payment between two or more third-party payers is called coordination of benefits (COB).

Medicare Secondary Payer (MSP)

Although the majority of the time when a patient has Medicare coverage, Medicare is the primary insurance (meaning the provider submits the claim to Medicare first), there are instances that result in Medicare secondary payer (MSP) status. There are very strict reporting rules governing MSP. From the provider's perspective, for example, if they assume Medicare is the primary payer and get reimbursed by Medicare as such but subsequently get paid by another insurance company as though that company was primary, they must notify Medicare and they must refund Medicare the difference between what Medicare paid and what it should have paid under MSP. An example of MSP is the working aged. Anyone who is over 65 and covered by an employer group health plan (EGHP) through their own or a spouse's plan must have the provider submit the claim to the EGHP first and then to Medicare with a copy of the EGHP's explanation of benefits. For a complete manual of MSP reporting requirements, see http://www1.cms.gov/manuals/downloads/msp105c03.pdf.

Medicaid

Medicaid is designed to provide health insurance coverage to people who have limited income and who qualify for coverage. It is partially funded by the federal government and partially by individual state governments. Each state has some flexibility on what is offered as long as it meets the minimum federal requirements.

Dual Eligibility—Medicare and Medicaid

Dual eligibility pertains to people who have Medicare and Medicaid. Medicare pays first and then, Medicaid processes any remaining costs. Physicians must write off any amount not covered by the combination of payments. Some states do have a small ($1 to $5) copayment that the patient must pay to the practice at the time the service is rendered.

Coordination of Benefits (COB): A system whereby the order of payment is coordinated among various payers when the patient is covered by more than one third-party payer so that the total combination of multiple payments never exceeds the charges for each service.

Medicare Secondary Payer (MSP): A term used to describe any situation in which a Medicare-eligible person has other coverage that must process benefits as the primary payer and then any balances may be submitted to Medicare for processing.

Medicaid: A jointly funded health care plan between the federal government and each state that was designed to provide health insurance coverage to people who have limited income and who qualify for coverage.

Dual Eligibility: A situation in which a patient has both Medicare and Medicaid coverage and no other insurance.

COMMERCIAL HEALTH INSURANCE

Commercial Health Insurance: A third-party insurance plan that does not receive any funding from the government for administration or payment of benefits.

Commercial Health Insurance, in simple terms, is private insurance that is paid for by other than the government. For example, group health insurance is made available by many employers for their employees. The employer contracts with any one of a large number of companies that provide health insurance. The employer pays the premiums directly (with or without employees contributing a share) to the commercial third-party payer and, in turn, has an annual agreement to receive specified coverage without a change in per-person premiums for the full year of the contract. Other commercial insurance is purchased by individuals who need health benefits. The one exception is that employees of the federal government are offered various commercial insurance options for which the federal government pays the premiums. Both government and commercial health care plans can be traditional or managed care plans.

One important concept is that commercial plans can vary significantly from patient to patient. For example, one patient covered by Aetna may have completely different benefits than another patient with Aetna insurance. Even members of the same group such as employees and retirees of General Motors may have different benefits than other members of that same group. For example, GM may have a higher level of coverage for executives than for nonexecutives. Also, some groups offer a choice of options to its employees, so money may be applied to preventive medicine coverage for one employee while a different employee may choose to use that share of his or her premium for dental insurance.

Most government third-party payers, on the other hand, have some standardization for people who have each type of government coverage. For example, people with traditional Medicare Part B have the same benefits and same share of cost nationwide.

MANAGED CARE

Managed Care Organization (MCO): The concept of managed care is to negotiate discounted rates with providers who treat patients covered by that managed care organization (MCO) and to improve quality of patient care by increasing coverage for preventive medicine and early detection screenings. The providers who agree to specific packages are considered part of that MCO's network.

Recent statistics indicate that over half of all people in the United States who have health insurance are covered through a managed care plan. The concept of managed care is to negotiate discounted rates with providers who treat patients covered by that managed care organization (MCO) and to improve quality of patient care by increasing coverage for preventive medicine and early detection screenings. The providers who agree to specific packages are considered part of that MCO's network.

There are several types of managed care plans, many of which combine characteristics of indemnity plans with characteristics of managed care plans. Remember from Table 5.1 indemnity plans typically base their allowed charges on either RBRVS or UCR and offer physicians a chance to participate with the plan. A participating physician agrees to accept the allowed amount as payment in full (without balance billing the patient for the difference between allowed amount and billed charges for any given service or procedure), and to submit claims directly to the third-party payer in exchange for any reimbursement being sent directly to the provider instead of the patient. Managed care plans, on the other hand, negotiate set rates for services with a network of physicians. These rates are generally referred to as a fee schedule.

Health Maintenance Organizations (HMOs)

Health Maintenance Organizations (HMOs), as the name implies, focus on the maintenance of health in individuals. This focus means that HMOs encourage healthy lifestyles and early detection of diseases through routine physical exams and screenings. The HMO model is arguably the first managed care model and also the most pure of the managed care philosophy. The HMO is based on a network of physicians and hospitals. Typically, each covered member chooses a primary care physician (PCP) who acts as a gatekeeper. This means that in order to see a specialist, the member must schedule an appointment with his or her PCP and obtain a referral to a network specialist—with some exceptions when a specific type of specialist, who is in the network, is not available within a certain distance of a member's home. The HMOs keep an updated list of network physicians—both PCPs and specialists. Some HMOs allow women two PCPs—a general practitioner and a gynecologist. Children may have a pediatrician as a PCP. In most cases, out-of-network providers are not covered at all unless the care is provided on an emergency basis. Also, with the exceptions of gynecologists and pediatricians, even network specialist services will not be reimbursed without a referral from the PCP. If a nonemergency hospitalization is scheduled, most of the time the physician must obtain prior authorization or precertification from the HMO for the services to be covered. HMO coverage is typically very comprehensive and the member only pays a per-visit copayment (generally between $10 and $30) for care in a physician's office. There are no deductibles or coinsurance and often no lifetime maximum benefits.

There are four basic models of HMO plans:

1. Group model in which the MCO has a contract with a single- or multispecialty medical group in each region in which it operates. The contracted group may offer its services exclusively to the MCO's HMO members or to both HMO and non-HMO patients. The most common type of reimbursement is based on what is called capitation or a combination of capitation for routine medical services and a fee schedule for certain specialized surgery or other procedures. A capitated rate means that all patients who are members of the group model HMO are added to a roster that is updated regularly by the HMO and sent to the group practice. The HMO reimburses the practice a fixed amount per patient per month, whether or not the patient receives any services that month. For example, the practice may receive $25 per month per patient on the roster. If there are 200 patients on the roster, the practice receives a check in the amount of $5,000.00 that month. If the average amount charged in a month for an office visit for non-HMO patients was $100.00 and the practice served 25 patients that month, then they would be up an average

Fee Schedule: A preset, specific dollar amount that will be charged or reimbursed for each type of service or procedure performed (generally based on individual CPT codes).

Health Maintenance Organization (HMO): HMOs are a type of managed care organizations that focus on the maintenance of health in individuals. HMOs encourage healthy lifestyles and early detection of diseases through routine physical exams and screenings. The HMO model is the first managed care model and also the most pure of the managed care philosophy.

Primary Care Physician (PCP): A physician/medical doctor who provides both the first contact for a person with an undiagnosed health concern as well as continuing care of varied medical conditions, not limited by cause, organ system, or diagnosis.

Gatekeeper: In managed care, a gatekeeper is the primary care physician who must refer patients to specialists or other medical services instead of patients being able to schedule appointments directly with a specialist.

Group Model: A HMO managed care model in which the MCO has a contract with a single-multispecialty medical group in each region in which it operates.

Capitation: A type of managed care that reimburses a physician or group a set amount of money each month for each member of the plan who lists the practice as their primary care physician, regardless of whether that patient received care that month.

Staff Model: A HMO where physicians are employed and all premiums are paid to the HMO and in which covered insurers must select a primary care physician, who has control over referrals to other physicians in or out of the group.

Network Model: In a Health Maintenance Organization (HMO), a network model of managed care is a large network of physicians in each geographic area—both single-specialty and multispecialty based on physician practices—who provide services to HMO members and nonmembers but who have a negotiated fee schedule with the HMO for its members.

Independent Practice Association (IPA): A HMO managed care model in which some number of independent physicians form a group that is then able to negotiate with a HMO to offer its members a network of general practitioners and specialists as though they were a network model. The difference is that the IPA is not a "group" for other purposes.

Preferred Provider Organization (PPO): A managed care organization of medical doctors, hospitals, and other health care providers who have agreed with an insurer or a third-party administrator to provide health care at reduced rates to the insurer's or administrator's clients.

Point-of-Service Plan: A type of managed care health insurance system that combines characteristics of both the HMO and the PPO in which members do not make a choice about which system to use until the point at which the service is being used.

of $2500.00. On the other hand, if they saw more than 50 HMO patients of the 200 on the roster (e.g., flu season), they would lose money. Typically, this sharing of the risk works out as a win-win situation for both the HMO and the practice.

2. **Staff model** is a model in which the physicians are salaried employees of the HMO and the HMO owns its own facilities (usually clinics and hospitals). Members are only covered when health care services are provided by these salaried physicians in one of the HMO's facilities unless there is either a "travel" provision for members who get sick or injured while out of their HMO's region and/or a provision for emergency services that couldn't be provided by an HMO-owned facility.

3. **Network model** is generally based on a large network of physicians in each geographic area—both single-specialty and multi-specialty physician practices—who provide services to HMO members and nonmembers but who have a negotiated fee schedule with the HMO for its members.

4. **Independent Practice Association (IPA)** model is a model in which some number of independent physicians form a group that is then able to negotiate with a HMO to offer its members a network of general practitioners and specialists as though they were a network model. The difference is that the IPA is not a "group" for other purposes. For example, they don't operate as a physician group for tax purposes.

In addition to HMOs, other main types of managed care plans include preferred provider organizations and point-of-service (POS) plans.

Preferred Provider Organizations

Preferred provider organizations (PPOs) are technically indemnity plans with some managed care characteristics. PPOs have a network of physicians who have negotiated rates with the PPO but the PPO members are able to choose any physician they desire each time they need medical care. The difference is that the member pays higher rates when treated by a physician (or hospital) that is not in the network. For example, a member may have an annual deductible of $100.00 in-network or $200.00 out-of-network and 20% coinsurance in-network and 30% coinsurance out-of-network costs. Also, the patient may be responsible for the difference between allowed and charged amounts with out of network but not in network.

Point-of-Service Plans

Point-of-service (POS) plans are a combination of HMO and PPO models of health care. In this case, network physicians have a HMO-style agreement with the POS for a fee schedule and the patient only has to pay a per-visit copayment. However, the member is free to seek services from nonnetwork providers but are responsible for deductibles, coinsurance, and the difference between allowed amount (usually UCR) and billed charges.

From the perspective of the practice manager, knowing how these options work provides a framework for decision making regarding negotiating managed care contracts based on the geographic location, the demographics of the communities served and the size and specialization of the practice.

HEALTH CARE REFORM

Health care reform legislation was passed in 2010. The intent of Health Reform is to make coverage of health care costs more affordable to employers who purchase insurance for their employees and to individual health care consumers, reduce health care costs, and to improve both quality and accessibility of health care in the United States by

- Limiting or eliminating abuse on the part of the insurance industry by implementing consumer protection laws.
- Regulating the insurance industry by making sure premiums are kept reasonable and by preventing third-party payers from denying coverage based on preexisting conditions or based on the expense involved in treating certain diseases.
- Implementing tax cuts, reducing premiums, and reducing out-of-pocket costs to make insurance affordable to middle-class Americans and small businesses.
- Providing protections for those who lose their jobs or start a new business so people know they will be able to purchase quality and affordable coverage in a competitive market that keeps costs down.
- Strengthening Medicare coverage by lowering the cost of prescription drugs and preventive care while concurrently increasing the money that is available to the government for the administration of Medicare benefits.
- Increasing the financial health of the federal government by reducing the deficit significantly over the 20 years between 2010 and 2030.

From the perspective of physician practice management, the most significant issues for the administrator to be aware of and to follow for changes that impact physician billing and reimbursement are incentives, penalties, and cutbacks to Medicare patients. One of these is Medicare's sustainable growth rate (SGR) formulas. These formulas are adjusted annually and are targeted to help control Medicare's cost of physician services. For years, the formulas have resulted in a reduction of payments to physicians who treat Medicare beneficiaries, often with delayed implementations after costly congressional debates and threats of litigation. As health care reform unfolds, there is pressure on Congress to ensure that the methods by which CMS reimburses physicians is also reformed. According to a May 2010 article in the NEJM.

On April 15 (2010), Congress voted to postpone a 21% reduction in Medicare fees that was to have gone into effect April 1, but a longer-term solution is not yet in sight.

The problems with the Medicare physician payment system are twofold, and each dimension poses complex political difficulties. First,

Sustainable Growth Rate (SGR): The maximum rate at which a company can grow revenue without having to invest new equity capital. For Medicare, SGR pertains to a formula of reimbursement for services that calculates the amount Medicare is able to pay out in benefits based on projected existing and new revenue for the period under consideration and still sustain itself.

Medicare is captive to an arbitrary, if elegantly conceived, formula for total payments to physicians—the sustainable growth rate (SGR). In the alternate reality of the Congressional budget process, the SGR will reduce Medicare's physician payments, which already trail those from private insurers, as far into the future as the eye can see. Second, there is widespread consensus that the relative fees in the current system are a significant cause of the growing imbalance in supply and utilization between primary care and specialty services in the U.S. health care system. That imbalance, in turn, is widely perceived as a major cause of both excessive costs and inadequate quality of care.

The enactment of health care reform after many considered it irreversibly derailed by the Senate election in Massachusetts has suggested to some that perhaps the U.S. political system is not so hopelessly gridlocked after all. Health care reform, some believe, might be a harbinger of a more sensible and productive approach to solving serious policy problems. Untying the political knots enmeshing Medicare physician payment will test that optimism.[1]

Accountable Care Organization (ACO): A type of health care reform in which the third party payer groups providers of different specialties and assigns that group a set of patients. The model ties provider reimbursement to both quality measures and reduction in total health care costs by eliminating redundant tests and treatments by coordinating the care of each patient between hospital care and various physician specialists and generalists.

Another part of health care reform that a savvy office administrator must follow is physician incentives such as physician payment reforms to enhance primary care services and encourage doctors to form "accountable care organizations" to improve quality and efficiency of care to Medicare beneficiaries.

The following Web sites provide regularly updated details of health care reform: http://www.healthreform.gov/about/index.html and http://healthcarereform.nejm.org/?cat=73.

SUMMARY

One of the responsibilities of a practice manager is to effectively manage the main sources of revenue for the practice—third-party payers. Financial health is critical as a means to enable the practice's team to provide exceptional health care to a loyal base of patients. The manager must stay proactive in monitoring external forces, such as federal health care reform initiatives, that impact the way in which both governmental and commercial third-party payers operate and how to implement mandated changes in the most cost-effective, team-oriented, patient-eentric manner.

CHAPTER REVIEW QUESTIONS

1. List one reason it is important for a practice administrator to know how third-party payers operate and to monitor changes in these operations.

_____

_____

_____

2. Why is it important for every member of the team to be aware of options that can save the patient money without compromising quality?

_____

_____

_____

3. What is the basic difference between government and commercial third-party payers?

_____

_____

_____

4. What type of managed care model is basically a traditional or indemnity plan but with the managed care concept of networked physicians a key element?

_____

_____

_____

5. What are the basic models under the HMO concept?

_____

_____

_____

6. Briefly name and describe the four parts of Medicare.

_____

_____

_____

7. Give an example of a patient over the age of 65 who may have Medicare as the secondary payer rather than the primary payer.

_____

_____

_____

8. What is the name of the formula that is used annually to determine any increases or cutbacks in the reimbursement physicians receive for the services and procedures they provide?

_____

_____

_____

REFERENCE

1. Vladeck, BC. Fixing Medicare's Physician Payment System. Available at: http://healthcarereform.nejm.org/?p=3375. Accessed June 7, 2010.

Workbook for
Chapter 5

Workbook:
Chapter 5 Managing Third-Party Payers

5.A: INTERNET SCAVENGER HUNT

Go to the following Web site and answer the questions below the link. http://www.aaahc.org/eweb/StartPage.aspx (HMOs may seek AAAHC accreditation)

- What is AAAHC?
- What is the first year AAAHC began accrediting ambulatory health care organizations?
- What is the fundamental purpose of AAAHC?
- What types of ambulatory health care organizations are accredited by AAAHC?

5.B: COMPARE AND CONTRAST BENEFITS BETWEEN THIRD-PARTY PAYERS

Go to the Web site: http://humana.com.
  Note the site contains several types of plans. Note the site also explains how each group plan works. Now go to any other third-party payer and see what types of group plans they offer.

- On the Humana site, what are the types of group plans? (Hint: There are 7.)
- On the site you chose, is there an equivalent to each type of Humana plan? If so, what is it?
- Which type of plan offers a combination of benefits from both an HMO model and a PPO model of group plan?

Now, on either website (Humana or the one you selected), find any two summary plans for the current year, print them out, and compare the benefits. Write a list of questions you would ask if you were trying to decide between these two plans you researched. Also, what questions would you ask if you were trying to compare one of these HMOs to one of the PPOs mentioned earlier (and also on the top of the med plan-benefit charts Web page).

5.C: CHART OF COMMON TYPES OF MANAGED CARE

Complete the chart below, which depicts some of the types of managed care plans discussed in this chapter. Mark a Y for yes and N for no in each column for each row.

| Benefits | Types of plan | | | | | |
	PPO	HMO-group model	HMO-staff model	HMO-network model	HMO-IPA model	Point-of-service plan
Are benefits paid for non-emergency, nonnetwork providers?						
Can a member go to a network specialist without a referral from a primary care physician?						
Is capitation a common form of reimbursement under this type of plan?						
Is there a deductible?						
Is there a copayment?						
Is the network physician able to see both managed care and nonmanaged care patients?						
Does the physician work for the MCO?						
List one unique aspect for each type of MCO listed						

5.D: CHART OF MEDICARE AS SECONDARY PAYER

Complete the following chart by placing an "X" in either the Primary box or the Secondary Payer box.

Scenario	Medicare primary	Medicare secondary
Patient is 67 years old and retired from General Motors. GM provides a health benefits package to retirees.		
Patient is 72 and works as an executive director of General Motors		
Patient has Medicare and a Humana Medigap plan		
Patient is age 66, retired and being treated for a back injury before he retired and successfully filed a workers' compensation claim for the injury. He now needs back surgery as a complication of the original injury		

5.E: EXPERT PANEL

Read the following real-life scenario. Your instructor may have you break into teams or respond as an individual expert. Each team or individual needs to research what options are available for an employer who is looking at a way to provide good benefits without increased costs to either the employees or to the practice. Assume for this assignment that your current health insurance is a traditional plan in which there is an annual $200 deductible and 20% coinsurance regardless of which doctor you go to. Don't try to compare drug and hospitalization benefits—just assume that if you find a good option for regular physician care, that plan is also a better deal for other benefits. Document how you would go about the task of comparing health care options if you were one of the employees. Once each team or individual action plan or proposal is prepared, the instructor may ask students to choose the top three solutions and describe why they are the best.

Sunshine Medical Group, a group of 25 employees located in a metropolitan area, has elected to purchase traditional health benefits from a large, private, third-party payer, since the practice opened 5 years earlier. It is time to negotiate the contract for coverage for the next calendar year and the proposal from the company is almost $85 per employee, per month, higher than the practice has been paying. The current amount per employee, per month, is $515.00 and the new amount is $599.00. The representative has suggested that charging a higher copayment and deductible for employees will lower the premium. The physicians and practice manager would rather find a reputable managed care *plan, possibly even an HMO since there are a lot of choices in their area, than to have to pass on any extra costs to the employees or reduce current benefits. They also don't feel the proposed increase is the best use of the practice's funds. The practice manager calls the employees together to present the situation and ask each employee to research options over the next 10 business days and return to a meeting to share their findings/proposals.*

6

Managing the Revenue Cycle and the Financial Health of the Practice

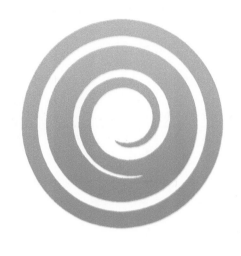

LEARNING OUTCOMES

Upon completion of this chapter, the student should...

- Illustrate the six steps in the revenue cycle
- Identify where in the revenue cycle various processes take place
- Analyze a denial of payment and a refund request from a third-party payer and determine whether or not each is valid
- Execute an appeal to a third-party payer in response to an invalid denial or refund request
- Explain what happens when claims are generated and submitted to a claims clearinghouse
- Explain the process of coordinating benefits between more than one third-party payer
- Write a legally sound collections letter to a patient
- Differentiate between the various types of common financial statement discussed in this chapter and explain the purpose of each

KEY TERMS

Adverse Benefit Determination
Assets
Balance Sheet
Cash Flow Statement
CMS 1500
Credits
Debits
Employee Retirement Income Security Act (ERISA)

Income Statement
Modifiers
National Correct Coding Initiative (NCCI)
National Uniform Claim Committee (NUCC)
Outpatient Code Editor (OCE)
Ratio
Summary Plan Description
Unbundling
Upcoding

⊗ OVERVIEW

Simply stated, the revenue cycle is everything that happens from the time a specific patient encounter is scheduled through the time that any services performed as the result of that appointment have been reimbursed for the full amount to which the practice is legally and ethically entitled. There are also some additional reports and analyses that occur retrospectively that are indirectly tied to the revenue cycle. As with every aspect of practice administration, effective management of the revenue cycle helps to assure the financial health of the practice which, in turn, contributes to the team's ability to focus on the patient without being distracted by worries about layoffs or having fully adequate equipment, supplies, and technology to optimize the provision of exceptional care. The savvy administrator must also manage peripheral financially related processes such as working with an accountant, helping the physicians understand financial statements, and knowing how to identify problematic areas or opportunities for improvement.

There are six main steps that are directly involved in managing the revenue cycle. These steps include

- Step 1: Patient registration, patient check-in, clinical encounter, and checkout
- Step 2: Correct coding and billing
- Step 3: Claims generation and transmittal
- Step 4: Processing payments and coordination of benefits (COB)
- Step 5: Preparation and transmittal of patient statements
- Step 6: Collections and finalizing payments

⊗ STEP 1: PATIENT REGISTRATION, PATIENT CHECK-IN, CLINICAL ENCOUNTER, AND CHECKOUT

There are two perspectives that are important for the practice manager to consider in Step 1 of the revenue cycle. The first is the patient's direct experience and the second is the role the revenue cycle plays in providing the secure financial environment that enables the team to focus on the patient.

The patient's direct experience in these processes has been discussed in earlier chapters from a patient-centric perspective of providing exceptional customer service with regard to acknowledging the patient's arrival, minimizing patient waiting time, keeping the patient informed when there is an unpredictable delay, and generally making the waiting area comfortable. The one aspect of the patient's direct experience that is integral to the revenue cycle and also offers a significant opportunity to increase patient loyalty is data collection.

There is a certain amount of demographic and clinical information that must be collected and maintained for every patient. One pitfall of this process is that many practices do not make collection of this data efficient for either the patient or the practice. In other instances, it is efficient for the practice but not for the patient. A savvy manager avoids inefficiency on the part of the patient to preserve patient loyalty and on the part of the practice to avoid bottlenecks in the workflow. Another aspect of data collection is that the more times the same data element is written or typed, the more likely that an error will be made which means that at some point, the inconsistency will have to be researched and corrected which is time consuming.

Forms play a big role in data collection and can make or break the overall success of this process for the patient, the practice, or both. The first rule is to make sure to audit every form used in the practice to determine if there are forms that duplicate information found on other forms. The only duplicate information that should occur on any forms is the minimum amount of data necessary to positively identify the right patient for every form—usually an account or medical record number and the patient's name are sufficient. Forms that collect redundant or unnecessary information should be redesigned and either combined with one or more other forms or shortened. Once the initial patient information is input (Chapters 1 and 10 elaborate on various options of inputting data based on whether the office uses a paper medical record or an electronic health record), the practice management system stores it so that appropriate information that hasn't changed since the previous visit is automatically retrieved when the patient medical record number, account number, or last name is keyed into a search field on the appropriate computer screen. The database that is part of any practice management software enables the appropriate data to be automatically supplied once the patient has been selected. For example, if the insurance specialist needs to generate a statement to the patient, the system would automatically supply the patient address, etc., in the correct location of the form.

If the office must have all prescriptions in a certain format, and the practice doesn't have a Web site or a patient portal that the patient can access in advance to supply the necessary information, then mail the forms to the patient in advance of the visit so he or she can complete the form one time from the source(s) and not have to write anything more than once. If a standardized form is not necessary, have the patient bring the information to the visit in any format they choose and then copy or scan whatever the information is on for inclusion in the medical record. Also, on a related note, don't make established patients fill out the same forms over again each time they are in the office. If they have been seen at the practice in the past year, ask them if there is any change in their contact information or insurance coverage since the last visit. If so, have the patient complete only those sections of the appropriate form. If the office has a paper record, the updated information can be attached to the original form and then the data can be input as an update into the practice management system. If it is an electronic health record, the updated information can be either scanned or input into the system by the most appropriate team member (e.g., receptionist for demographic information and nurse or medical assistant if they've seen another doctor or been in the hospital since the last encounter).

Regardless of what practice management system an office uses, or what format is used for keying in scheduling and billing information, there are certain data elements required. Some systems allow for additional

> **TIP**
>
> The second rule is don't ask a patient to bring a complete list of current medications and medical history only to have the patient or a team member transfer all of that information onto one or more standard forms.

HEALTH INSURANCE CLAIM FORM

APPROVED BY NATIONAL UNIFORM CLAIM COMMITTEE (NUCC) 02/12

CARRIER

PICA   PICA

1. MEDICARE (Medicare#)   MEDICAID (Medicaid#)   TRICARE (ID#/DoD#)   CHAMPVA (Member ID#)   GROUP HEALTH PLAN (ID#)   FECA BLK LUNG (ID#)   OTHER (ID#)   1a. INSURED'S I.D. NUMBER   (For Program in Item 1)

2. PATIENT'S NAME (Last Name, First Name, Middle Initial)   3. PATIENT'S BIRTH DATE MM DD YY   SEX M   F   4. INSURED'S NAME (Last Name, First Name, Middle Initial)

5. PATIENT'S ADDRESS (No., Street)   6. PATIENT RELATIONSHIP TO INSURED   Self   Spouse   Child   Other   7. INSURED'S ADDRESS (No., Street)

CITY   STATE   8. RESERVED FOR NUCC USE   CITY   STATE

ZIP CODE   TELEPHONE (Include Area Code) ( )   ZIP CODE   TELEPHONE (Include Area Code) ( )

9. OTHER INSURED'S NAME (Last Name, First Name, Middle Initial)   10. IS PATIENT'S CONDITION RELATED TO: 11. INSURED'S POLICY GROUP OR FECA NUMBER

a. OTHER INSURED'S POLICY OR GROUP NUMBER   a. EMPLOYMENT? (Current or Previous) YES NO   a. INSURED'S DATE OF BIRTH MM DD YY   SEX M F

b. RESERVED FOR NUCC USE   b. AUTO ACCIDENT? YES NO   PLACE (State)   b. OTHER CLAIM ID (Designated by NUCC)

c. RESERVED FOR NUCC USE   c. OTHER ACCIDENT? YES NO   c. INSURANCE PLAN NAME OR PROGRAM NAME

d. INSURANCE PLAN NAME OR PROGRAM NAME   10d. CLAIM CODES (Designated by NUCC)   d. IS THERE ANOTHER HEALTH BENEFIT PLAN? YES NO *If yes*, complete items 9, 9a, and 9d.

READ BACK OF FORM BEFORE COMPLETING & SIGNING THIS FORM.
12. PATIENT'S OR AUTHORIZED PERSON'S SIGNATURE I authorize the release of any medical or other information necessary to process this claim. I also request payment of government benefits either to myself or to the party who accepts assignment below.

SIGNED _____ DATE _____

13. INSURED'S OR AUTHORIZED PERSON'S SIGNATURE I authorize payment of medical benefits to the undersigned physician or supplier for services described below.

SIGNED _____

PATIENT AND INSURED INFORMATION

14. DATE OF CURRENT ILLNESS, INJURY, or PREGNANCY (LMP) MM DD YY QUAL.   15. OTHER DATE QUAL. MM DD YY   16. DATES PATIENT UNABLE TO WORK IN CURRENT OCCUPATION FROM MM DD YY TO MM DD YY

17. NAME OF REFERRING PROVIDER OR OTHER SOURCE   17a.   17b. NPI   18. HOSPITALIZATION DATES RELATED TO CURRENT SERVICES FROM MM DD YY TO MM DD YY

19. ADDITIONAL CLAIM INFORMATION (Designated by NUCC)   20. OUTSIDE LAB? YES NO $ CHARGES

21. DIAGNOSIS OR NATURE OF ILLNESS OR INJURY Relate A-L to service line below (24E)   ICD Ind.   22. RESUBMISSION CODE   ORIGINAL REF. NO.

A. B. C. D.
E. F. G. H.
I. J. K. L.

23. PRIOR AUTHORIZATION NUMBER

24. A. DATE(S) OF SERVICE From MM DD YY To MM DD YY	B. PLACE OF SERVICE	C. EMG	D. PROCEDURES, SERVICES, OR SUPPLIES (Explain Unusual Circumstances) CPT/HCPCS MODIFIER	E. DIAGNOSIS POINTER	F. $ CHARGES	G. DAYS OR UNITS	H. EPSDT Family Plan	I. ID. QUAL.	J. RENDERING PROVIDER ID. #
1									NPI
2									NPI
3									NPI
4									NPI
5									NPI
6									NPI

PHYSICIAN OR SUPPLIER INFORMATION

25. FEDERAL TAX I.D. NUMBER   SSN EIN   26. PATIENT'S ACCOUNT NO.   27. ACCEPT ASSIGNMENT? (For govt. claims, see back) YES NO   28. TOTAL CHARGE $ 29. AMOUNT PAID $ 30. Rsvd for NUCC Use

31. SIGNATURE OF PHYSICIAN OR SUPPLIER INCLUDING DEGREES OR CREDENTIALS (I certify that the statements on the reverse apply to this bill and are made a part thereof.)

SIGNED _____ DATE _____

32. SERVICE FACILITY LOCATION INFORMATION   a. NPI   b.

33. BILLING PROVIDER INFO & PH # ( )   a. NPI   b.

NUCC Instruction Manual available at: www.nucc.org   **PLEASE PRINT OR TYPE**   APPROVED OMB-0938-1197 FORM 1500 (02-12)

Figure 6.1 CMS 1500.

CMS 1500: A standardized form originally from the Center for Medicare and Medicaid Services but used to submit claims to most third-party payers so that physician and other eligible practitioners get reimbursed for services covered by the third-party payer.

information but none have less than the data needed on a standard form for filing claims. This is good news in that the billing form, which is a CMS 1500 as seen in Figure 6.1, may be used as a guide for designing data collection forms that are needed to obtain the information necessary to get reimbursed. For information on completing any of the fields on the CMS 1500, visit the Web site for the National Uniform Claim Committee (NUCC) at www.nucc.org.

Once the demographic information is collected and updated as needed, the next part of this step in the revenue cycle is the collection of information related to the clinical aspect of the encounter. The form used to obtain the history from a new patient has already been discussed. Sometimes a medical assistant or nurse actually completes the form based on verbal responses from the patient regarding all medical and surgical history plus certain information regarding family history that may be an indicator of risk factors for inherited diseases. The physician may further clarify answers with the patient.

If the patient's history is on file with the practice, and the physician reviews the medical record to see if any previous history is pertinent for the current encounter, in addition to discussing the history of the present illness or condition with the patient, then the physician needs to document the details of what he or she reviewed (both from previous records or verbally with the patient) in the medical record. This process will support billing for the proper level of history performed and deemed medically necessary based on the diagnosis or diagnoses pertinent to the current episode of care.

The remainder of the clinical information is input by members of the team. For example, a nurse or medical assistant may weigh the patient, record blood pressure, read the patient's blood sugar, etc., and record the results in the patient health record. Ideally, the practice uses an EHR and the results are input efficiently into a template so the results can be captured in a graph to look at trends. Then, the physician must document (or dictate) the subjective history, the objective physical exam, the assessment, and the plan for treatment (SOAP order) as described in Chapter 1.

The patient is then given any prescriptions, educational information, orders for outside tests or diagnostic studies, and a date and time for the next appointment.

National Uniform Claim Committee (NUCC): A voluntary committee created to develop a standardized data set for use by the noninstitutional health care community to transmit claim and encounter information to and from all third-party payers. It is chaired by the American Medical Association (AMA), with the Centers for Medicare and Medicaid Services (CMS) as a critical partner.

> **TIP**
>
> Although somewhat common, it is not advisable to hand an established patient a form containing comprehensive questions about past, family, and social history. This practice is frustrating for the patient and may also result in a questionable audit if the practice considers asking questions about each body system as representing a comprehensive history for billing purposes.

STEP 2: CORRECT CODING AND BILLING

As mentioned previously, in some practices, the physicians do all or most of their own coding. In others, a professional coder reviews all appropriate information from the medical record and codes the record. Still other offices have an electronic health record module that performs computer-assisted coding. Regardless of who codes the records, the administrator must know, at the very least, how coding works and how to ensure the practice is in compliance with coding and billing guidelines. On one end of the spectrum, a practice that doesn't know exactly how to code correctly, but wants to play it safe, is probably not receiving the full amount to which it is legally and ethically entitled. On the other end, the fines for incorrect coding are significant enough to force a practice into bankruptcy and, in extreme cases, result in criminal charges against the owners of the practice. The legal ramifications of noncompliance are discussed in a later chapter as is how medical coding assists in assessing and improving practice performance. The focus of this section is the role of correct coding in the revenue cycle. Simply stated, medical coding is the process of translating medical information found in the medical record (e.g., a history and physical report) into alphanumeric codes representing standard descriptions that list all the reasons for an encounter with a health care professional (e.g., routine physical exam) and all the services and procedures that were performed during an encounter.

Table 6.1 contains a brief description of some terms that impact the coding step in the revenue cycle.

Regardless of which option a practice uses to code medical records, including a certified coder or certified medical biller and coder, a qualified outside person should spot audit the codes periodically because sometimes experienced coders either interpret something incorrectly or miss an update in coding guidelines. Also, provide opportunities for coders to participate in professional development and continuing education activities.

There are consultants and businesses dedicated to auditing, but it may be just as effective and less expensive to ask the director of Health Information Services at a local hospital if one of the coders is available after hours to conduct an audit on a contract basis. If there is another similar practice in the area and the two administrators work well together, an arrangement may be negotiated in which each practice's

Modifiers: A two-character suffix added to the end of a CPT or HCPCS code to change or provide more specific information to the basic code description.

Table 6.1	Medical Coding Terminology	
Terms	Explanation of Impact on Revenue Cycle
Current Procedural Terminology (CPT-4)	CPT-4 is published and maintained by the American Medical Association (AMA). CPT codes represent evaluation and management services, anesthesia, surgery, laboratory and pathology, radiology, and medicine-related services and procedures. The RBRVS and UCR reimbursement methods described in the previous chapter are calculated based on individual CPT codes and therefore drive physician reimbursement from third-party payers.
Healthcare Common Procedural Coding System (HCPCS)	HCPCS is a coding system used by CMS to meet the needs of Medicare and Medicaid reimbursement although other third-party payers have adopted HCPCS. CMS purchases the rights to use CPT as HCPCS Level I and then maintains Level II HCPCS codes, which are codes that provide more detail than CPT codes and used to code services, drugs, supplies, home medical equipment etc., not adequately covered in CPT.
Modifiers	Modifiers are used as suffixes to CPT and HCPCS Level II codes to designate special circumstances. The code itself is the same but the modifier may describe that the procedure did not require the standard amount of time or resources but there is no other code to describe that procedure so a modifier is added. Some modifiers are descriptive and don't impact reimbursement such as LT for left side and others result in either an increase or decrease in reimbursement.

Table 6.1	Medical Coding Terminology (*continued*)
Terms	**Explanation of Impact on Revenue Cycle**
International Classification of Diseases-9th Edition–Clinically Modified for use in the United States (ICD-9-CM)	Although CPT and HCPCS Level II codes drive reimbursement, a third-party payer will deny or reduce reimbursement for any CPT or HCPCS code that isn't justified as medically necessary. ICD-9 codes are used for that purpose. ICD-9-CM consists of three volumes, but Volume 3 is only used by hospitals to code procedures reflecting utilization of the facility for operations and other procedures. Volumes 1 and 2, however, are used to code any health encounter. Volume 1 is a tabular listing (i.e., numeric order) of codes and Volume 2 is an alphabetic index used to guide the coder to the most accurate tabular code. ICD-9-CM contains signs, symptoms, conditions, diseases, and other reasons for a patient having an encounter with a health care provider. For example, there is a diagnosis code that describes the reason for the encounter as a routine physical exam on a healthy person. ICD-9-CM also contains codes to supplement the diagnosis by supplying details on how and where an injury or poisoning occurred (e.g., motor vehicle accident on a public highway). In 2015, ICD-10 codes will replace ICD-9 codes. Volume 3 of ICD-9 will be replaced by ICD-10-PCS or Procedural Coding System but like Volume 3, the PCS codes only impact facility coding.
National Correct Coding Initiative (NCCI) and Outpatient Code Editor (OCE)	Dating back to 1996, CMS implemented the NCCI to increase control over appropriate payments for Medicare and Medicaid patient services and built many of these guidelines into the OCE which edits for compliance with these guidelines.
Unbundling	In CPT, there are many instances in which a procedure can be performed independently of other procedures and therefore a CPT code exists but there are also codes that represent a package of services commonly performed together. In this case, it is unethical to "unbundle" the package by coding each component separately instead of selecting the packaged code. For example, there are lab panels in which one code represents several tests. If all of these tests are performed, the panel code must be used. If a practice submits each test under its individual code instead, thereby unbundling the panel, the practice could be severely fined for not complying with the rules.
Upcoding	Upcoding is choosing a code that pays more when that code is not a true reflection of the level of services performed. It is also not using a modifier that will reduce payment when the situation calls for such a modifier. An example is choosing a high evaluation and management code for an office visit when either the physician did not fulfill the criteria for that level of code or the physician did fulfill the criteria but the full criteria wasn't justified (e.g., highest level of history and physical exam on an established patient) by the patient's diagnosis.

National Correct Coding Initiative (NCCI): A CMS initiative that includes a policy manual that promotes the accurate coding of claims and is based on input from a diverse group of coding and reimbursement experts. The manual is updated annually.

Outpatient Code Editor (OCE): It is a software program used by CMS and most claims clearinghouses that identifies errors and inconsistencies on claims that are then electronically returned to the sender to correct before CMS will process the claim for reimbursement.

Unbundling: There are codes that combine procedures commonly performed together (such as all of the laboratory tests that are typically done to determine a person's overall heart health) into one code. Unbundling is coding each individual code separately instead of using the combination code. Unbundling is not legal or ethical.

Upcoding: The act of choosing a higher code than warranted by the patient's condition.

coder would do a random audit of the other practice's coded records—perhaps quarterly. Audits are even more critical if physicians do their own coding, a computer-assisted coding software package is used, or a noncertified coder is used.

One other extremely important aspect of correct coding is physician documentation. Often, physicians don't document as thoroughly or precisely as necessary to clearly describe all of the elements needed to select the most accurate code. From a physician's perspective, the primary purpose of documentation is to ensure continuity of patient care which is, indeed, the most important aspect of medical documentation. However, administrators need to reinforce the concept with all physicians that documentation can make or break the financial health of a practice as well. Therefore, correct coding involves good documentation practices and a process that ensures the documentation is coded properly.

STEP 3: CLAIMS GENERATION AND TRANSMITTAL

Practice management systems collect and store all of the data elements required on the CMS 1500 form illustrated in Step 1. The fields on the CMS 1500 form that reflect the purpose of the encounter (ICD-9-CM codes) and the services rendered (CPT and HCPCS codes) are Fields 21 and 24, respectively. At the end of the description below, there is an illustration of these fields completed for a given scenario.

Field 21 contains space for up to four ICD-9-CM codes. Note that ICD-9-CM codes are comprised of three, four, or five alphanumeric characters. If there are more than three characters, there is a decimal after the third character. One exception is E codes that describe the external causes of injuries. The format for these codes is E000 or E000.0. In the case of E codes, the fourth digit is actually input right above the decimal point on the CMS form. If there are five characters on the E code, the fifth character is input without a decimal, even though the ICD-9 codebook has a decimal. Remember, these forms are either sent electronically or mailed and scanned into a third-party payer system so the items like decimal points are to help with ease of readability by the user but not read by the computer system. The claims processing systems know by field location what the proper format of each data element is. Some encoders and practice management systems omit the decimal but, when printed on a CMS form, the decimal is included.

In Field 24 on CMS 1500 forms, up to six services per claim form may be submitted on one form. Starting from line number 1, the dates of service (both from and to) are required for each line. Many practice management systems default to the current date and have to be changed. Then, if there is more than one line, the system defaults the dates on line 2 to the same dates input on line 1. This is often correct but there are exceptions. For example, a physician may go to the hospital to admit a patient, which involves documenting a history and physical and initial orders. Then, the next day, the physician may have spent quite a lot of time with the patient checking progress and submitting orders. The third and fourth days may have required a less intense visit for checking progress and orders. Finally on the fifth day, the physician discharges the patient. Continuing with this example, the next field is a code for place of service. A complete list of place of service codes can be found at http://www.cms.gov/MedHCPCSGenInfo/Downloads/Place_of_Service.pdf. The place of service code when the physician is admitting, treating, or discharging a hospital inpatient is 21. The next field, No. 24C (EMG), is only required by certain payers but the options are a Y if the claim is for emergency services and an N if not. Field 24D is the CPT or HCPCS Level II code and any applicable modifiers—up to four, two-digit modifiers. Field 24E is a link between the diagnosis and the procedure on each line. Each procedure code can be justified for medical necessity by linking up to four diagnosis codes per procedure code. The linkage is left justified and can use any combination of up to four codes indicated by 1234 (no commas). The billing specialist must be very careful with linkages. For example, if a patient comes to the office, the physician is not allowed to code both an evaluation and management service and a surgical procedure on the same day unless the procedure was done for a separately identifiable reason than the evaluation and management service. For example, if the surgery was to suture a laceration but the patient also had an upper respiratory infection, the physician could code for both as long as the E&M code has a modifier (25) indicating the service was for a distinctly different reason than the surgery, and the E&M code is linked only to the diagnosis requiring the E&M service and the surgery code is linked only to the diagnosis requiring the surgical procedure. Field 24F indicates the amount the practice charges for the procedure or service code listed on each line. Finally, Field 24G designates units or days of service.

Figure 6.2 is an example of Fields 21 and 24 completed for the scenario above in which a physician performs a high-level admission to the hospital for a patient on day 1 (CPT 99223), performs a high-level subsequent care service the next day (99233), mid-level subsequent care services ((99232 × 2) on days 3 and 4, and a low-level discharge service (99238) on day 5. The patient has been admitted due to a severe

21. DIAGNOSIS OR NATURE OF ILLNESS OR INJURY (Relate Items 1, 2, 3 or 4 to Item 24E by Line)¬

1. 796.2   3. 493.92

2. E9457   4. ____ . ____

24. A. DATE(S) OF Service From — To MM DD YY MM DD YY	B. PLACE OF SERVICE	C. EMG	D. PROCEDURES, SERVICES or SUPPLIES (Explain Unusual Circumstances) CPT/HCPCS MODIFIER	E. DIAGNOSIS POINTER	F. $charges	G. Units
1 010112 101012	21	N	99223	123	200.00	010
2 010212 010212	21	N	99233	123	175.00	010
3 010312 010412	21	N	99232	123	150.00	020
4 010512 010512	21	N	99238	123	150.00	010

Figure 6.2 CMS 1500 with Fields 21 and 24 completed.

adverse reaction (severely elevated blood pressure) to a prescribed drug (Albuterol, for asthma). The diagnosis codes describe high blood pressure without a diagnosis of hypertension (796.2) due to adverse reaction to Albuterol properly administered (E945.7) in a patient with an acute exacerbation of asthma (493.92). Note that all three diagnoses are linked to all services in this case. Also note the "from" and "to" dates on the third line and the multiple units or days of service on this line which the payer would multiply by the dollar amount charged so, in this example, it would calculate $300.00.

Once all of the data required to generate an electronic or printed copy of the CMS 1500 form for an encounter have been entered (or retrieved from the database) into the practice management system, the system holds the claim until the billing specialist is ready to generate a group of claims (usually called a batch) for transmission.

CLAIMS CLEARINGHOUSES

As mentioned in the first chapter, a medical claims clearinghouse enables practices to electronically submit all of their claims for a given billing cycle (e.g., daily or weekly) to the clearinghouse. At the clearinghouse, claims run through a series of logic edits so that an error can be rejected and sent back to the practice to fix, which prevents the third-party payer from denying the claim—a more costly process. Most claims clearinghouses charge by the claim with an option for them to print out any claim that can't be routed to the payer electronically and mail it for a higher per-claim cost. For large practices, another option is to purchase clearinghouse software which is costly, but then there is no per-claims cost. Many practice management systems come with an option for claims clearinghouse services through a certain vendor as part of the monthly or annual monthly maintenance fees. These services may be discounted due to the number of practices using a specific vendor through a contract with the practice management system software vendor.

STEP 4: PROCESSING PAYMENTS AND COORDINATION OF BENEFITS

Most practice management systems have an initial set of codes that are designed to explain the reason for a balance to be written off, submitted to a secondary payer, or billed to the patient. The existing messages can be edited for customization by the practice and new codes can be added by the practice. It is critical that any message that will be read by the patient for any reason (e.g., patient statement or collections letter) is the most precise code for the situation and is worded in a manner that contributes to the overall practice goal of a loyal patient base.

If all of the previous steps have been accurately and consistently performed, then there shouldn't be any surprises in the amount of payment received from any third-party payer. However, management of denials is covered in Chapter 7

Box 6.1

Opportunities to Build Loyalty Are Present in Most Office Tasks

From the perspective of the administrator, the two most important aspects of payment processing and COB is to make sure there are well-written policies and procedures in place to guide the billing specialist in payment verification and to make sure that any message that will appear on a patient statement regarding the patient's financial responsibility is both appropriate and patient centric.

Assuming there is a payment, the typical action at this step is for the billing specialist to apply the payments in the practice management system. Assuming the payment is correct, there is often a legitimate outstanding balance. The policies and procedures should specify what to do for each reason a medical procedure was not paid in full by the third-party payer. One example is there is a legitimate balance but there is also a secondary payer for this patient so the action is to apply the payment information from the first payer and then submit a claim with the first payer's explanation of benefits to the secondary payer. This process is called coordination of benefits (COB). Another example is writing off the difference between billed and allowed amounts if the practice has agreed to accept the payer's allowed amount as the full amount of reimbursement. Yet another example is that the patient owes a legitimate balance. Some sample, patient-centric messages for patient balances are shown under the patient statements step of the revenue cycle.

Troubleshooting Aged Claims

CMS and most other third-party payers consider submitting a duplicate claim (intentionally or not) to be a process that falls under the fraud and abuse guidelines. Years ago, if a practice hadn't gotten a response from a third-party payer, the insurance specialist would simply resubmit the charges. On the practice side, this process added to the per-claim cost of claims transmission in addition to not solving whatever problem caused the delay in the first place. To reduce this extra cost, some practices would add the aging charge to a new claim the next time they see that patient. Either way, if the third-party payer wound up paying both services for any reason, then the practice had to incur the expense of processing a refund to the insurance company. CMS recognized that it was inefficient to pay duplicate claims on their end too. The solution was to add submission of duplicate claims or duplicate lines of service to the list of fraudulent or abusive billing practices, thereby penalizing or even prosecuting the offenders.

Managing these aging claims without resubmitting as duplicates involves analyzing a system-generated report generally known as aging analysis or outstanding accounts receivables by age. It is helpful to request this report by third-party payer to identify trends that might indicate a payer that is consistently late in paying claims. With this information, and with consideration for patients affected, the practice may want to discuss the situation with the payer. If there is not a satisfactory solution, the practice may choose to call any patients who have this coverage and give them substantial advanced notice—6 months, for example—that the practice intends to discontinue participating with this payer and let the patient know why. Then, let the patient know that this simply means the practice will no longer participate or accept assignment for this insurance but the staff will be happy to make sure the patient has everything he or she needs to submit his or her own claims to the payer in the future. Also, let patients know that if they exercise this option, they will need to pay for services in full at the time of any subsequent medical visits, but that a payment plan may be an option.

Starting with the oldest claims, the billing specialist will contact the payer/provider services department armed with a list of aging claims from that payer. Then, the specialist will walk through with the representative, claim by claim, to determine what is holding the claim up. If it's the payer and they can tell what's wrong, they usually promise to expedite the processing. Other times, though, they inform the billing specialist that the claim is pending peer review which means they will probably be requesting notes and reports from the practice to make a determination of medical necessity. Make sure they tell the billing specialist what they need while they are on the phone, exactly where to send any required supporting documentation, and how to ensure it will be routed in a manner so that the examiner/medical professional at the insurance company knows the documentation has been received for review and adjudication. Sometimes the insurance company will indicate that some or all of the practice's aging claims are being manually processed due to editing caused by incomplete or unclear information being submitted such as missing modifiers, discrepancies in dates of service between a hospital bill and the physician's hospital-based services, and missing a code that identifies cause of an injury. Sometimes it turns out the billing specialist missed a requirement and can not only get all of the aging claims processed by supplying the missing information but also make sure the problem is corrected on subsequent claims.

STEP 5: PREPARATION AND TRANSMITTAL OF PATIENT STATEMENTS

Ideally, a practice that has successfully built a loyal patient base has established a give-and-take relationship with the patient in which the patient perceives the overall value of having exceptional physicians and staff members is so great that it is a priority to pay the practice whatever is owed once any third-party payers have processed the claims. Whether or not this is true of ALL patients in the practice, great care must be taken by the practice administrator to ensure that all patient statements are accurate, that there is a clearly visible message thanking the patient for his or her selection of this practice among the many choices patients have, and all messages regarding balances owed to the practice describe the exact reason for the balance. Another important aspect of the patient statement is to offer the patient an opportunity to call the practice if he or she needs to discuss an extension to the due date or a payment plan.

Reason for Unpaid Balance	Action	Message
Copayments are the patient's responsibility and are intended to be collected at the time of the office visit or consultation. Sometimes, however, the patient doesn't have the money at that time or else, the money was inadvertently not collected at that time. Another scenario is that a copayment has been increased by the payer since the last visit and that increase was not caught at the time of service resulting in an insufficient copayment being collected the day of the service.	If the full, correct amount of copayment was not collected at the time of service, the amount due will be reflected on the next cycle of patient statements.	Please note that your managed care plan charges a copayment in the amount of $25.00 per visit. It is customary to collect this amount at the time of the office visit. We are sorry for any inconvenience but we failed to collect this copayment (or, the full amount of this copayment) on January 12, 20XX. Please remit payment at your convenience within 30 days or call our office within that time period at (111)222-1212 and we'll be happy to assist you with any alternative arrangements you may require or to answer any questions. Thank you, again, for choosing our practice.
Billed charges exceed allowable charges	If the practice participates with the payer, then this difference must be written off. If the practice doesn't participate, the practice may submit the balance to the patient. However, the administrator should make sure the patient is aware of this policy BEFORE any services are rendered. If the patient agrees to pay more to go to this practice than to a participating physician, then, the practice has to decide whether or not	We have received payment from your insurance company. As we discussed at the time of your visit on January 12, 20XX, our practice does not have an agreement with your plan to accept their allowed amount as payment in full. We are diligent in keeping our charges reasonable but some payers do not take this into consideration, therefore, we cannot participate with all plans. We do appreciate your loyalty to our practice. Please remit payment at your convenience within 30 days or call our office within that time period at (111)222-1212 and we'll be happy to assist you with any alternative arrangements you may require or to answer any questions. Thank you, again, for choosing our practice.
Deductible and/or coinsurance is the patient's responsibility and is not typically collected at the time of service since it is hard to calculate the exact amount and having to either refund or collect additional funds from the patient is not prudent.	These balances are rarely challenged and generally anticipated by the patient	We have received payment from your insurance company. As we discussed on January 12, 20XX, our policy is to wait until after any third party payers have processed your claim so we can bill you for the exact amounts of deductible and/or coinsurance. Now that we have that information, please remit payment at your convenience within 30 days or call our office within that time period at (111)222-1212 and we'll be happy to assist you with any alternative arrangements you may require or to answer any questions. Thank you, again, for choosing our practice.

Figure 6.3 **Actions and messages for outstanding balances.**

Some suggestions for patient-centric messages based on the reasons for the balance are listed in Figure 6.3, and a sample patient statement is illustrated in Figure 6.4.

STEP 6: COLLECTIONS AND FINALIZING PAYMENTS

As discussed previously, even an exceptional leader who successfully coaches an excellent, patient-centric team must occasionally deal with a situation in which an employee is not a good match for that team. Likewise, a highly patient-centric practice will have to deal with some number of patients who are nearly impossible to satisfy.

(Dated and on Letterhead)

Dear. Mrs. Williams:

Thank you for choosing our practice to serve your medical needs. We are privileged to have you as a patient.

We have received a correct payment from your insurance company in the amount of: $XXX.XX for your minor surgical procedure in our office on March 23, 20XX. We have also written off the difference between your insurance plan's allowed amount and our original billed charges. Your share of cost for deductible and coinsurance is $XX.XX. Your prompt remittance of this balance will be greatly appreciated. If you have any questions or would like to discuss payment options, please call our office at your earliest convenience. Thanks again for your loyalty to our practice.

Sincerely,

Figure 6.4 Sample patient statement.

In general, a patient-centric practice has fewer problems with patients being late or not showing up for appointments, fewer patients who threaten litigation, and fewer patients who don't meet their financial obligations to the practice than those practices that are not team oriented and patient focused. However, when a patient is an exception to this general rule, it is sometimes necessary to initiate a collections process.

The Big Picture

Before a practice can make the best decisions about patient collections, it is important to understand that health care is in a constant state of change. Some of these changes leading up to health care reform include the dynamics of employers' purchasing health coverage for their employees. Every year, health care costs rise, which means that third-party payers find it necessary to increase premiums for equivalent coverage. Employers, on the other hand, don't necessarily have the ability to incur more costs so they have to decide how to keep the employees covered without spending much more money than the previous year. The most typical solution is to negotiate contracts with payers in which the employees pay substantial deductibles and coinsurance or copayments. This solution by itself creates a financial hardship on the typical patient who is also possibly paying part of their own premium and a huge premium if they have dependents on their employer's plan. To make it worse for providers, the patient's share of cost may vary by encounter based on factors such as the type of provider, the provider's network status, and the type of service. Therefore, it makes it nearly impossible to know the patient's share of cost at the time the service is rendered. Trying to estimate that share of cost is not usually cost-effective because either the practice will have to process a refund to the patient or bill the patient for the difference between the amount collected and the amount of patient liability. It is also not conducive to the patient-centric approach that requires every step of the patient–provider relationship to be as accurate and efficient as possible.

The shifting of significantly more of the financial burden for health care coverage to the employee has resulted in an average physician having an annual increase in bad patient debt in the neighborhood of $10,000.00. Furthermore, these working people often don't qualify for Medicaid even if they don't earn very high wages.

One bit of good news is that these issues are being addressed nationally because without some remedy, some providers are on the verge of taking drastic actions such as only providing nonemergency care to patients who are willing and able to make a significant payment toward full billed charges at the time of service or who have proof of exceptionally good medical coverage.

Financial Policy

Meanwhile, the practice needs to have a very clearly but kindly worded financial policy posted at the receptionist desk. It's also wise to explain the policy to new patients when they schedule an appointment so they know what to expect in advance. Whatever the policy is, a good suggestion is to say something like "The focus at Sunshine Medical is on providing exceptional care to each and every one of our valued patients. We make every attempt to deliver healthcare as economically as possible but due to the fact that we are only able to serve patients when we are reimbursed for our services in a timely and accurate manner, we do need your cooperation as requested. We do try to accommodate individual financial needs by discussing payment options but our policy is to collect all copayments at the time service is rendered. We accommodate billing most insurance companies for the patient but the patient must know that ultimately, the cost of our services is the patient's responsibility if the insurance company denies payment for any reason other than the service not being medically necessary. We will make an attempt to verify in advance if we learn from an insurance company that they don't cover a service that we deem medically necessary so the patient or guardian can make an informed decision before the service is rendered. Thank you for your support of this practice—we're here for you and hope to be able to meet your medical needs for as long as you desire."

The Collections Process

In the unfortunate event that a patient has not responded to overdue statements, the following is a brief description of the key aspects of

TIP

Check the state medical bill collection laws which vary regarding hours in which one is allowed to call a patient, what the state laws are regarding calling the patient's place of employment regarding collections, etc., and do not threaten the patient or speak to anyone else unless the practice has formal documentation of a legal guardian of the patient and the staff member making the call is positive that is to whom he or she is speaking.

collections with the pros and cons of contracting with an agency presented. Typically, once the first statement has been sent to the patient, the practice should submit a second request after 30 days. Then, the billing specialist should try calling the patient. It is essential for the specialist to be prepared with all verified payment information and knowledge from the third-party payer about why the payment (or denial) is correct. It's a good idea to draft a simple form to help keep the billing specialist on track in case the patient isn't very receptive. It's also a good idea to only make the calls when a manager is available so that if the patient becomes argumentative, the billing specialist will be able to tell the patient that if the patient prefers, the practice manager will explain the situation. Sometimes the patient demands to speak to a manager immediately and it's very nice to be able to say, "Mrs. Jones, our practice manager, Mary Smith will be happy to discuss your account with you."

The form for telephone calls should contain, at a minimum, the following:

- The patient's name
- Account number
- Financially responsible party if other than the patient
- Telephone numbers (convenient if a callback is necessary)
- The dates of visit(s)
- Amounts paid or denied by insurance
- Whether the patient has made any attempt to contact the practice since the second notice
- Caller signature line with date and time in case of legal action

Sixty days from the initial statement, a formal, certified letter should be sent to the patient. Somewhere between 70 and 80 days from initial statement, a second certified letter should go out to the patient. Finally, after 90 days, the account should be turned over to a collection agency. Some practices turn the accounts over to an agency after 30 days but since collection agencies generally are paid based on a substantial percentage of what they collect, the practice should at least try to handle the account for the first 90 days on a trial basis. If they are successful over half of the time, then they should continue this process. If <50% successful, it may be advantageous to use a collection agency after the first 30 or the first 45 days. There is merit in making the collections agency the "bad guys" from the patient's perspective.

See Figure 6.5 for some sample wording on the first (60 days) and last (70 to 80 days) certified letters asking for payment before the account is turned over to collections.

Employee Retirement Income Security Act (ERISA): Law enacted in 1974 to protect an employee's pension plan but as employers started to add health insurance as a benefit of employment, health benefits were placed under the protection of this law.

DENIAL, APPEALS, REFUNDS, AND ERISA

Steven M. Verno, CMMB, CMMC, NREMTP, an expert in the claims processing, denials, appeals, and refunds that fall under the Employee Retirement Income Security Act (ERISA) laws, has graciously contributed this section.

(First Letter on Letterhead and Dated)

Dear Mr. Smith:

As indicated on your latest patient statement, your health insurance plan has correctly paid their share of the cost of your office visit on January 23, 20XX. We have subsequently written off the difference between our usual billed charges for this service and your payers allowed amount because we agreed to participate with their company. The balance represents your 30% coinsurance of $175.00. Since this amount is overdue, please contact our office within 10 business days to make arrangements for payments if needed or else please remit the full amount due to our office within 10 business days. We accept VISA, Mastercard and Discover and have included the information we need below for you to complete and return in the self-addressed, stamped envelope we've completed for your convenience if you chose this option. Otherwise, please drop a check, money order or cash by our office within this same timeframe.

(Final Letter on Letterhead and Dated)

Dear Mr. Smith:

 The purpose of this letter is to notify you that your long over-due account is being transferred to a collection's agency. As a courtesy, if you contact this office to make payment arrangements or remit payment in person or postmarked NOT LATER THAN April 10, 20XX, no action will be taken to negatively affect your credit scores. However, on April 10, 20XX, further legal collections actions will be initiated.

Figure 6.5 Excerpt from first and final letters of collection.

ERISA was enacted in 1974 to protect an employee's pension plan but as employers started to add health insurance as a benefit of employment, health benefits were placed under the protection of this law. ERISA is a federal law. Health benefits provided by an employer who is not a federal employer or a church employer come under the jurisdiction of ERISA (Reference Title 29 United States Code (USC) 18, 1144(a) and U.S. Supreme Court Cases of Davilla vs. Aetna and Calad vs. Cigna). Therefore, any adverse benefit determination such as a denial of services or a request from a payer for a refund of previously paid benefits (Reference: Title 29 Code of Federal Regulations (CFR) 2560.503-1, see http://www.gpoaccess.gov/cfr/index.html) falls under the jurisdiction of ERISA. The patient or the patient's legal representative can file a claim or appeal an adverse benefit determination.

Adverse Benefit Determination: A determination by a third party that a service for which a claim was received is not payable or that a previously paid service was paid in error and must be refunded.

Practice administrators must know that when routine procedures for handling denials or refund requests are unsuccessful, ERISA may be used to appeal on behalf of the patient. For example, a payer (or a legal representative of that payer) may try to use ERISA to its advantage by sending out a retroactive denial and request for refund to the provider years after the payment was made. If the provider tries to cite state law for timely filing (many states have laws that define the maximum length of time an insurance company has to request a refund for retroactive adverse benefit determinations), the insurance company may correctly inform

Summary Plan Description: A document containing a comprehensive description of a retirement plan that must be filed with the Department of Labor that includes the terms and conditions of participation and which is distributed to all potential participants in advance of enrollment.

the provider that since ERISA is a federal law, then the states have no jurisdiction. However, a knowledgeable practice administrator will know the steps to follow in these instances. For example, since the provider was paid originally due to the patient assigning benefits to that provider, the payer often requests a refund directly from the provider instead of the patient, thereby bypassing the patient's right to appeal an adverse benefit determination. ERISA requires a revised explanation of benefits be sent to the patient as defined in Title 29 CFR 2560.503-1. The member then has 180 days from the date of the denial to submit an appeal as defined in their summary plan description. Every payer is required to provide every member a copy of the member's summary plan description which must contain key information such as the appeals process. Many payers have these summaries on their Web site. Furthermore, the payer must inform the member of the adverse benefit determination (current or retroactive) and all policies used to deny the benefit as well as what is needed to submit the appeal. The patient is entitled to full disclosure to use in their appeal. Once all appeals processes have been filed, the patient is entitled to seek resolution in federal court. It could be possible the benefit denial may be deemed to be wrongful; therefore, no refund to the payer is due.

Therefore, the first step upon receiving a request to refund previously paid benefits is to inform the insurance company (or their representative) to contact the patient so that the patient can exercise their appeal rights as defined under ERISA. Also, inform them they are prohibited from offsetting any future payments due the practice from another patient pending a federal court order. (By offsetting payments, the payer may be creating additional adverse benefit determinations on the patient(s) whose benefits are offset and whose benefits are also under ERISA jurisdiction). A sample response is shown in Figure 6.6.

Then, refer any phone calls to the patient. If the patient hasn't authorized the practice to represent them, in writing, separately from the assignment of benefits that only authorizes the insurance company to make a direct payment to the provider instead of to the patient for health benefits, then the practice is not legally able to discuss benefit issues with the insurance company or their representative. However, the team member making the call can explain to the patient that if the patient wishes to have the practice represent them in any ERISA-protected proceedings (combined with an assignment of benefits) the patient can sign a letter, an example of which is shown in Figure 6.7

If a practice has any questions during this process—especially with regard to correspondence from a third-party payer that seems to be either bypassing patient rights or threatening the provider with collections—the administrator should contact an attorney.

MANAGING ADDITIONAL FINANCIAL ASPECTS OF THE PRACTICE

If the reader is starting to believe a practice manager or administrator has to be a financial and legal expert, it does seem that way. In reality, though, the practice manager needs to know when to seek the advice of an attorney or a public accountant; when to bring in an expert to

Dear XYZ Insurance Company (or ABC Law Firm on Behalf of XYZ Insurance Company):

We thank you for your follow-up letter and your identification that our patient, James C. Smith's health benefits are under ERISA jurisdiction (therefore state statute of limitations does not apply). In case you are not aware, when retroactively denying benefits that the member believed to be provided as a benefit of employment, an adverse benefit determination (ABD) has been performed. An ABD is defined in Federal Regulation, specifically, 29 CFR 2560.503-1. When an ABD has been performed retroactively, you or your client is required by Federal Regulation to send the member, an updated Explanation of Benefit (EOB) form, as regulated by Federal Regulation, specifically 29 CFR 2450.503-1. By sending us this claim for an alleged overpayment due to an adverse benefit determination, it could be possible that you or your client may be in violation of Federal ERISA laws (the same law cited by you in your explanation that your request for refund of a payment that exceeded state statute of limitations was valid since ERISA takes precedence over state laws) because the member is not being provided the opportunity to (a) file an appeal which is also protected by Federal law or (b) to file a lawsuit in Federal Court.

Rather than filing a complaint with the Secretary of Labor, the Federal Trade Commission, the Office of Insurance Regulation and the Internal Revenue Service, we will provide you with the opportunity to correct this wrong that we believe has been performed against the member whose federally protected health benefit has been denied so that the member can exercise their appeal rights. If the member elects to pursue this issue in Federal Court, we will await the court decision before we take any additional action. The refund demand could be dismissed by the court. We caution you and suggest that you advise your client against offsetting the amount you are requesting from a claim currently in progress. Offsetting could be deemed to be an additional adverse benefit determination.

A copy of this letter is being sent to the member with our recommendation that they inform their plan sponsor (their employer) of the adverse benefit determination and that they consider seeking legal counsel as to their appeal rights and their right to seek a cure in Federal Court.

Figure 6.6 Response to request for refund on a previously paid benefit.

audit medical coding and when to use their expertise combined with the expertise of the team, to solve problems, make decisions or handle processes without needing outside advice.

Regarding additional financial aspects of managing a medical practice, most practices use the services of an accountant. However, the manager is usually responsible for analyzing certain financial reports with or without help from the accountant so the manager can present summaries in meetings with the physicians or, when requested, the board of trustees for larger medical practices. Managers use the results of this analysis to assist with decision making such as whether or not to propose a new position, performance improvement, and problem solving. The budget process was discussed previously but other financial reports are important tools in keeping the practice in good financial health.

Managers should have a general idea of the cost of doing business by functions. For example, the manager should know the total cost to the practice for performing an MRI if they offer that procedure.

Two of the most useful financial statements in any business are the balance sheet and the income statement.

The Balance Sheet

A balance sheet is a statement that shows a snapshot on a given date at a given time, of what a medical practice owns, known as assets, any liabilities and any owner's equity or capital. Since this information

Balance Sheet: A summary of the financial balances—assets, liabilities, ownership equity as of a given date of a medical practice or any business.

Assets: The total resources of a medical practice including cash, accounts receivables, property, equipment that could be sold for cash, and any other entity which can be legitimately assessed a value.

SUNSHINE MEDICAL GROUP
123 Main Street
Anywhere, USA 12345
(999)555-1212

Date: _____

Patient Name: _____

Patient Address: _____

Patient City: _____

Patient State: _____Patient Zip Code: _____

Employer:_____

Member Health Plan ID:_____

I hereby certify that the insurance information that I have provided Sunshine Medical Group is true and accurate as of the date of service. I certify that benefits, to pay any and all medical claims, are available as of the date of service and under the jurisdiction of the federal Employee Retirement Income Security Act (ERISA). If authorization is needed to provide me with medical care, I certify that I have obtained said authorization from my insurance company in order to seek medical care from Sunshine Medical Group.

I understand that intentionally providing false insurance information may be considered as fraud. I am fully aware that having health insurance does not absolve me of my responsibility to ensure that my medical bill is paid in full. I also understand that my insurance company may not pay 100% of the amount of the medical claim and I may be responsible for any and all amounts not payable by my insurance company as outlined in my summary benefits plan.

Pursuant to 29CFR2560.503-1, I hereby authorize Sunshine Medical Group to submit clasims, appeals, and information requests for any and all documents, policies, procedures and internal decisions that were used to perform an adverse benefit determination of my employer sponsored health benefits protected under the jurisdiction of 28 USC 18, 1003(a) and 1144(a), on my behalf, as if I were submitting any appeals and requests to the insurance company listed on the copy of the current insurance cared and explanation of benefit form I have provided Sunshine Medical Group, in good faith. My signature hereby directs my insurance company to provide Sunshine Medical with the information requested as if I were making said request myself. Sunshine Medical is also authorized to file grievances on my behalf when XYZ insurance Company refuses to comply with informational requests made on my behalf.

I fully agree and understand that the submission of a claim does not absolve me of my responsibility to ensure the claim is paid in full. I hereby instruct and direct XYZ insurance Company to pay by check, made out and mailed to Sunshine Medical Group, 123 Main Street, Anywhere, USA 12345.

This is a direct assignment of my rights and benefits under this policy. His payment will not exceed my indebtedness to the above mentioned assignee and I have agreed to pay in a current manner, any balance of said professional service charges over and above this insurance payment. Upon receipt of said check, I authorize Sunshine Medical to deposit checks received on my account when made out to me in the event XYZ Insurance Company prohibits payments be made payable directly to the provider.

I authorize the release of any information directly pertinent to my case to any insurance company, adjuster or attorney involved in my case.

I authorize Sunshine Medical to be my personal representative. I fully understand and agree that I am responsible for full payment of the medical debt if my insurance company has refused to pay 100% of my benefits within 90 days of any and all appeals or request for information. I also agree that any fines levied against my insurance company will be paid to Sunshine Medical for a acting as my personal representative. A photocopy of the Assignment shall be considered as effective and valid as the original.

_____

Signature of Patient and, if different, Policyholder

_____

Date

(Lines for two separate witnesses to sign and date should also be included)
[sample copyrighted by Steve Verno 2004 and updated in 2010].

Figure 6.7 Sample patient authorization to represent patient and assignment of benefits.

changes every time the practice performs any type of transaction such as collecting a copayment from a patient, it is important to look at the date and time of the report. The assets of the practice are entered (usually in a specialized accounting software package) on the left side of the balance sheet and are referred to as debits (not to be confused with a checking account which is opposite of an accounting system), while liabilities and owner's equity are entered on the right side as credits. Every time there is an increase on the left (assets), there must be a corresponding decrease on the right (liabilities and owner's equity) and every time there is a decrease on the left, there must be a corresponding increase on the right. Therefore, an increase in assets is a debit (increase on left; corresponding decrease on right). On the other hand, a decrease in assets is a credit (decrease on the left; corresponding increase on the right). Likewise, a decrease in liabilities and owner's equity is a debit while an increase in liabilities and owner's equity is a credit in the accounting ledger and on the balance sheet at that snapshot in time. The name balance sheet refers to the fact that totals of asset must always equal the totals of liabilities plus owner's equity and therefore the left side of the balance sheet must be balanced with the right side. So, assets always equal liabilities plus owner's equity.

The Income Statement

The income statement is a report of a medical practice's revenue and their expenses, including any applicable taxes. This report will help the practice analyze the cost of providing various services but also is a tool that from the top down shows revenues (from patients, insurance companies, and miscellaneous revenue); total expenses (such as electric bill, rent or mortgage payments, malpractice insurance, equipment lease or maintenance, payroll expenses including taxes and health insurance, janitorial, office supplies, and travel).

From the income statement, a manger can figure out the cumulative profits.

So, the income statement shows the flow of cash into and out of the practice during whatever period of time the statement covers (monthly, quarterly, or annually by year). The net income, also known as retained earnings, for a period, is reflected under owner's equity on the balance sheet because equity shows profits that stay invested with the practice as opposed to being paid out as bonuses or in stock.

Other Financial Statements and Financial Management Concepts

When the income statement is combined with the statement of retained earnings for a period, the resulting statement is usually known as a flow of cash or cash flow statement. This statement shows the flow of cash, often by categories such as cash received from patients and insurance companies, cash spent on payroll, and other expenses. There is also a category that shows money invested in capital expenses such as large equipment and a category that shows business financial transactions such as loans and debt payments. At the end, there is a

Debits: In accounting or bookkeeping, using a double-entry system, there are accounts: assets, expenses, liabilities, owner's equity, and income. Assets plus equity must be equal to liability plus owner's equity plus income. Debits are entries on the left and increase a debit account (e.g., assets and expenses) and decrease a credit account (liabilities, income, and owner's equity). Credits are on the right side and increase a credit account.

Credits: In accounting or bookkeeping, using a double-entry system, there are accounts: assets, expenses, liabilities, owner's equity, and income. Assets plus equity must be equal to liability plus owner's equity plus income. Debits are entries on the left and increase a debit account (e.g., assets and expenses) and decrease a credit account (liabilities, income, and owner's equity). Credits are on the right side and increase a credit account.

Income Statement: A report of a medical practice's revenue and their expenses, including any applicable taxes. This report will help the practice analyze the cost of providing various services but also is a tool that from the top down shows revenues, total expenses, etc.

Cash Flow Statement: A financial statement that demonstrates how changes in the accounts and income on the balance sheet affect the inflow and outflow of cash.

line for net cash increase and for both the beginning and ending cash for the practice. Managers need to analyze the cash flow to identify any trends that may need to be addressed such as increases in expenses without corresponding increases in revenue which, if not analyzed and corrected, may cause a negative balance in ending cash. An example might be adding a medical assistant due to a couple of months of increased patient services but then realizing that the increase was a bubble due to seasonal issues such as allergies and that the patient load reverts back to normal on the third month after hiring the new medical assistant.

Another aspect of managing the financial health of the practice is to look at a few common ratios and rates. The first one is an accounts-receivable aging report which was discussed earlier in this chapter from a management perspective but from a financial view, it basically is a tool to estimate the efficiency of the revenue cycle. Since the odds of collections decrease significantly (from a payer or a patient) with the passage of time, this report helps determine if there is an opportunity to improve the billing process since billing errors cause denials, delays in payment, and problems collecting money from a patient when they aren't confident they owe that amount.

Ratio: The number of times something occurs divided by the number of times it could have occurred (including the number of times it did occur) multiplied by 100 with the result being the percentage of times the something being measured actually happened.

A ratio is the number of times something occurs divided by the number of times it could have occurred times 100 (to convert the decimal to a percentage). For a common example, let's say the manager wants to determine the ratio of how much money is collected by the practice for a given month versus how much was billed. The manager would run a report that showed the total charges for a given period and the amount collected as of 90 days later. Let's say the amount billed was $100,000 and the amount collected was $88,000.00. Take the number of times (amount in this case) that an activity actually happened divided by how many times (amount) it could have happened for a collection ratio. $88,000.00/$100,000.00 × 100 = 88%. Benchmarking against other similar practices to see if this rate is acceptable is discussed in Chapter 7.

Other formulas useful in a medical practice to provide a marker for when something is abnormally high or low include the average amount billed per patient (total amount billed divided by the total number of patients during that same period, times 100), compared with the amount a given doctor makes per patient (physician salary for the period divided by the number of patients treated during the same period, times 100). For example, if the average amount billed per patient turns out to be $92.00 and the amount it costs a physician to treat an average patient is $75.00, then one can determine the efficiency of a given doctor (as compared to other doctors in the practice). Don't lose sight of the fact, though, that this ratio only looks at individual physician efficiency, not net profits per patient. Similar formulas can be used to determine the average cost of a specific procedure, such as an x-ray or all of the procedures in a department. Just remember to think about what data is necessary to know and why and then make sure that everything that should be included in either the numerator (top number in a fraction or division formula) or the denominator (bottom number in a fraction) is considered.

SUMMARY

The revenue cycle is the lifeblood of a medical practice. A medical office team with exceptional team members and a loyal patient base must have a consistent source of revenue in order to operate. The revenue cycle contains six basic steps and several peripherally related functions. The steps, each of which must be consistently performed efficiently and accurately, include (1) patient registration, check-in, clinical encounter, and checkout; (2) coding and billing; (3) claims generation and transmittal—including claims clearinghouses; (4) processing payments and COB; (5) preparation and transmittal of patient statements; and (6) collections and finalizing payments. The peripheral functions include management of denials, appeals, and refunds in addition to report generation and analysis. Finally, the practice manager is responsible for managing the revenue itself through the budgeting process to meet the expenses of the practice and plan for capital improvements.

CHAPTER REVIEW QUESTIONS

1. Define the steps in the revenue cycle.

_____

_____

_____

2. Identify some of the benefits of effective management of the revenue cycle.

_____

_____

_____

3. What are some of the steps a knowledgeable practice administrator will follow when seeing to a denial of payment and a refund request from a third-party payer?

_____

_____

_____

4. Explain the limited role of a provider in executing an appeal to a third-party payer in response to an invalid denial or refund request from the insurance company (or their representative).

_____

_____

_____

5. Explain what happens when claims are generated and submitted to a claims clearinghouse.

_____

_____

_____

6. Explain the process of coordinating benefits between more than one third-party payer.

_____

_____

_____

7. Discuss the points of writing of a legally sound collections letter to a patient.

_____

_____

_____

8. Differentiate between various types of common financial statements discussed in this chapter and explain the purpose of each.

_____

_____

_____

Workbook for
Chapter 6

Workbook:
Chapter 6 Managing the Revenue Cycle and the Financial Health of the Practice

6.A DRAW A DIAGRAM: DRAW A DIAGRAM SHOWING THE STEPS AND ACTIVITIES IN THE REVENUE CYCLE, IN SEQUENCE

Review the details of the sequence and what functions are in the steps in the revenue cycle from your textbook. Draw a diagram with each step of the revenue cycle contained in a box. Place the boxes in order from Step 1 through Step 6. Document key activities that occur in each step. Use the format provided:

Step 1: (Title)	Step 2: (Title)	Step 3: (Title)
Key Activities:	Key Activities:	Key Activities:
Step 4: (Title)	Step 5: (Title)	Step 6: (Title)
Key Activities:	Key Activities:	Key Activities:

6.B INTERNET SCAVENGER HUNT: CODING AND BILLING RULES

Go to the Web site: https://www.cms.gov/nationalcorrectcodinited/
What is the OCE?
What is the main purpose of the NCCI?
What is a MUE?
What year was NCCI implemented?

6.C: FILL IN A CMS 1500 CLAIM FORM

HEALTH INSURANCE CLAIM FORM

APPROVED BY NATIONAL UNIFORM CLAIM COMMITTEE (NUCC) 02/12

| | PICA | | | | | | | | | | PICA | |

1. MEDICARE ☐ (Medicare#)   MEDICAID ☐ (Medicaid#)   TRICARE ☐ (ID#/DoD#)   CHAMPVA ☐ (Member ID#)   GROUP HEALTH PLAN ☐ (ID#)   FECA BLK LUNG ☐ (ID#)   OTHER ☐ (ID#)   **1a. INSURED'S I.D. NUMBER** (For Program in Item 1)

2. PATIENT'S NAME (Last Name, First Name, Middle Initial)

3. PATIENT'S BIRTH DATE MM ┊ DD ┊ YY   **SEX** M ☐ F ☐

4. INSURED'S NAME (Last Name, First Name, Middle Initial)

5. PATIENT'S ADDRESS (No., Street)

6. PATIENT RELATIONSHIP TO INSURED   Self ☐ Spouse ☐ Child ☐ Other ☐

7. INSURED'S ADDRESS (No., Street)

CITY   STATE

8. RESERVED FOR NUCC USE

CITY   STATE

ZIP CODE   TELEPHONE (Include Area Code) ( )

ZIP CODE   TELEPHONE (Include Area Code) ( )

9. OTHER INSURED'S NAME (Last Name, First Name, Middle Initial)

10. IS PATIENT'S CONDITION RELATED TO:

11. INSURED'S POLICY GROUP OR FECA NUMBER

a. OTHER INSURED'S POLICY OR GROUP NUMBER

a. EMPLOYMENT? (Current or Previous)   YES ☐ NO ☐

a. INSURED'S DATE OF BIRTH MM ┊ DD ┊ YY   **SEX** M ☐ F ☐

b. RESERVED FOR NUCC USE

b. AUTO ACCIDENT?   YES ☐ NO ☐   PLACE (State)

b. OTHER CLAIM ID (Designated by NUCC)

c. RESERVED FOR NUCC USE

c. OTHER ACCIDENT?   YES ☐ NO ☐

c. INSURANCE PLAN NAME OR PROGRAM NAME

d. INSURANCE PLAN NAME OR PROGRAM NAME

10d. CLAIM CODES (Designated by NUCC)

d. IS THERE ANOTHER HEALTH BENEFIT PLAN?   YES ☐ NO ☐   If yes, complete items 9, 9a, and 9d.

READ BACK OF FORM BEFORE COMPLETING & SIGNING THIS FORM.
12. PATIENT'S OR AUTHORIZED PERSON'S SIGNATURE I authorize the release of any medical or other information necessary to process this claim. I also request payment of government benefits either to myself or to the party who accepts assignment below.

SIGNED _____   DATE _____

13. INSURED'S OR AUTHORIZED PERSON'S SIGNATURE I authorize payment of medical benefits to the undersigned physician or supplier for services described below.

SIGNED _____

14. DATE OF CURRENT ILLNESS, INJURY, or PREGNANCY (LMP) MM ┊ DD ┊ YY   QUAL.

15. OTHER DATE QUAL.   MM ┊ DD ┊ YY

16. DATES PATIENT UNABLE TO WORK IN CURRENT OCCUPATION FROM MM ┊ DD ┊ YY   TO MM ┊ DD ┊ YY

17. NAME OF REFERRING PROVIDER OR OTHER SOURCE   17a.   17b. NPI

18. HOSPITALIZATION DATES RELATED TO CURRENT SERVICES FROM MM ┊ DD ┊ YY   TO MM ┊ DD ┊ YY

19. ADDITIONAL CLAIM INFORMATION (Designated by NUCC)

20. OUTSIDE LAB?   YES ☐ NO ☐ $ CHARGES

21. DIAGNOSIS OR NATURE OF ILLNESS OR INJURY Relate A-L to service line below (24E)   ICD Ind.

A. _____ B. _____ C. _____ D. _____
E. _____ F. _____ G. _____ H. _____
I. _____ J. _____ K. _____ L. _____

22. RESUBMISSION CODE   ORIGINAL REF. NO.

23. PRIOR AUTHORIZATION NUMBER

24. A. DATE(S) OF SERVICE						B. PLACE OF SERVICE	C. EMG	D. PROCEDURES, SERVICES, OR SUPPLIES (Explain Unusual Circumstances) CPT/HCPCS ┊ MODIFIER	E. DIAGNOSIS POINTER	F. $ CHARGES	G. DAYS OR UNITS	H. EPSDT Family Plan	I. ID. QUAL.	J. RENDERING PROVIDER ID. #
From MM	DD	YY	To MM	DD	YY									
1													NPI	
2													NPI	
3													NPI	
4													NPI	
5													NPI	
6													NPI	

25. FEDERAL TAX I.D. NUMBER   SSN ☐ EIN ☐

26. PATIENT'S ACCOUNT NO.

27. ACCEPT ASSIGNMENT? (For govt. claims, see back)   YES ☐ NO ☐

28. TOTAL CHARGE $

29. AMOUNT PAID $

30. Rsvd for NUCC Use

31. SIGNATURE OF PHYSICIAN OR SUPPLIER INCLUDING DEGREES OR CREDENTIALS (I certify that the statements on the reverse apply to this bill and are made a part thereof.)

SIGNED _____   DATE _____

32. SERVICE FACILITY LOCATION INFORMATION
a.   b.

33. BILLING PROVIDER INFO & PH # ( )
a.   b.

NUCC Instruction Manual available at: www.nucc.org   **PLEASE PRINT OR TYPE**   APPROVED OMB-0938-1197 FORM 1500 (02-12)

CARRIER

PATIENT AND INSURED INFORMATION

PHYSICIAN OR SUPPLIER INFORMATION

Complete the above CMS form manually. You can make up all the information except the following: Patient was in a car accident on 0110XX near a walk-in clinic. Since she was not hurt badly, after the report was filed, she drove to the clinic and was seen on the same date. The doctor coded the following on the superbill (for place of service, go to the Web site indicated in your text for a complete table):

ICD-10 codes: s91.001A (open wound of ankle), V43.92 (auto accident without collision, injuring driver of car); I10 (hypertension).

CPT/HCPCS: 9920125 for a blood pressure check and problem focused history and physical related to the hypertension but not the motor vehicle accident; 14301 to repair wound of lower leg using adjacent tissue transfer.

6.D ACTIVITY: ANALYZE A REMITTANCE ADVICE

Look at the excerpt from the above remittance advice (RA). Search the CMS website for remittance advice and see the remark codes listed at www.wpc-edi.com/reference/codelists/healthcare/remittance-advice-remark-codes. Then answer the following questions:

What is the denial code and description for Jack Rap's procedure code 94760 on the RA above?

What is the procedure code for Benny Fischer's two services dates on the above RA?

What is the total amount charged for I.M. Hurt's two services from January 17th?

What is the total amount paid on the services for Jack Rap?

How much was applied to deductibles for Benny Fischer?

How much total coinsurance will you bill to the patients for all services on the above RA, assuming you accepted assignment for these services?

6.E: YOUR TURN: WRITE A COLLECTIONS LETTER

Using the collections letter in the text as a guide, draft a letter that will be sent to the patient 60 days after the initial statement was sent.

7

Managing Quality and Performance Improvement

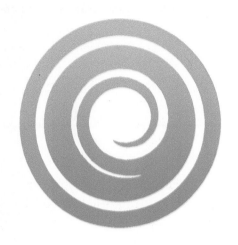

LEARNING OUTCOMES

Upon completion of this chapter, the student should...

- Explain what total quality management (TQM)/continuous quality improvement means from the perspective of a medical practice
- Document medical practice examples of each of the six aims of quality health care put forth by the Institute of Medicine
- Describe reengineering and work simplification in a medical practice
- Explain how benchmarking works
- Describe the tools commonly used in performance improvement and create a plan–do–check–act (PDCA) model for a given practice management scenario
- Explain how utilization management fits under TQM projects
- Explain how risk management fits under TQM projects
- Describe the practice manager's role in physician credentialing by a hospital or other medical facility including how the facility uses the National Practitioner Data Bank (NPDB)

KEY TERMS

Benchmarking
Brainstorming
Continuous Quality Improvement (CQI)
CPT Category II Codes
Decision Matrix
National Practitioner Data Bank (NPDB)
Pay-for-Performance (P4P) Medical Care

Physician Quality Reporting Initiative (PQRI)
Plan–Do–Check (or study)–Act (PDCA/PDSA) Cycle
Potentially Compensable Event (PCE)
Reengineering
Tax Relief and Health Care Act (TRHCA)
Total Quality Management (TQM)
Work Simplification

◎ OVERVIEW

Practice-wide immersion in quality is arguably the single most critical element of building a loyal patient base. Although quality is a broad and somewhat subjective term, there are some aspects of total quality management (TQM) that are critical for a manager to know and to implement in order to continuously monitor, assess, and improve practice performance in terms of safety, patient care, and nonclinical services. The physicians and the practice manager instill awareness, by every single member of the team, of what constitutes quality in his or her own tasks, in addition to how each function impacts and is impacted by all other functions. Therefore, as has been pointed out in numerous articles and books, quality outcomes require a foundation of strong leadership communications and teamwork.

Our patients have choices and are therefore customers or consumers just like any other business. As an added challenge, visiting a physician for treatment is an entirely different experience than visiting a resort. So, while leaders in both businesses need to be concerned about patient loyalty, the patient often has a completely different mindset about consuming health care services than about consuming hospitality services.

In medical practice, a TQM approach includes consideration of all aspects of quality as well as risk management, utilization management (UM), and provider credentialing.

This chapter explores methods of defining, measuring, assessing, and improving quality as well as methods and tools that contribute to the overall effectiveness of achieving continuous performance improvement and increased staff and patient loyalty to the practice—regardless of the size of the practice.

◎ TOTAL QUALITY MANAGEMENT AND PERFORMANCE IMPROVEMENT

Total quality management (TQM) and continuous quality improvement (CQI) are sometimes used interchangeably with CQI seeming to be more frequently used in health care. Regardless of which term is preferable, TQM/CQI is a "structured organizational process for involving personnel in planning and executing a continuous flow of improvements to provide quality care that meets or exceeds expectations…. CQI is simultaneously two things: a management philosophy and a management method."[1]

From a macro perspective, quality in health care is currently assessed based on the Institute of Medicine's contention that all health care stakeholders (from the individual patient through anyone who purchases coverage for health care services to health care providers) should pursue the following six aims—"healthcare should be:

1. Safe
2. Effective
3. Patient-centered
4. Timely
5. Efficient
6. Equitable"[2]

Total Quality Management (TQM): An integrative philosophy of management for continuously improving the quality of products and processes that contends that the quality of products and processes is the responsibility of everyone who is involved with the creation or consumption of the products or services offered by an organization.

Continuous Quality Improvement (CQI): A formal method of quality improvement that continuously assesses all aspects of performance and seeks to improve any process, in order of highest impact to lowest impact, so that the practice is continuously improving individual and overall outcomes.

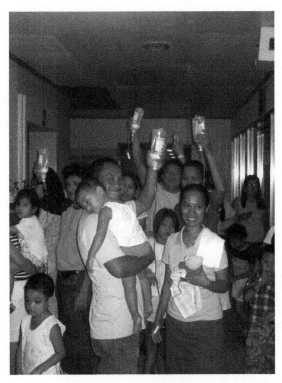

Figure 7.1 Diverse group of people in a waiting room.

Most of these terms are self-explanatory; however, equitable, in this case, refers to a broader than literal perspective. By equitable, it means safe, quality medical care should be accessible to all regardless of geographic location, degree of wealth or poverty, race, color, gender, religion, or any other socioeconomic factor (Fig.7.1).

From the micro perspective of improving health care in medical practices, a practice manager must be familiar with the above aims and then be able to focus on how to facilitate the achievement of these goals. Notice that these goals do not all pertain exclusively to the clinical aspects of a practice. For example, the patient-centered health care model in medical practice is dependent on every aspect of the patient's experience from the first phone encounter—perhaps with a receptionist—through every single time that the patient relies on any member of the team for any service, including requests to obtain copies of medical records, referrals, patient education, and the entire revenue cycle. The loyal patient perceives the medical practice as a miniature health care delivery system comprised of a team of motivated, competent, happy, helpful, compassionate, efficient professionals, regardless of whether they are asking a question about insurance or having surgery.

PERFORMANCE ASSESSMENT AND IMPROVEMENT METHODS AND TOOLS

There are many tools and methods for achieving performance improvement. A few of the most commonly used of these tools and methods are described below.

Reengineering and Work Simplification

Reengineering: The analysis and design of workflows and processes within an organization to help rethink or redesign for efficiency.

As mentioned in Chapter 2, reengineering falls under the organizing function of management and is also a performance improvement philosophy. Reengineering is a strategy in which every process of an entity, a medical practice in this case, is analyzed from the perspective of a new beginning with the goal of drastically improving the performance of the practice as a whole. It always produces change and since some people resist change, a successful project requires the practice manager not only to embrace change but to facilitate it. It is crucial to have the support and participation of the physicians (or at least one or two key physicians) and to inspire the team to be creative and to think critically. In a reengineering project, each step of the medical practice workflow is examined carefully to determine if that process is necessary, and if so, is there a more efficient way to accomplish it. Increasing the efficiency of a process or group of processes might include using different technology or doing certain tasks in a different sequence or cross-training. All policies, procedures, and forms should be assessed in this thorough performance improvement process. Step by step and as a whole, a successful re engineering project will result in positive changes that improve quality, increase efficiency, and decrease any risks such as being fined for incorrect billing practices or being sued for malpractice.

If a practice is going to change from paper medical records to electronic health records, reengineering is a very important step because without critically analyzing steps in the paper medical record workflow, a practice may wind up with an automated version of inefficient processes and therefore not realize the full benefits of an electronic health record system.

Work Simplification: A scientific study of work processes with a view to making that process more efficient and effective by making them more simple and thereby raising productivity and reducing labor, materials, space, time, and energy in the process of producing goods or delivering a services.

Work simplification is a component of reengineering when the entire workflow is being analyzed but is also useful on its own when a comprehensive restructuring is not necessary. Work simplification is organizing work to eliminate waste. To help remember the steps in work simplification, think of the acronym SCRAP:

- Simplify
- Combine tasks to avoid duplication
- Reduce distances people have to move to get their jobs done
- Arrange work to flow smoothly
- Promote participation

Anytime there is a bottleneck or an increase in overtime, or a drop in morale or an increase in expenses, employ the work simplification process to solve the problem or improve a process.

Benchmarking

Benchmarking: Comparing a practice's performance or work processes against either a national standard representing best practices or an otherwise similar practice that is known to have better performance outcomes especially with regard to quality, timeliness, and cost.

Simply stated, benchmarking in a medical practice is the comparing of outcomes. Comparisons can be made with another similar (size, specialty, and geographic location) practice or with aggregate data representing regional or national averages from similar practices. Since the intent of benchmarking is to improve outcomes, the comparison practice or aggregate data must be at a higher performance level than the practice seeking improvement.

Benchmarking can be done for clinical or nonclinical outcomes. An example of a clinical outcome for an orthopedic practice might be postsurgical complication rates after total hip replacement surgery. An example of a nonclinical process to benchmark is the percentage of charges written off as bad debt.

To benchmark an outcome, select the outcome that needs to be improved; identify the similar practice that is performing better; collect, analyze, and interpret the data that has been collected; and use the findings to improve the practice's performance in whatever process is analyzed. A sample data collection form for benchmarking practice costs is shown in Figure 7.2. Once the data is collected, there are free tools available online that will compare the data from the practice being analyzed against other similar practices based on a national norm. The results are based on a percentage. If the practice is in the 50% range, it means that the practice is performing on an average basis. Below 50% is a strong indicator of a need to improve and above 50% means that while there is always room to improve, the practice is performing relatively well in the area analyzed.

The following tools, brainstorming, decision matrixes, and a plan–do–check–act cycle can be used to improve performance based on benchmarking data. These tools help identify a possible solution to a performance issue or an idea for improving performance in any area of the medical practice.

Brainstorming, Decision Matrixes, and the Plan–Do–Check–Act (PDCA) Cycle

One of the most common performance improvement methods that is also relatively easy to use is a plan–do–check (or study)–act (PDCA/PDSA) cycle. This method was originally introduced in the 1920s by Walter A. Shewhart. The cycle was subsequently modernized and made popular by William E. Deming. Before this model can be implemented

Plan–Do–Check–Act (PDCA) Cycle: A recurring four-step management process typically used in business; a successive cycle that starts off small to test potential effects on processes, but then gradually leads to larger and more targeted change.

Data Collection Form for Benchmarking Practice Costs by Physician Practice Name: Number of Physicians:	
1. Total Account Receivables (A/R) per Physician	$
2. Total Medical Revenue per Physician	$
3. Total Support Staff (cost) per Physician	$
4. Total General Operation Cost per Physician	$
5. Total Operation Cost per Physician (Sum of 3+4)	$
6. Total Revenue After Operation Cost per Physician	$

Figure 7.2 Benchmarking data collection form.

> ## Box 7.1
>
> ### Getting the Team Involved in PDCA
>
> The savvy leader knows that once a process has been identified through benchmarking as a target for performance improvement, the next critical step is to get the team involved. Announce the results of the benchmark to everyone on the practice team. Celebrate the fact that the practice is above the comparable practice(s) in all patient safety and clinical areas. Then, explain the area in which the benchmark indicates need for improvement. Identify the key people who have any direct or indirect impact on the process to be improved. Initiate a brainstorming session with these team members to determine any potential causes for a high patient call back rate and ideas for improvement.

Brainstorming: A technique involving a group of people who generate creative ideas in a spontaneous manner in an attempt to solve a problem or make a decision.

to help improve a specific process, the problem area needs to be identified. For example, if a practice benchmarks key indicators and determines it is performing better than comparable practices in patient safety and other clinical outcomes but it has an *average of 10% higher patient calls regarding test results*, then the PDCA method can be used to reduce patient calls and improve patient loyalty.

Brainstorming is the process of using a group of people to generate fresh ideas. The first step is to select a facilitator—often the manager (Fig. 7.3). The facilitator first describes the current flow of work for the identified process and explains why it has been selected as a target for performance improvement. In the example described above under the PDCA method, the practice would use these tools to determine how to reduce patient calls regarding status of test results. To brainstorm solutions to the specific identified patient call volume, the facilitator would describe the current flow of ordering tests and reporting results to the patient. The facilitator has either a flip chart or a dry erase board on which to record the ideas generated. Then, the facilitator explains to the team that this is a nonjudgmental process. The facilitator further describes the objective—reducing patient calls for test results in this example. The facilitator then asks each person to spontaneously, without evaluating the idea first, say aloud any idea that comes to mind that may help improve the process. The facilitator jots down whatever is said encouraging each person to take a turn. The facilitator continually nods to each person around the table until nobody has any additional

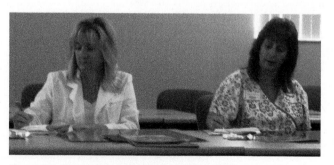

Figure 7.3 Group brainstorming with facilitator taking notes.

suggestions. At that point, the manager asks the team to help group the ideas into categories based on similarities. In this case, there may be a category that contains technology such as adding a module on computerized physician order entry to the existing electronic health record system or purchasing an e-referral Internet service. Another category might be related to communicating time frames to the patient. Yet another might be ideas for making the workflow more efficient. See Figure 7.4 for an example of the results from a brainstorming session about test results.

Once the ideas have been categorized and any synonyms removed, a decision matrix will help identify the exact solution that will be implemented using the PDCA/PDSA cycle. A decision matrix is a table

Decision Matrix: A graphic tool used to evaluate and prioritize a list of options using weighted criteria determined by the team. For example, a decision matrix can be used to choose an electronic health record vendor or to solve a problem.

Ideas in the order generated	Categories of Ideas
1. Buy the new module available in the EHR that can do computer physician order entry 2. Appoint one person to call patients with test results once doctor authorizes each result 3. Purchase an e-referral service 4. Let patients know it will be up to a week before the office calls so they don't keep calling the office 5. Pick one time per day to call patients with that day's processed results and let the patient know at the time they have the test done that they will be called between X and Y time not later than the 5th business day after the test. 6. Have the doctors look at results daily between X and Y times and authorize the nurse to call the patients within an hour thereafter. 7. Ask patients to wait 5 business days and then call in between 3-5 in the afternoon to receive results 8. Tell the patients that if they don't hear from the office in a week, the results were good. 9. Hire a part-time person to come in every day and call patients with all results approved by a doctor 10. Change the workflow so there is a set time or range of time every day to process results and call patients 11. Have doctor email results to patient if negative or a note to call the receptionist to schedule an appointment regarding results if results are positive for a disease 12. Whenever a patient calls in, instead of taking a message, just stop everything and get the results if available 13. Ask the doctors to review results 1-2 a day every day and then route the chart to the nurse immediately – the nurse will then call the patient immediately	Ideas are grouped into categories the group agrees upon. For example: Category – Technology (#1, #3 & #11) Category – Communications (#4, #5, #7, #8) Category – Workflow (#2, #6, #10, #12 and #13) Category – Staffing (#9) Because there is more than one proposed solution for the first 3 categories, the group can decide together which idea within each category is favored. Assuming the group decided that if they are going with technology, purchasing a license for a web-based e-referral system is best; if communications, then number 5 is preferred; and of workflow options number 6 is preferred. Then, chose the weight of each element that will go into making the final decision such as cost, patient relations, ease of implementing change and staff efficiency. Determine a weight for each of these as indicated in the next illustration. Assign each solution a rating 1-5 and then multiply the rate by weight for each category. Total the points for each proposed solution and the highest point solution will be chosen to implement.

Figure 7.4 Results from a brainstorming session on processing test results.

in which the criterion is listed in rows and the potential solutions are listed in columns. A decision matrix can be used for selecting a candidate for a job, selecting the best vendor when purchasing a new system or equipment, or deciding the best solution for a problem. See Figure 7.5 for a sample decision matrix based on the test results scenario given. The team decides a value (usually on a scale of one to five with five being the most important) for each of the criteria identified as factors to consider before making a decision. Then, the team evaluates each solution and ranks that solution on a scale of one to five for each of the individual criteria listed. Finally, the value is multiplied by the rating for each of the solutions, for each of the criteria and the columns are totaled with the highest total being the solution chosen to implement a PDCA cycle.

To use the PDCA method, a circular rather than linear process, the team does the following:

- Plan. The planning step includes documenting any relevant history and the current process or workflow. Then, the plan outlines the proposed process, anticipated results, and any additional assumptions pertaining to the process.

- Do. This is the step in which the plan is implemented as a test, on a small scale, to determine if the actual implementation of the plan is going to work.

- Check or study is the step in which the results of experimental implementation are analyzed to determine if the actual results match those in the plan.

- Act is the final step in which, if the test produces the desired results, the new process is implemented fully as a new process. If, however, the results were not as successful as planned, the team must go back to

Category	Wt.*	E-refer Rate**	E-refer Value***	Communications Change-Rate	Communications Value	Wrkflw Rate	Wrkflw Value	Inc Staff Rate	Inc Staff Value
Cost to implement	5	1	5	5	25	5	25	2	10
Ease of implementation	4	4	16	4	16	5	20	2	8
Impact on Patient Satisfaction	5	5	25	5	25	3	15	3	15
Impact on efficiency	4	5	20	4	16	3	12		16
TOTAL			66		82		72		49

*On a scale from 1-5, the weight is the amount of importance the team places on that category in comparing from a list of options with 5 being the most important (e.g. 5 is lowest cost)

** Rate is how well the solution meets the criterion in each category

*** Wt times rate in each category is value of that solution for each category with the column being totaled at the bottom – choose the solution with the highest total value. The change in communications is the best solution – rated highest because it actually combines improved, more efficient workflow with the improvement in communications with the patient.

Figure 7.5 Sample decision matrix.

Case Study

PERFORMANCE IMPROVEMENT TO REDUCE PATIENT PHONE CALLS FOR RESULTS OF TESTS

Part I: Nancie is the practice manager. This is her first attempt at using the performance improvement tools discussed in this chapter. She did an excellent job on the benchmark portion which correctly identified that the practice was performing well in most areas but below average in the volume of calls received by patients requesting test results.

Nancie called the staff together to brainstorm potential solutions to this performance issue. She had the right idea but she also had already made up her mind what she thought would work so, when the team started to take turns calling out ideas, she debated with them and then wrote down a modified version of the idea. When someone said something she thought was really good, she stopped the brainstorming session to discuss the suggestion in more detail. It didn't take long for some of the staff to decide that she was going to do what she wanted to do anyway so a couple of people encouraged her to describe what she believed the solution to be even though there were only a few ideas on the board and most of those were related to Nancie's idea. She pointed to her modified notes on the dry erase board and explained that the next step, if everyone was out of ideas, was to apply the suggestions to a decision matrix.

What should Nancie have done to make this process more effective? She may have truly had the best idea from the start but without a spontaneous, nonjudgmental team session, she may have missed out on an even better suggestion or an improvement upon her idea. So, she needed to follow the process as described earlier in this chapter. Also, the next step is a decision matrix but if you don't have more than one idea, it defeats the purpose of evaluating the idea with the best value overall for the practice.

Part II: Assume that the brainstorming session was done properly and that there were several suggestions to consider. The team would then use a decision matrix to determine the best solution. For the purposes of this case study, the solution that was most feasible for this practice was to redo the entire test results reporting workflow and to communicate more effectively with the patients. Nancie then initiates the PDCA cycle.

Plan: Currently, patients call the office within a couple of days after having a test performed (laboratory test, pathology for biopsy, or a diagnostic imaging procedure). A receptionist takes a message because the medical assistant or other clinical team member is usually busy with a patient. Often, the messages are all placed on the appropriate team member's work area at the end of the workday. The next morning, the team member checks for each patient's results. If not yet received from the lab or imaging center, the team member places the message for follow-up the next day but doesn't have time to call the patient. The next day, the patient, quite annoyed at not having heard anything the previous day, calls again. The process of message taking starts over but now, the medical assistant has two messages from the same patient so they wind up checking for results twice. If they have the results but they aren't normal, then the medical record must be pulled, the lab results and patient message clipped to the outside of the folder, and the folder placed in the physician's inbox. This means another day may pass before the patient receives a call. If the results are normal, protocols permit the medical assistant or a nurse to finally call the patient (who is now downright testy) with the good news that the results are normal.

The identified solution, assuming a paper-based medical record and assuming that the practice can't afford to purchase an electronic referral system, is (1) notify each patient that they can expect a call from the practice on or before the fifth business day after the test is done and explain if they call the office before the fifth business day, it will delay the patient notification process but they should call if they haven't heard from the office by the end of the fifth business day; (2) schedule a specific time each day during which a clerical support team member pulls the paper medical record for each test result received, paperclips the lab result to the outside of the folder, and places these documents into a special bin; and (3) a medical assistant or nurse either calls the patient to schedule an appointment with the physician or lets the patient know the results were normal, files the lab result(s) appropriately, and returns the paper record for re-filing.

Do: Implement the planned solution for blood tests only to test the plan.

Check: Check the phone message logs to determine if any of the pilot patients called the office before the office notified them of the results. If so, determine if the call was made prior to the fifth business day?

Act: If this process reduces the number of calls, implement it for all tests.

What would you have done in Nancie's case to take better advantage of the PDCA cycle?

To optimize the use of the PDCA cycle, Nancie should have determined the number of patients who typically call back before the test results are available. She should also have conducted an informal survey of patients who have had tests recently to determine what their expectations were regarding how soon the office would contact them with results and their degree of satisfaction with the process. Then, she should have started the new procedure on approximately half of the patients having blood tests representing both new and established patients but kept the existing procedure in place for the other half of the patients. She should also have documented the expected results in the plan. Then, during the "check" phase, she could distribute the original survey to both groups of patients (the pilot group and the group for which the pilot was not implemented). These additional steps would help determine more precisely how effective the new process is. She should also make sure the team is kept informed of the findings so when they are asked to implement a new procedure full scale, they realize that they helped improve a process that resulted in higher patient loyalty and more control over the process as individuals.

determine if the plan needs to be revised and retested or if there was an error made in implementing the pilot. In either case, the PDCA cycle can be used until both the plan and the small-scale implementation produce the desired outcomes.

ASSESSMENT AND IMPROVEMENT OF CLINICAL PERFORMANCE AND PATIENT SAFETY

Evidenced-based medicine refers to the use of the most current and best research evidence in treating patients. "This research is incorporated into clinical practice guidelines-statements of the right things to do for patients with a particular diagnosis or medical conditions."[3]

THE PHYSICIAN QUALITY REPORTING INITIATIVE AND PAY FOR PERFORMANCE

In 2006, the Tax Relief and Health Care Act (TRHCA) was enacted, authorizing CMS to establish the Physician Quality Reporting Initiative (PQRI). PQRI included a financial incentive program to encourage certain professionals to report, on a voluntary basis, quality measures using CPT Category II codes and modifiers. CMS collects these data as part of a plan to use a pay-for-performance (P4P) strategy that will encourage the provision of high-quality, cost-effective, and safe care to all patients.

In 2007, the first year of implementation, there were 74 unique reporting measures in the areas of preventive care, management of chronic conditions, management of acute conditions, and utilization of resources. Basically, a code from Category II, with modifiers as appropriate, indicates that a requirement was or was not met. If not met, the reason is indicated by unique modifiers that explain, for example, that the protocol was taken into consideration but not followed because of medical, patient-based, or system reasons. The difference is, without this system, there isn't an efficient way to determine if national protocols of safe, quality patient care that are developed from evidence-based medicine are being followed or not. Also, without a defined system in place, if the protocols aren't being followed, nobody knows if it's because of lack of awareness by a physician or because the physician had a legitimate reason why the protocol was not followed in certain instances. Finally, for continuing quality improvement, CMS needs a method to assess the effectiveness of both the protocols and of programs to make physicians aware of new protocols. As with any continuous quality program, the protocols will be modified as new evidence is gathered that leads to improvements. See Figure 7.6 for an example of a Category II code and modifier that indicates that the quality measure of "tobacco use assessed" was considered but excluded from implementation due to the patient refusing to participate[4].

Theoretically, P4P isn't intended to replace existing reimbursement methodology, and initially there were no plans to penalize physicians and other providers who chose not to participate in this reporting process.

Tax Relief and Health Care Act (TRHCA): Provided key changes to health care savings accounts and modified, extended, and added new provisions regarding tax credits for several different groups.

Physician Quality Reporting Initiative (PQRI): A 2006 effort at public reporting of health care quality, this program provides incentive payments to physicians who report quality data; however, to date these results are not publicly available for use by consumers.

CPT Category II Codes: Supplemental tracking codes in the CPT manual that help measure performance compared with national protocols.

Pay-for-Performance (P4P) Medical Care: A compensation system whereby providers are rewarded for meeting preestablished quality and efficiency targets for delivery of health care services; opposite of fee-for-services payment model.

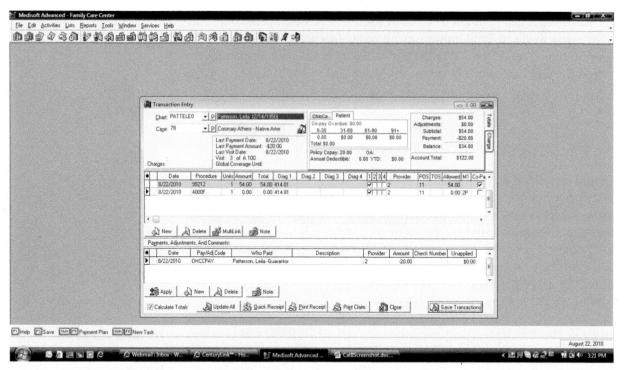

Figure 7.6 Screen print of a CPT category II code added to encounter data. (Screen print from NCG Medical's Perfect Care's Integrated EHR with Practice Management software donated to Lake–Sumter State College for academic use.)

In other words, the philosophy behind P4P is to improve medical care for all by encouraging providers to become more aware of and practice evidence-based medicine with regard to quality and safety protocols and not as a system of reimbursement with penalties.

In the private sector, a program called Bridges to Excellence is an example of one of several P4P projects that give incentives to health care providers who demonstrate they have implemented comprehensive strategies and tools (e.g., information technology) to improve the management of patients and deliver safe, timely, effective, efficient, equitable, and patient-centered care. An example is a per-patient incentive for every diabetic patient who successfully meets the targets of a provider-implemented disease management program.

Two important aspects of all public and private P4P models that are critical for practice managers to understand is that patient satisfaction is measured along with outcomes of clinical treatment, and an electronic health record system with disease registries and solid reporting mechanisms are integral to success

⊗ ASSESSMENT AND IMPROVEMENT OF NONCLINICAL PERFORMANCE

As with the scenario described earlier in this chapter in which the reporting of test results to the patient was improved, nonclinical performance can be improved through benchmarking, analyzing the practice management reports to determine processes for potential improvement, brainstorming, using a decision matrix, and implementing a plan–do–check–act cycle for each targeted process.

Categories include claims aging with various third-party payers, claims denials, requests by third-party payers for a refund, aging patient accounts, percentage of write-offs, collections, patient wait time (on hold for telephone calls or in the physical waiting room), patient no-shows, bottlenecks, etc.

UTILIZATION MANAGEMENT FROM A QUALITY PERSPECTIVE

The goal of a UM plan is to make sure the patient is receiving quality care at the most appropriate level of service. When the physician is conducting hospital rounds, this process is driven by hospital utilization review specialists. In the office, the physician often has to determine initially whether to schedule the patient for an inpatient service or whether that patient's overall status would enable the same procedure to be done as a day-surgery patient at an ambulatory surgery center. On a less obvious scenario, the physician must determine which tests are the most appropriate to diagnose and treat a patient with the minimum amount of expense. Third-party payers maintain that the purpose of UM audits and denials for services the payer does not feel are medically necessary is to ensure that every health care provider considers all aspects of delivering safe, effective health care in the most economical setting. Therefore, they are as concerned with a physician attempting major surgery on a high-risk patient in an outpatient setting as they are with a physician admitting an otherwise healthy 25-year-old to the inpatient setting for minor surgery.

The bottom line is that the more cost-effective our health care delivery system becomes, the more health care we can provide without costs increasing for patients and eliminating wasteful practices means additional money to spend on those services necessary to improve every patient's health status.

RISK MANAGEMENT FROM A QUALITY PERSPECTIVE

Managing risk essentially means eliminating or minimizing any unplanned payout of funds which are referred to as potentially compensable events (PCEs). Examples include fines for incorrect coding and billing procedures, legal fees to defend against a medical malpractice suit, and workers' compensation claims and patient or visitor injury while on the property owned by the practice.

Risk management protocols are driven by the tenets of exceptional quality because if every function (clinical, nonclinical, building and equipment maintenance, etc.) is consistently done well, there will be no errors resulting in the practice being sued or being fined. Obviously, the better a practice is at TQM that includes continuous quality assessment and performance improvement, the more loyal the patients and the higher the morale among the team will be.

An aspect of risk management that falls under the responsibility of any hospitals in which physicians in your practice have privileges is the

Potentially Compensable Event (PCE): An adverse event that occurs in the delivery of health care or services with resulting injury to the patient including any adverse event or outcome, without legal fault, in which the patient experiences any unintended or unexpected negative result.

The Data Bank at a Glance

NPDB	HIPDB
Background	
The National Practitioner Data Bank was established under Title IV of Public Law 99660, the Health Care Quality Improvement Act of 1986, and is expanded by Section 1921, as amended by section 5(b) of the Medicare and Medicaid Patient and Program Protection Act of 1987, and as amended by the Omnibus Budget Reconciliation Act of 1990. NPDB is an information clearinghouse to collect and release all licensure actions taken against all health care practitioners and health care entities, as well as any negative actions or findings taken against health care practitioners or organizations by Peer Review Organizations and Private Accreditation Organizations.	The Healthcare Integrity and Protection Data Bank was established under section 1128E of the Social Security Act as added by Section 221(A) of the Health Insurance Portability and Accountability Act of 1996. HIPDB was implemented to combat fraud and abuse in health insurance and health care delivery and to promote quality care. HIPDB alerts users that a more comprehensive review of past actions by a practitioner, provider or supplier may be prudent.
Who Reports?	
• Medical malpractice payers • State health care practitioner licensing and certification authorities (including medical and dental boards) • Hospitals • Other health care entities with formal peer review (HMOs, group practices, managed care organizations) • Professional societies with formal peer review • State entity licensing and certification authorities • Peer review organizations • Private accreditation organizations	• Federal and State Government agencies • Health plans
What Information is Available?	
• Medical malpractice payments (all health care practitioners) • Any adverse licensure actions (all practitioners or entities) revocation, reprimand, censure, suspension, probation any dismissal or closure of the proceedings by reason of the practitioner or entity surrendering the license or leaving the State or jurisdiction any other loss of license • Adverse clinical privileging actions • Adverse professional society membership actions • Any negative action or finding by a State licensing or certification authority • Peer review organization negative actions or finding against a health care practitioner or entity • Private accreditation organization negative actions or findings against a health care practitioner or entity	• Licensing and certification actions Revocation, suspension, censure, reprimand, probation Any other loss of license - or right to apply for or renew - a license of the provider, supplier, or practitioner, whether by voluntary surrender, non-renewal, or otherwise Any negative action or finding by a Federal or State licensing and certification agency that is publicly available information Civil judgments (health care-related) • Criminal convictions (health care-related) • Exclusions from Federal or State health care programs • Other adjudicated actions or decisions (formal or official actions, availability of due process mechanism and based on acts or omissions that affect or could affect the payment, provision, or delivery of a health care item or service)

Figure 7.7 The data bank at a glance (from http://www.npdb-hipdb.hrsa.gov/topNavigation/aboutUs.jsp).

The Data Bank at a Glance	
NPDB	**HIPDB**
Who Can Query?	
• Hospitals • Other health care entities, with formal peer review • Professional societies with formal peer review • State health care practitioner licensing and certification authorities (including medical and dental boards) • State entity licensing and certification authorities* • Agencies or contractors administering Federal health care programs* • State agencies administering State health care programs* • State Medicaid Fraud Units* • U.S. Comptroller General* • U.S. Attorney General and other law enforcement* • Health care practitioners (self query) • Plaintiff's attorney/pro se plaintiffs (under limited circumstances)** • Quality Improvement Organizations* • Researchers (statistical data only) * eligible to receive only those reports authorized by Section 1921. **eligible to receive only those reports authorized by HCQIA.	• Federal and State Government agencies • Health plans • Health care practitioners/providers/suppliers (self-query) • Researchers (statistical data only)
Who Cannot Query?	
The Data Bank is prohibited by law from disclosing information on a specific practitioner, provider, or supplier to a member of the general public. However, persons or organizations can request information in a form that does not identify any particular organization or practitioner.	

Figure 7.7 *(continued)*

provider credentialing process. Although managers are not directly involved in this process, they are often called upon by physicians to complete the application for appointment or reappointment paperwork at hospitals where the physicians in the practice have privileges. The file generally contains, at a minimum, the application itself; copies of all relevant licenses, diplomas, board certifications, permits (e.g., permit to prescribe controlled substances), certificate of liability insurance, and a current printout of the National Practitioner Data Bank (NPDB) query results; and a set of references from faculty or medical executives. The NPDB was created by the Health Care Quality Improvement Act (HCQIA) of 1986 and is a database containing information on every practitioner regarding any adverse quality of care information available about each practitioner. Figure 7.7 shows an overview of the NPDB as well as the more recently established (through HIPAA) Healthcare Integrity and Protection Data Bank (HIPDB).

The credentialing file also contains a listing of which privileges the hospital has authorized. This process is conducted by the hospital because the hospital can be sued if a physician makes a mistake, so part

National Practitioner Data Bank (NPDB): A computerized database of all payments made on behalf of physicians in connection with medical liability settlements or judgments as well as adverse peer-review actions against licenses, clinical privileges, and professional society memberships of physicians and other health care practitioners.

of their risk management responsibilities include verifying that each physician is current in any continuing medical education requirements and that the provider's license has not been suspended or called under questioning by authorities.

SUMMARY

A practice manager plays a large role in the overall performance of all functions in a medical office. TQM or CQI in medical practice is a strategy that pertains to both clinical and nonclinical functions in a medical office in an attempt to consistently deliver safe, effective, patient-centered, timely, efficient, and equitable health care. Efficient health care delivery requires management of the utilization of health care services as well as the efficient operations of all nonclinical functions in a medical office. An efficient practice is one in which there are no wasted steps that take away from each person's primary role in the practice, including getting reimbursed for the care that is delivered. Safe and equitable health care requires effective management of risk. Any PCE, either clinical in nature or nonclinical, is ideally either eliminated or minimized by an effective TQM philosophy that is well communicated throughout the practice. An area of risk management that practice managers often assist physicians with completing is the physician credentialing process.

There are methods and tools that a practice manager can use to facilitate CQI. Some of the more common of these methods include benchmarking, reengineering, work simplification, brainstorming, using a decision matrix, and implementing a PDCA cycle.

Creating an environment in which everyone is tuned into the goals of knowing the right things to do and then doing them right results in a high morale team and a very loyal patient base.

CHAPTER REVIEW QUESTIONS

1. Define what is meant by CQI. What is another name for this process?

_____

_____

_____

2. List the six aims put forth by the Institute of Medicine that pertain to any health care stakeholder. What is meant by the aim of "equitable" health care?

_____

_____

_____

3. Describe the concept of reengineering as a performance improvement method.

_____

_____

_____

4. What are the elements that comprise work simplification?

_____

_____

_____

5. Give an example each of a clinical function and a nonclinical function that can be benchmarked to determine if these functions are opportunities for improving performance.

_____

_____

_____

6. List what is included in the plan step of a PDCA cycle.

_____

_____

_____

7. At which step in the PDCA cycle would a manager have to revisit the plan to determine if it needs revision? If that determination is made, what happens next?

_____

_____

_____

8. What tool can be used after the results of a brainstorming session in order to evaluate and select the best solution to a problem?

_____

_____

_____

REFERENCES

1. McLaughlin, CP, Kaluzny K. Continuous Quality Improvement in Health Care: Theory, Implementations and Applications. 3rd ed. Sudbury, MA: Jones and Bartlett; 2006.
2. Institute of Medicine, Committee on Quality of Health Care in America. Crossing the Quality Chasm: A New Health System for the 21st Century. Washington, DC: National Academy Press; 2001.
3. Abdelhak M, Grostick S, Hanken, MA et al. Health Information: Management of a Strategic Resource. 3rd ed. St. Louis, MO: Saunders/Elsevier; 2007.
4. Falen TJ, Noblin A, Ziesemer B. Learning to Code with CPT/HCPCS. Baltimore, MD: Lippincott Williams & Wilkins; 2010.

Workbook for
Chapter 7

Workbook:
Chapter 7 Managing Quality and Performance Improvement

7.A: TEAM PROJECT: DEVELOP A PATIENT SURVEY TO IDENTIFY POTENTIAL AREAS OF IMPROVEMENT

Assume you are an experienced practice manager who accepted a position with a midsized family practice. The physicians are all highly respected. You realize shortly that the patients that are coming to the practice are putting up with inefficiency and poor customer service just because they have a lot of faith in the physicians themselves. As an experienced administrator, you understand that if the practice could develop a team approach to turning the practice into one that is fully patient centered, the practice would grow by word of mouth and revenue would stabilize as patients started to realize the value they were getting for their money. You've spent the first 3 months working on morale because nobody seemed to like working there when you started and they seemed to be a talented but self-absorbed group of individuals. Your efforts at team building have paid off quickly and now absenteeism has dropped to an all-time low, all employees are working together. Morale is up. Now it's time to figure out what the existing patients consider important because, although there has been some improvement, you know that patients are not showing signs of becoming loyal patients. You call the team together and assign sub-teams to work on developing survey questions that address all aspects of a customer's experience with the practice.

For this assignment, each student is on a team. Each team has a different area assigned to them. Each team must develop at two to three questions and a rating scale that will help the practice as a whole figure out how to become more patient centric in all of the areas listed below.

The areas are as follows:

1. *Time from requesting a nonemergency appointment to actually getting that appointment*

2. *Waiting time between scheduled appointment time and time actually seen*

3. *Amount of times and information that the patient must either answer questions or complete forms*

4. *Test results issues*

5. *Customer Service*

6. *Financial policy (what is collected upfront, billing issues, patient statements)*

7. *Referrals to specialists*

7.B WORKSHEET: IDENTIFY TRENDS AND SUGGESTIONS FROM PATIENT SURVEY RESULTS

Each student will complete the survey from the first assignment (7.A) and then identify any trends. Then, each student will write one recommendation for each area and list the order in which the recommendations should be addressed.

7.C: VIDEO ACTIVITY (HOW NOT TO PROBLEM-SOLVE THROUGH BRAINSTORMING)

 (See video clip on thePoint Web site to complete this activity.)

1. The video clip is based on the following case scenario (Part I Only) presented in the chapter:

    Part I: *Nancie is the practice manager. This is her first attempt at using the performance improvement tools discussed in this chapter. She did an excellent job on the benchmark portion which correctly identified that the practice was performing well in most areas but below average in the volume of calls received by patients requesting test results.*

    Nancie called the entire staff together to brainstorm potential solutions to this performance issue. She had the right idea but she also had already made up her mind what she thought would work so, when the team started to take turns calling out ideas, she debated with them and then wrote down a modified version of the idea. When someone said something she thought was really good, she stopped the brainstorming session to discuss the suggestion in more detail. It didn't take long for some of the staff to decide that she was going to do what she wanted to do anyway so a couple of people encouraged her to describe what she believed the solution to be. She pointed to her modified notes on the dry erase board and explained that the next step, if everyone was out of ideas, was to apply the suggestions to a decision matrix.

    _____

    _____

    _____

2. View the video clip. (SCRIPT HERE)

    _____

    _____

    _____

3. Identify any mistakes you think were made by Nancie.

_____

_____

_____

4. Jot down ideas for how Nancie could have handled this situation more effectively at the same time as she used the principles of "controlling" to resolve the issue while maintaining high team morale.

_____

_____

_____

5. Now, using the same scenario, write how you would have handled that situation had you been Nancie. Include any dialogue from the team meeting. Be prepared to either submit your findings and solution or to role-play your solution with a classmate.

_____

_____

_____

7.D: EXPERT PANEL

Read the following real-life scenario. Your instructor may have you break into teams or respond as an individual expert. Each team or individual needs to create a dialogue depicting how a real-world conversation may go in which the manager, Ellen, addresses the quality issues in the scenario with Sam.

Ellen has recently hired an experienced certified medical assistant, Sam. Sam gets off to a good start with regard to taking vital signs, drawing blood, preparing specimens for lab analysis, and bringing the patients to the examining rooms.

Toward the end of the probationary period, Sam started to make some mistakes. He mixed up the x-ray results from two patients with severe shoulder pain—one had arthritis and the other a torn rotator cuff; he allowed several lab specimens to get contaminated causing the patients to have to return to the office so another specimen could be obtained; and he tried to make the patients think they had caused the problems.

7.E TEAM PROJECT: USE THE PLAN–DO–CHECK–ACT METHOD TO IMPROVE A DEFINED PROCESS

Take one of the solutions proposed in 7.B and implement that solution using the PDCA method. Document the plan, show what was tested, analyze the test results, and recommend whether or not to implement the solution into daily operations.

8

Customer Service, Patient Loyalty, and Marketing

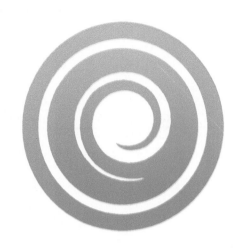

✥ OVERVIEW

Imagine how it would feel, as an established patient, to look forward to an appointment with your doctor even if you know there is a chance that you'll be seen by one of the other physicians in the practice. What would make you feel that way? Different people may have varying responses to that question, but there are core factors that most people would agree contribute to a feeling of loyalty to both a physician and to the physician's medical practice. These factors include, but are not limited to confidence

- That every single person in the practice is highly competent
- That all employees communicate effectively
- That the wait will be short and pleasant
- That your health information will be kept confidential and secure
- That you will be treated with respect and dignity over the phone, in person, and in written correspondence
- That each person in the practice values you as a person
- That any referrals for tests or specialists will be followed up by your physician to ensure the best possible continuity of care

Behind the scenes, a practice that delivers the consistently exceptional patient services described above has a management philosophy of taking care of each team member as though the employees are customers because people must be valued and feel secure before they can sincerely value others. Patient-centric culture, once achieved, perpetuates itself because the high morale of the team combined with loyal patients creates a unique work experience that generates greater enthusiasm and energy.

Progress toward achieving patient loyalty should be periodically measured and the results used for continuous improvement. Once a practice is well on its way to building a loyal patient base, effective marketing will assist the natural growth that occurs with an outstanding reputation.

✥ FIRST IMPRESSIONS—TELEPHONE ETIQUETTE, PROCEDURES, AND OPTIONS

If a manager were to have a staff meeting to brainstorm ideas for improving patient loyalty in the category of telephone services, a good place to start would be to have everyone suggest various things they personally like and don't like about the telephone aspects of dealing with their own physicians and physician office staff.

Typically, the most common issues involve

- Rudeness
- Being placed on hold for long periods of time
- Not receiving a return phone call after leaving a message

- Dealing with lengthy or even confusing choices when an automated phone answering service is used
- Being transferred more than once—especially if information has to be repeated after initially telling the first person the same details—or the patient has to leave a message after having been transferred one or more times.

Solutions will vary based on the size of the practice. Regardless of which protocols a practice adopts, every practice must ensure that anyone who may ever have to answer the phone, even infrequently, understands which team members primarily perform or are cross-trained in the key functions of the practice and how the information in an office flows so they can either answer the question directly or transfer the patient to the best available person. Also, everyone in the office needs to be committed to timely return of phone calls when a message is necessary, so that the patients can be told when to expect a return phone call.

Some suggestions to draw from when making a decision about telephone policies, procedures, and equipment for a specific practice include the following:

- A simple automated answering system that first alerts patients that if they are calling about a medical emergency, to please hang-up and dial 911 and proceeds to providing the days and hours of operation. Then, the patient should be given brief, clear options such as if you are calling to schedule, change, or confirm an appointment, please dial 1; if you are calling about health insurance or medical records, please dial 2; if you would like to speak to a nurse or medical assistant about test results or any other question regarding your health, please dial 3, or please stay on the line and someone from our office will be with you as soon as possible.
- Always ensure the phone is answered before it rings a fourth time.
- If a patient must be placed on hold, be sure that every team member knows to ask if it is all right to place the patient on hold and receives a positive response before actually placing the caller on hold.
- All team members should be careful not to eat or drink anything while speaking on the phone.
- All phones should be in an area where the surrounding noise level isn't so loud that it detracts from being able to hear the patient clearly or from the patient being able to hear clearly—a good-quality headset is best for people who answer the phones frequently (Fig. 8.1).
- Anyone speaking to a patient must always remember to listen carefully and with utmost respect and patience—even if the patient seems to be speaking aimlessly.
- Have a well-defined call routing or call transfer procedure based on the type of call. The call routing procedure explains step by step, based on the position of the person answering the phone, when to handle the call, when to transfer it and to whom, and when to take a message. Figure 8.2 provides an example.

> **TIP**
>
> This option requires that someone is almost always available to answer the phone in each applicable department and, for the rare occasion when the phone cannot be answered, the caller should be instructed to leave his or her name, reason for the call, and the best number to reach the caller followed by a message stating the approximate time the call will be returned. For example, the message might be, "If your call is received before 3:00 P.M., it will be returned by 6:00 P.M. the same day. All other calls will be returned the following business day between 8:00 and 10:00 A.M." It is imperative to meet the promised turnaround time for return calls.

Call Routing or Call Transfer Procedure: A procedure that contains a list of every known type of phone call the office might receive and then describes the action the person receiving the call should take for each type.

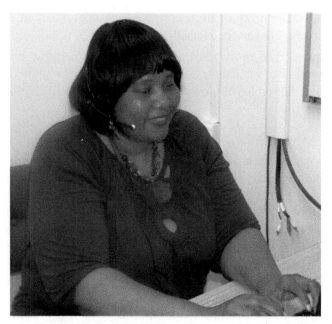

Figure 8.1 Receptionist with headset.

Electronic Prescribing: A form of computerized order entry in which the clinician uses a computer to submit an order for a prescription or refill. The order passes through patient safety edits and, once cleared, is pending in the pharmacy computer to fill the order.

Computerized Physician Order Entry (CPOE): A process in which a clinician inputs orders for patient care into a computer system that is connected to the appropriate recipient such as a pharmacy, a laboratory or an imaging center. The order is filled or the test is conducted and the results of the test are returned electronically to the clinician.

Patient Portals: Health care-related online applications that allow patients to interact and communicate with their health care providers, such as physicians and hospitals.

Personal Health Records (PHRs): A health record where health data is maintained and controlled by individual users themselves and which conforms to recognized interoperability standards enabling data to be shared at the patient's discretion.

Communications Services Company: A company that contracts with a medical office to provide various levels of communications support using technology or actual manpower. For example, a communications company is able to remind patients when an appointment is scheduled for the following business day. The services can be very limited or comprehensive.

In addition to the above strategies for handling phone services, Chapter 10 will introduce and describe technology such as secure email messaging, texting, Web-based interactive patient education capabilities, electronic prescribing or e-prescribing, computerized physician order entry (CPOE), which is an electronic test ordering and results-reporting system, patient portals, personal health records (PHRs), and other technology-based tools that may minimize the sheer number of calls typically received by the practice.

Another strategy to significantly reduce phone calls and increase patient loyalty is to contract with a communications services company that can actually use your physician and team's voices to notify patients, in a manner that is compliant with HIPAA rules, of any messages the practice chooses to broadcast—such as notifying all patients scheduled for an appointment on a certain day that a physician has been called out of state for a personal emergency—or routine messages such as appointment reminders. The vendors generally offer up to three contact numbers and an e-mail option to communicate professionally with your patients. A couple of examples are found at www.DrDial.com and www.notifymd.com.

FACE TO FACE WITH THE PATIENT

When a consumer has choices, what are some of the things that lead that consumer to purchase an expensive item at a particular store, even if that store is farther away than a competitor's business, when there are several choices in the same vicinity that carry the same brand at approximately the same price? If the consumer has never shopped at any of the stores before, chances are, he or she will just pick one and buy the item. The next time they need a similar item, they may pick a different store simply

Reason for Call	Transfer to or Take Message	Notes
Patient with any financial/ billing questions	Transfer to available insurance or billing specialist	If patient is irate, receptionist should say, "I appreciate your frustration, Mr/Mrs X. May I place you on hold so I can locate our manager to speak with you?
Patient with legal questions regarding release of medical records	Transfer to available health information technician if applicable, otherwise to manager	Ok to take a message in this case if someone who knows the legal guidelines for release of information is not available but be sure to tell the patient when he or she can expect a return phone call
Patient with request for copies of medical records	Receptionist (or anyone in practice who answers the call) should be able to respond directly to how the patient can obtain records or have them sent to another provider by completing a release of information form	If the records are needed for continuity of health care, it is sometimes necessary to have the release form faxed to the practice by the other provider and subsequently fax the required parts of the record to the provider following the guidelines in Chapter 9
Patient calling in self-test results such as blood sugar level or blood pressure per clinician's request; requests for prescription refills; questions regarding whether or not test results have been received by the practice	Receptionist should be able to pull the patient medical record, carefully record the information from the patient on a message pad or other note, verify patient contact information in case a clinician needs to call the patient back, attach the note to the record and route the record to the appropriate clinician (may be a physician or a physician extender)	If a physician extender is available, an alternative is to have the receptionist transfer the call directly if the practice determines that is a preferable protocol
Patient with questions about abnormal test results that have been received	If a physician or physician extender is available, the best recourse is to transfer the call so the clinician can let the patient know if they need to come in to discuss the results in person	If a clinician is not available, the receptionist may take a message but assure the patient that a physician or nurse (or PA) will call them back as soon as possible and not later than, e.g. 5:00 p.m. the same day since this situation can be very stressful for the patient
Patient with Scheduling Questions	Whomever answers the phone should be able to deal with these questions directly	All team members should know how to look up and enter scheduling information on the practice management system
Physician or Physician/Hospital representative calling for physician orders or to discuss a current patient with the patient's primary care physician	Unless the appropriate physician is in an examination room with a patient, he or she should be paged to take the call immediately	If the physician is in an exam room, the caller should be asked to either hold until the physician is out of the exam room or, a detailed, urgent message should be taken with assurance to the caller that the physician will call back immediately
Patient Complaints	Should be routed to the practice manager	If manager is not available, all team members should be trained to assure the patient that his or her problem is very important to the practice and that the manager will return the patient's call as soon as possible. The person taking the call should be sure the manager is going to be back in the office later the same day or else ask the patient if the patient would like to speak to someone else or wait until the next day to speak with the manager

Figure 8.2 A sample phone call routing procedure.

because the second store is more convenient to where the customer is on the day of the purchase. However, if that customer has previously shopped at one of the stores that happened to be the farthest away from home and the experience was such that the consumer felt like everyone in the store treated him or her like the most important person in the world at that point in time, and like there is no place else the employee would rather be at that moment, the customer will go out of his or her way to return for future purchases as well as recommending the store to others. The same is true of "purchasing" health care services. If a patient has had the type of encounter with a physician's practice as described above or has heard from a trusted friend that the friend had such an experience, that patient will most likely drive farther to establish a relationship with the practice that is consistently focused on the patient.

One way to develop the kind of patient-centric culture that promotes a loyal patient base in a medical practice is to have every team member interact with every patient, every encounter, with a focus based upon the mental framework of, "at this moment in time, there is no other place I'd rather be and no other person with whom I'd rather be." Although this philosophy seems unrealistic, it isn't meant to be taken literally. It is a point of reference to make team members aware of the fact that if they strive to attain this level of focus on the patient, it will result in a positive shift toward the idealistic goal and the patients will feel important. If patients feel highly respected and important each time they speak with a member of the practice team, they will develop a sense of loyalty. For whatever reason, even people who like their jobs tend to lose sight of the fact that no matter how good they are at what they do, the job doesn't exist without customers. Having loyal patients in a positive environment enables employees to optimize their skills and to grow professionally. In health care, the customer is more sensitive than customers in other businesses because they are not on a vacation or shopping spree but seeking help they need to stay as healthy as possible. They are justifiably self-absorbed when they don't feel well and they are not in as much control as they are when they are consumers of nonhealth care services or products.

As a manager, it is important to be vigilant with regard to team interactions with patients so that if a problem develops, it can be addressed and resolved immediately.

THE WAITING GAME

There are several aspects of practice management that will minimize the average amount of time a patient has to wait between arriving on time for a scheduled appointment and being seen by a physician or other practitioner. There are also techniques to make any time spent in the waiting room as pleasant as possible for the patient and for anyone who is waiting with the patient.

Minimizing Patient Waiting Time

Every member of the team must remember that part of showing respect for patients is recognizing that their time is as valuable as the physicians' and every other team member's time. No matter what patients do with their time, the key is IT'S THEIR TIME. So, loyal patients are patients who know that everyone who works in their physicians' offices, including the physicians, values every patient's time as much as they do their own time.

One of the delicate aspects of keeping the schedule on track is to address patients who cause delays either because they are late or because they ask the physician or other team members about several conditions that were not mentioned when the appointment was scheduled.

A culture of accountability that involves the patient equally with the practice management team will contribute significantly toward the goal of consistently keeping the schedule on track. A practice policy that is well written, well communicated, and consistently enforced supports this desired culture of accountability.

Figure 8.3 provides a sample policy that should be brought to the attention of every patient and reinforced to both patients and team members at every opportunity. Note that this single policy addresses everyone's commitment to personal accountability to the schedule and to the financial health of the practice.

Beyond establishing a culture of personal accountability by every single person including each physician and each patient, other strategies to reduce the amount of time a patient is kept waiting include the

Culture of Accountability: A concept that promotes each individual in a medical practice, including each patient, to willingly accept accountability to fulfill their obligations. So, a receptionist is accountable for positive patient communications, providing accurate information to patients and inputting accurate information into the computer system, taking good messages, etc., while a patient is accountable for arriving on time for appointments, meeting all financial obligations in a timely manner, and letting the receptionist know before the actual appointment is scheduled, all of the things that patient would like to discuss with a practitioner so the receptionist can schedule the most appropriate amount of time.

To Our Patients…

It is our commitment to provide you with excellent care. To this end, we ask you to share in our team philosophy of personal accountability.

This means that every member of your practice team is committed to providing each of our patients with exceptional healthcare that focuses on the uniqueness of each individual patient.

To fully and consistently achieve this goal, each of the members of the practice team commit to:

- Efficiently and accurately performing every duty
- Ensuring adequate time is spent with each patient without any patient having to wait longer than 10 minutes from the time their appointment is scheduled to the time it begins.
- Treating each patient with respect and dignity
- Listening carefully to each patient to be sure we hear and address each of your questions or concerns
- Assisting the patient in the payment process for each service

Please assist our team's efforts to serve you by personally committing to:

- Scheduling your appointment in advance but when your condition necessitates a same-day visit, please understand that you may have to wait until we can see you without inconveniencing the patients who are scheduled that day.
- Being as specific as possible about all of the questions you have of our physicians when you schedule your appointment so we can allot the most appropriate amount of time for your visit.
- Using our web-based registration system that will eliminate the need for you to complete any forms once you arrive, if you have access to a computer, or, letting us know in advance that you would like help using the computer in our waiting room once you do arrive at your appointment (arrive 15 minutes before your scheduled appointment in this case).
- Always bring your insurance card each visit even if your policy hasn't changed.
- Come prepared to pay any projected share of cost or to discuss a payment plan with our staff
- Read your health insurance plans summary of benefits and bring it with you if you have questions
- Please let us know immediately if there is anything we can do to better serve you

We are Honored to Have You as a Patient

Figure 8.3 Policy to promote a personal accountability culture.

intelligent use of available technology or contracting certain services out to a reputable service vendor or a combination of the two. As detailed more in Chapter 10, intelligent use of technology includes identifying and defining a need, researching and analyzing the available options, narrowing down the options and obtaining a proposal from the vendors of most interest, selecting the vendor, planning and communicating to the team how to best implement the new technology, training every user, and implementation and close postimplementation monitoring to ensure the technology is working as planned.

Some of the same technology and contracted services mentioned under telephone protocols earlier in this chapter can also assist with minimizing patient waiting times. For example, offering secure e-mail messaging, texting, patient portals, PHRs and online scheduling, and registration options and other innovative technologies capture the patients' needs more thoroughly than having the patient call in to a busy receptionist to schedule an appointment. Another advantage is that all of the registration information for new or established patients can be collected with the advantage of online patient help screens and drop-down menus to reduce errors, reduce patient wait times, and increase patient loyalty.

In addition, there are services such as those offered through MicroMD at www.micromd.com and Navicure at www.navicure.com that assist with the full revenue cycle—an important aspect of which is to have patients arrive on time, armed with all of the information they need, for each visit. These services as well as those mentioned previously can also call patients from a waiting list with physical addresses close to the practice to see if they would like to come in the same day due to a cancellation.

Focus on the Patient–Waiting Room Considerations

A waiting room needs to be comfortable for a largely diverse patient population including children a mom has to bring with her to an appointment or children who are patients. Some patients will be hesitant to sit right next to a stranger, while others want to sit as close to the friend or family member accompanying them as possible. Some patients can't stand to be idle, while others cherish a peaceful, uninterrupted chance to just sit in a comfortable chair. What's an office manager to do—especially without spending a fortune?

Chairs with arms and washable padding or upholstery are practical for the typical, nonobese, patient who comes to your practice without anyone else. For example, assume that your waiting room needs to accommodate up to 10 patients at any given time and that there needs to be room for up to six additional people for those patients who bring someone with them. There should be at least six chairs with small tables between them so that strangers aren't elbow to elbow. The small tables should contain a variety of current magazines including a health-related option (Fig. 8.4). There should be soft lighting that is adequate to read by but not glaring for those who just want to relax. Six more similar chairs can be lined up against another wall with a little space in between but easy to move closer together or farther apart. There should then be two loveseats or oversized chairs in corners with room to set a child carrier on each side. These seats will make obese patients more comfortable

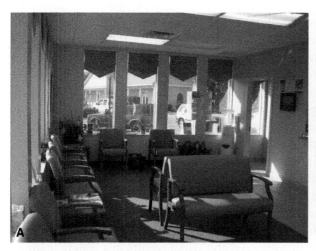
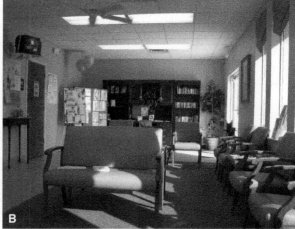

Figure 8.4 **A,B:** Well-designed waiting rooms.

or allow a child to sit on a parent's lap or even a couple to sit together. Finally, if there is space, yet another corner can be dedicated to small children with a few toys that can be easily sanitized regularly. A television might seem like a good idea but it can create more disturbance than it's worth. If the option is available then someone who is hard of hearing may want to turn the volume up which will disturb patients who are quietly talking to a family member or who simply are trying to think. It's also difficult to choose what type of program people are interested in watching. A better option is to have wireless available and perhaps a couple of laptops that can be used by patients—also providing an option if they bring their own computer.

Periodically, a team member should go around the waiting room and ask if anyone needs anything. In a busy practice, it's hard to keep track of patients in the waiting area but it's an important part of the overall goals of any practice.

PATIENT EDUCATION AND FOLLOW-UP

Following up with patients and ensuring strong coordination of care among a patient's multiple providers is critical to patient safety as well as optimal patient health outcomes. In Chapter 10, using technology to assist in continuity of patient care is thoroughly described but with or without technology, patient education and follow-up is as important as initial patient care.

A patient is significantly more likely to carefully follow medical advice if the patient thoroughly understands the reason for the advice. Conversely, a patient is likely to forget or simply ignore advice—even directly from a trusted physician—when the benefits, risks, and alternatives are not fully described and understood. Therefore, educating the patient is a critical element of optimizing the outcomes of each patient encounter with a health care professional. The practice should provide written and online patient education options for the most commonly treated conditions. Additionally, the key aspects of patient education need to be presented verbally to the patient before the patient leaves the office each time.

Many patients have multiple chronic conditions and therefore are regularly seen by specialists as well as a primary care physician. Once patients have been educated not only about each of their chronic conditions but also about the importance of prescribed medications, various lab or imaging tests and communicating pertinent information to all of their providers, the practice team needs to ensure the patient isn't just turned loose until the next visit. For example, if the patient is scheduled for a lab test later in the week, a medical assistant or nurse should flag the medical record to follow up a day or so after the scheduled test to make sure the office receives a copy of the lab results, views them, lets the patient know that the results were either normal or that the patient needs to schedule an appointment to discuss abnormal results with the physician and then either file normal results or re-flag the record to make sure the patient does come in to discuss abnormal results in a timely manner.

Other follow-up includes making sure the primary care physician receives updates from each specialist the patient encounters between primary care visits because specialist care may impact a primary care physician's recommendations for medications and other treatment and avoid duplication of tests.

Patient education leads to patients who are partners in managing their health care which increases compliance and patient follow-up prevents delayed diagnosis of problems, duplication of tests, and contraindications of prescribed medications plus follow-up increases the quality and safety of patient care. All of these factors contribute to the ultimate goal of loyal patients who are receiving the best possible care (Fig. 8.5).

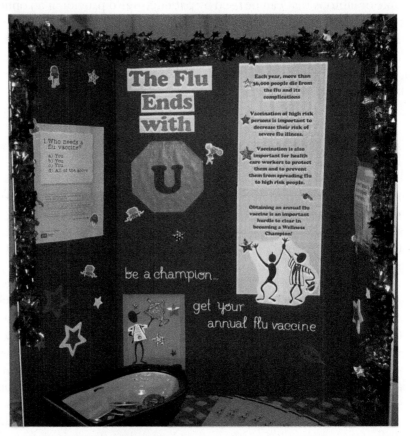

Figure 8.5 Patient education poster.

Box 8.1

Everyone Is Important in the Customer Service Chain

If a receptionist doesn't do a very good job, then a patient (or a lot of patients if left unchecked) may decide to seek medical care elsewhere. Loss of external customers or patients means loss of business which eventually results in the failure of a practice. As such, the receptionist is just as important to the success of the business as the patients. The same is true for every single member of the team, so everyone has to ensure they do their best to help each other focus on the patient.

OTHER CUSTOMERS—INTERNAL AND EXTERNAL

Every employee, including the physicians, is a customer of every other team member. Therefore, it is imperative that each member of the team is treated by the manager and other team members with the same degree of respect and concern that the manager desires for each team member to demonstrate with each patient.

If one person's behavior or lack of competence results in a loss of patients, every member of the team is negatively impacted. Likewise, each member of the team can only do for a patient what other members of the team make possible by doing their jobs exceptionally well. The following case study illustrates the far-reaching impact of one member of the team not performing well and not treating the other members as internal customers.

Case Study

CHAIN REACTION

Doctor Smith has poor documentation habits. Jill, the administrator, has spoken to the doctor previously explaining the fact that when he doesn't document adequately it causes continuity of care issues for the patients and also results in billing errors because the coder cannot select any codes that are not supported fully by the documentation. Incorrect billing has many negative outcomes such as making the practice vulnerable to being fined on one end of the spectrum and the practice not getting reimbursed the full amount to which it is legally and ethically entitled on the other. The impact on the patient is twofold as well: poor continuity of care based on poor documentation is a patient safety issue that could result in litigation against the practice, and incorrect insurance payments cause the patient extra time at best and extra money if the problem isn't resolved. If the service underpays, the patient may be unfairly responsible for additional out-of-pocket charges which is not conducive to creating a loyal patient. Today, Mrs. Jones, one of Dr. Smith's patients, calls the receptionist and demands to speak to the billing specialist. Due to a chain reaction that started with poor documentation of medical necessity by Dr. Smith, the patient received

an unexpected (and incorrect) bill from the practice. The billing special-
ist is frustrated with the physician because the physician doesn't seem to
understand, or even want to, the importance of documentation and takes
out that frustration on the patient who is getting angrier by the moment.
Enter the manager who is now stuck with an oblivious doctor, an irate and
soon to be ex-patient, a billing specialist who feels like the blame is being
misplaced on his already overburdened shoulders and nobody is happy.

How can this unpleasant work environment be corrected through a combination of internal and external customer service? First, Jill must speak with the external customer, the patient in this case, to regain the patient's loyalty and to restore the patient's confidence in the competence of the practice team—including Dr. Smith. The second customer is internal—the disgruntled billing specialist. She may ask him to please be patient while she addresses his concerns because she is confident of a team-oriented outcome. She must be careful not to criticize Dr. Smith or to seemingly take sides because the practice is only one team, not two.

As far as the impetus behind this cog in the team coherence, one strategy, assuming Dr. Smith is not the managing physician, is for Jill to document as much factual data as possible about the incidents involving patients with complaints about duplicative tests due to a specialist not seeing a needed test result in the documentation from Dr. Smith; other continuity of care issues; billing issues—whether or not the patient was involved—and any other situation that is due, in any part, to Dr. Smith's insufficient documentation. Then Jill should draft a chart showing estimated losses due to under coding and estimated potential losses due to fines for documentation not supporting billed codes and loss due to patients finding another primary care practice. Jill should then meet with the managing physician and explain that in addition to the chart she has drafted, morale has suffered tremendously making it nearly impossible for the rest of the practice team to provide the kind of patient-centric service to which it was capable. Ideally, Dr. Smith will see the light and join the team effort to build patient loyalty, or decide to find another practice. Meanwhile, Jill can refocus her team on the patients by explaining her understanding of the domino effect created when any member of the team forgets that each member is an internal customer of each other member.

Practices don't exist in a vacuum. Therefore, there are external customers to consider because patients view their entire episodes of care as an extension of their primary care providers. Therefore, it is critical for the team to be aware that hospital health information services and scheduling staff are treated with the same customer service focus as the patient because if those people find your office pleasant to deal with, they will be more responsive and friendlier to the patients you refer than they may be to other patients. Other external customers include suppliers so that patients aren't inconvenienced by the office running out of anything needed during a typical office encounter, any subcontractors such as after-hours answering services, specialists to whom the practice refers patients, and any other representative that the practice relies on to provide exceptional service to the practice or to its patients.

MEASURING PATIENT LOYALTY

First, a merely satisfied patient is not necessarily a loyal patient. Remember, a loyal patient will promote your practice to others as well as go out of his or her way to stay with your practice. Finding a reliable method in which to objectively measure patients who are loyal, patients who are satisfied, and patients who are not satisfied, and simultaneously generating meaningful feedback on opportunities to improve patient loyalty is challenging. Many surveys do not adequately differentiate between loyalty and satisfaction. This inadequacy is partly due to the number and title of ratings and partly due to the questions themselves. See Figure 8.6 for some sample survey questions. The same type of

---

1. Are you a new patient to this practice? _____Yes   _____No

2. If you are a new patient, how did you learn about our practice?

   _____NA   _____Word of Mouth   _____Website   _____Brochure

   _____Health Magazine   _____Hospital   _____Other (Please specify)

   _____

3. How long did you expect to wait between your scheduled appointment time and the start of your

   actual appointment? _____0-10 min   _____11-15 min _____>15 min

4. How long was your actual wait today? _____0-10 min   _____11-15 min _____>15 min

5. Please select the rating that best applies overall to our waiting room:

   _____Significantly exceeded expectations   _____Exceeded expectations

   _____Satisfactorily met expectations   _____Barely met expectations

   _____Did not meet expectations

6. Do you have any suggestions for us on how to improve our waiting room?

7. Based on your overall experience today, how likely are you to return to our practice when you need

   healthcare services?

   _____Extremely likely _____Somewhat Likely _____Possibly _____Not very likely

   _____Definitely not

8.

9. Based on your overall experience today, how likely are you to refer a friend to our practice?

   _____Extremely likely _____Somewhat Likely _____Possibly _____Not very likely

   _____Definitely not

Figure 8.6 **Sample patient survey.**

questions can be asked for any aspect of the practice—facilities, clinical services, front-office experience, and business services such as insurance processing. Furthermore, when presenting the survey, there should be no pressure on the patient to inflate numbers by giving them some sort of guilt about the impact of an "other than excellent" rating. A practice should not tie customer rankings to financial incentives because that increases the likelihood that team members will encourage high responses. According to Fred Lee, "It makes no sense to adopt scoring systems from the service leaders without adopting their rigor in protecting the subtle difference between customers who are likely to be loyal promoters of their services and those who are likely to defect, even though they said they were satisfied. They know that their future depends on the difference in the customer's mind between satisfaction and loyalty."[1]

MARKETING AND GROWING THE PRACTICE

A practice with a loyal patient following will perpetuate growth by word of mouth. However, if the practice grows too fast, it may become a victim of its own success. Growth management is as important as growth itself. In other words, if a practice follows all of the protocols described in this book and finds itself getting more and more requests for new patient appointments, the practice has to be sure not to burn out any of its team members who make this success possible. Therefore, the physicians and the manager should have a plan to consistently evaluate the need for additional employees and figure out how to make sure hiring a new clinician doesn't overburden the nonclinical team members. Once the practice experiences the balance of a team working well together to stay current with all aspects of patient care and business processes, the management team should be able to estimate how much total work each new patient will generate for each member of the team. At the point in which the management team determines that the practice needs an additional clinician, it may also consider adding a part-time receptionist and a part-time billing specialist. It is possible to use temporary help or offer over time until the additional patients being treated levels out but remember temporary help may not offer the same level of patient focus that each team member has learned to deliver. Hiring the right new people is also critical to the balance of the team as discussed in earlier chapters.

In today's competitive health care environment, a new practice or a practice that has experienced an extreme makeover due to new management requires an effective way to attract patients initially. Once the practice has established a loyal following, some of the same strategies that attracted patients in the first place will continue to supplement word-of-mouth recruiting of new patients while concurrently offering existing patients updates on the practice.

A well-designed, interactive Web site offering patient registration and scheduling software is arguably the single most cost-effective marketing and retention strategy available today. The initial investment of a Web designer experienced in medical practice marketing will pay for itself because a Web site must do more than list demographic information about the practice. A Web site that does justice to a patient-centric practice provides facts about the physicians' qualifications but also engages a viewer by highlighting what that practice has to offer that another practice with equally qualified physicians doesn't. That's where a group photograph of the entire practice team along with the philosophy of patient-centered teamwork to provide each patient with safe, effective, and individualized care for every aspect of every encounter with your practice makes a distinguished impression. Photos of the comfortable waiting area as well as an exterior shot of the building if it is attractive make the practice look inviting.

Remember that the Web is a powerful tool but most practices have discovered that fact so a practice's Web site must standout in ways that are important to prospective patients. An option to read a brief personal biographic sketch of each team member is a nice touch. For example, a physician's professional profile should include a few words on why he or she chose to study medicine and perhaps a personal philosophy about medical practice. Each team member should have a profile. Quotes from loyal patients touting the uniqueness of the practice make a favorable impression—especially when there is a variety to encompass not only the quality of care from the clinicians but the attentiveness and competence of the receptionist and other nonclinical team members.

Once the necessary demographics and unique aspects of your practice are in place to attract new patients, there are five more features that will not only be attractive to prospective patients but also a valued service to established patients. These features are discussed more fully in Chapter 10 and include

- Online patient registration for new patients and ability to update existing data
- Online patient scheduling for new or existing patients
- Online, secure e-mail messaging between clinicians and patients
- Patient education (links to disease-specific Web sites plus practice-generated information)
- Patient portals/PHRs

The practice will enjoy free marketing from any hospital in which the physicians have privileges in addition to any managed care organization with which the physicians have agreements. The manager should ask each of these organizations if they will please list the Web site address (URL) on all printed directories and a link to the practice Web site on all online directories.

Social media warrants mentioning because it is gaining in popularity among all businesses, even health care. Many health care providers are beginning to use social media such as Facebook and Twitter to attract new patients and to communicate new services to both established and prospective services. A practice should be cautious, however, when determining whether or not the benefits of social media outweigh potential risks. For example, if a customer does happen to

Social Media: The use of Web-based and mobile technologies to turn communication into interactive dialogue creating social interaction.

have a bad experience, which can happen in even the best of practices, that patient can post negative, uncensored comments about the bad experience from their perspective, even if their perspective is skewed. Of course, HIPAA compliance is vital if a practice does pursue social networking.

Finally, for the prospective patient who isn't likely to use a computer, more traditional marketing includes a newsletter or brochure containing the key features that are on the Web site and including the Web site address that can be distributed at local senior centers, the community areas of senior residential complexes, long-term care facilities, hospital waiting areas, and other key places to attract people who are less likely to use the Internet. A monthly newsletter is a nice touch to the Web site as well as paper copies. Other traditional advertising may include paid advertisements in local health magazines or even the newspaper but to be worth the cost, every ad has to contain a message that distinguishes the practice from other practices in the area. If the physicians are willing, name recognition through submitting a health column to local newspapers with the physician or practice byline is a good strategy.

SUMMARY

Customer service, patient loyalty, and marketing strategies encompass both internal and external customers. Internal customers refer to the fact that each team member is a customer of every other team member. If the physicians and the manager instill this important sense of meeting each other's needs, then each team member will be able to focus on external customers. External customers include patients, of course, but also people who can influence a practice's patients indirectly such as the receptionist at the imaging center where a patient of yours has to be referred. Patient loyalty is dependent on many factors, including competence of each person affiliated with the practice in any manner. In addition to a culture of team-based, patient-focused service and health care, the entire patient experience includes telephone encounters, the pleasantness and time spent in the waiting room, every face-to-face encounter, the manner in which the team interacts in the presence of a patient, what they hear from friends who have been to your practice, the professionalism of any correspondence from the practice, the accuracy of all treatment and business aspects, and the degree to which every member of the team treats the patient with respect, dignity and attentiveness.

Marketing will occur naturally once the practice is well established but some degree of marketing is still necessary. A practice that follows the principles delineated in this chapter will be able to combine marketing strategies with value-added service to the established patients via a well-designed Web site and some effective traditional tools such as brochures. The practice should grow naturally with a proactive manager at the helm of a patient-centric team.

CHAPTER REVIEW QUESTIONS

1. What are the most common complaints involving telephone encounters between a patient and a member of the practice team?

   _____

   _____

   _____

2. What is the mental framework from which every member of the team should consider each time the team member interacts with a patient?

   _____

   _____

   _____

3. What philosophy of respect will promote patient loyalty when the patient must wait between the scheduled appointment time and the time actually seen by a clinician?

   _____

   _____

   _____

4. In addition to establishing a culture of accountability for patients and the team and having a well-documented, well-communicated policy supporting that culture, what other tools are available to help keep the daily schedule on track so patients don't have to wait long once they arrive for a scheduled appointment?

   _____

   _____

   _____

5. Briefly describe the seating aspects of a well-designed waiting room.

   _____

   _____

   _____

6. Why is patient education and follow-up so important?

_____

_____

_____

7. Why is it important for members of the practice team to treat each other as much like customers as they do the patient?

_____

_____

_____

8. List some of the features of a practice Web site.

_____

_____

_____

REFERENCE

1. Lee F. *If Disney Ran Your Hospital: 9½ Things You Would Do Differently.* Bozeman, MT: Second River Healthcare Press; 2004.

Workbook for
Chapter 8

Workbook:
Chapter 8 Customer Service, Patient Loyalty, and Marketing

8.A: YOUR TURN: WRITE A POLICY AND A PROCEDURE FOR ANSWERING THE OFFICE TELEPHONE

Remember from earlier chapters that a policy ties to the overall mission of the practice and is a general guide to follow when possible. For example, if part of the mission of the practice is to build a loyal patient base, then the policies that guide the running of the practice should indicate the patient focus aspects such as "our policy regarding patient wait time is to consistently ensure patient wait time does not exceed 15 minutes over the scheduled appointment time." This policy alone may be supported by several procedures which are step-by-step guide to accomplishing a task that supports a policy. So one of the procedures tied to this policy might be a step-by-step guide to how to schedule the appointment in the first place so the patient is asked to please let the receptionist know other issues (not in detail but enough to get an idea of how much time to schedule) besides the main reason for the appointment the patient anticipates discussing with the physician or other clinician. The receptionist would educate the patient that the reason for the request is because the practice adheres to the "wait time not to exceed 15 minutes" policy but that it takes a team effort between the practice staff and the patient to consistently honor this policy.

Write a policy pertaining to the telephone aspect of building a loyal customer base, and then write one step-by-step procedure to support the policy. Procedures may include how to answer the phone and take a message or how to answer the phone and then determine the action such as transferring the call to a clinician or to the billing specialist.

8.B: VIDEO ACTIVITY: CHAIN REACTION

 (See video clip on thePoint Web site to complete this activity.)

- The video you are about to view is based on the following case scenario from the text: *Doctor Smith has poor documentation habits. Jill, the administrator, has spoken to the doctor previously explaining the fact that when he doesn't document adequately it causes continuity of care issues for the patients and also results in billing errors because the coder cannot select any codes that are not supported fully by the documentation. Incorrect billing has many negative outcomes such as making the practice vulnerable to being fined on one end of the spectrum and the practice not getting reimbursed the full amount to which it is legally and ethically entitled on the other. The impact on the patient is twofold as well: poor continuity of care based on poor documentation is a patient safety issue that could result in litigation against the practice, and incorrect insurance payments cause the patient extra time at best and extra money if the problem isn't resolved. If the service underpays, the patient may be unfairly responsible for additional out-of-pocket charges which is not conducive to creating a loyal patient. Today, Mrs. Jones, one of Dr. Smith's patients calls the receptionist and demands to speak to the billing specialist. Due to a chain reaction that started with poor documentation of medical necessity by Dr. Smith, the patient received an unexpected (and incorrect) bill from the practice. The billing specialist is frustrated with the physician because the physician doesn't seem to understand, or even want to, the importance of documentation and takes out that frustration on the patient who is getting angrier by the moment. Enter the manager who is now stuck with an oblivious doctor, an irate and soon to be ex-patient, a billing specialist who feels like the blame is being misplaced on his already overburdened shoulders and nobody is happy.*

1. View the video clip. (The clip opens with the billing specialist approaching the manager and saying, "Mrs. Jones is on the phone, irate because she got another erroneous bill from us—it's not my fault. I can only code what Dr. Smith documents and he's causing me to look like I'm making mistakes—I can't deal with his poor documentation anymore if I also have to take the blame for his sloppy work." The manager thanks the billing specialist, excuses her, and picks up the phone. The manager has no clue how to get the doctor to improve so she decides to place the burden on the patient's shoulders. The manager picks up the phone and tells the patient, "look, I understand you are upset but Dr. Smith is the problem here, not our billing specialist. If you like Dr. Smith, you just have to put up with the fact that he's a good doctor but he doesn't document enough information to justify payment for the services he performs. You could try one of our other doctors").

_____

_____

_____

2. Identify any mistakes you think were made by Jill.

_____

_____

_____

3. Jot down ideas for how Jill could have handled this situation more effectively by accepting responsibility for the problem as a "practice problem" not making the patient feel like her doctor isn't up to par or like the practice isn't a team.

_____

_____

_____

4. Now, using the same scenario, write how you would have handled that situation had you been Jill. Include any dialogue from both parties—Jill and Mrs. Jones. Remember, the goal in this exercise is to try to turn an irate patient into a loyal one until the documentation issue can be resolved internally without any patients being involved.

_____

_____

_____

8.C: TEAM PROJECT: BRAINSTORM IDEAS FOR IMPROVING THE WAITING AREA

The instructor will assign teams. The teams should brainstorm ideas for making a waiting room pleasant for a diverse group of patients and then be prepared to discuss the features of their waiting room.

8.D: YOUR TURN: CREATE A PATIENT EDUCATION FORM

Select any chronic disease and create a form that could be used on the practice Web site and printed for the patient to take home from an appointment. The form should provide a brief explanation of the disease, bullets about things to do and things to avoid, and follow-up recommendations (e.g., track blood pressure readings at rest and after activity each day for 1 week and then bring these readings to your follow-up appointment with the nurse next week). Also, find at least one link to add to the form containing more information on the condition or disease.

8.E: YOUR TURN: DEVELOP A SURVEY TO MEASURE PATIENT LOYALTY

Based on the information in the chapter and Internet research of sample surveys, design a brief survey that will distinguish between a loyal patient and one who is merely satisfied.

9

Managing the Legal Aspects of Health Information

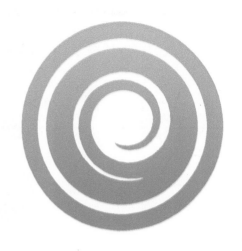

Information Security Officer
Legal Health Record (LHR)
Magnetic Stripe Security Badge
Minimum Necessary
Office of Civil Rights (OCR)
Organized Health Care Arrangement
Personal Health Records (PHRs)
Protected Health Information (PHI)
Provider Self-Disclosure Protocol (SDP)

Quality Improvement Organizations (QIOs)
Recovery Audit Contractors (RACs)
Red Flags Rule
Safe Harbor
Spoliation of Records
Stark Law
Treatment, Payment, and Operations
   Information (TPO)
Whistle-Blowing

OVERVIEW

It is said that the scope and speed of evolution of the electronic age far surpasses any previous era of human development. The analytical ability of electronic data processing is exceeded only by its capacity to store a seemingly endless supply of information. When we look for a rationale for the myriad rules and regulations in place attempting to guide the use of the electronic medical record, we need look no further than the headlines of any newspaper or electronic news source on practically any given day to find a lamentable story or two regarding fraud and misuse of the electronic medical record. We also live in an era that, at one and the same time, decries the absence of privacy yet clamors for the advantages of full and complete disclosure of information. Aside from avoiding any negative repercussions, medical office managers should remember the many positive reasons for maintaining an excellent medical record beginning and ending with exceptional patient care (see Figs. 9.1 and 9.2).

COMPLIANCE WITH HIPAA

The privacy and security of the medical record has never been of greater concern. Developments in modern technology including electronic communication, instantaneous transmission of data, and the inability to provide absolute protection of vital yet confidential information concerning the patient can exasperate the efforts of even the most vigilant medical office manager and cause nightmares for the medical practice.

What is Privacy:

Privacy has many different definitions ranging from informational privacy to personal autonomy.

1. Privacy is a complex set of rules and institutions which determine the limitations and availability of information.

2. Privacy is unwanted scrutiny under threat of real losses stemming from violations.

3. Absolute privacy is unattainable but there are good reasons for pursuing policies which might prevent the erosion of its boundaries.

4. With regard to personal health information, the sensitive nature of the information makes the loss of privacy all the more risky and potentially damaging.

Figure 9.1 What is privacy?

> ## Purposes of the health record:
>
> - Allows health care providers to provide continuity of care to individual patients
> - Planning patient care
> - Documenting communication between the health care provider and any other health professional contributing to the patient's care
> - Assisting in protecting the legal interest of the patient and the health care providers responsible for the patient's care
> - Documenting the care and services provided to the patient in support of reimbursement
> - Educate medical students/resident physicians and staff
> - Provide data for internal auditing and quality assurance
> - Provide data for medical research

Figure 9.2 Purposes of the health record.

Faced with the looming problems facing the medical record that the electronic revolution posed, the U.S. Congress in 1996 passed the Health Insurance Portability and Accountability Act (45 CFR 160, 164), commonly referred to as HIPAA. While the intent of the legislation included protection of health insurance coverage for workers and their families when they change or lose their jobs, HIPAA is most commonly associated with the establishment and implementation of security and privacy standards for medical records. By encouraging the adoption of electronic systems for the management of medical records, HIPAA also aspires to improve the efficiency and efficacy of the health care system in the United States. Federal oversight of the administrative simplification standards set forth in HIPAA is relegated to the Centers for Medicare and Medicaid Services (CMS), an agency within the U.S. Department of Health and Human Services.

Medical office managers should initially approach HIPAA from two perspectives—the HIPAA Privacy Rule and HIPAA Security Rules.

- **HIPAA Privacy Rule.** The HIPAA Privacy Rule (hereafter referred to as "the Privacy Rule") was created to put into practice the patient privacy requirements within HIPAA and to protect identifiable patient health information.

  - The Privacy Rule applies to health care providers who transmit any health information pertaining to transactions of a financial or administrative nature in electronic form. Health plans or health care clearinghouses (entities that process billing transactions between a health care provider and insurance companies) are also subject to the provisions of the HIPAA Privacy Rule (46 CFR 160.103[3]). This part of the Privacy Rule applies to the electronic record only.

  - In addition to financial or accounting information, the Privacy Rule also applies to health information that can be used to identify the patient and is kept under the control of the medical provider regardless of its format. This information such as patient name, address, Social Security number, and insurance policy number is referred to as patient-identifiable health information

HIPAA Privacy Rule: A rule created to put into practice the patient privacy requirements within HIPAA and to protect identifiable patient health information.

Protected Health Information (PHI): Provision under HIPAA defining any information, in any format, about health status, provision of health care, or payment for health care that can be linked to a specific individual including any part of a patient's medical record or payment history.

HIPAA Security Rules: A rule created to protect ePHI (i.e., PHI that is created, stored, maintained, and communicated by the medical provider electronically).

or protected health information (PHI). The medical office manager must be aware of the fact that PHI must be kept private **regardless of the format in which the record is maintained.** So not just the electronic record but paper and even oral records are subject to this aspect of the Privacy Rule.

- HIPAA Security Rules. This part of HIPAA (hereafter referred to as "the Security Rules") applies only to the PHI that is created, stored, maintained, and communicated by the medical provider *electronically*. In other words, information such as patient name, address, and Social Security number must be protected under the Security Rules if it is stored in an electronic format—the Security Rules do not apply to paper records or oral communication.

HIPAA Privacy Rule and the Medical Office Manager

Part of the intent of the HIPAA Privacy Rule is to secure uniform protection of health care information throughout the United States. As stated above, virtually all medical practices are subject to the provisions of the Privacy Rule. There are some finely crafted exceptions both in practice as well as in substance but these are rare and should be considered only under the advice of legal counsel. Basically, the medical office manager should assume that all so-called patient-identifiable information is PHI and thus is covered by the Privacy Rule.

Patients enjoy a number of rights under the Privacy Rule designed to give them more control over their own health information. These include

Designated Record Set (DRS): Under the HIPAA Privacy Rule, DRS is any medical record or billing record, including any item or repository containing protected health information, that is used to make decisions about individuals and is collected, maintained, used, or exchanged by or for any covered entity.

- Patients have the right to access their own PHI in a designated record set (DRS) defined by the Privacy Rule as medical records and billing records about individuals maintained by or for a covered health care provider which is used, in whole or in part, by or for the covered entity to make decisions about individuals with certain exceptions (e.g., psychotherapy notes, certain research study notes, and notes related to certain anticipated legal actions).

- Patients have the right to request that the medical practice amend PHI in a DRS with certain exceptions such as when the medical provider did not originate the record or when the record is considered complete as is.

- Patients have the right to an accounting of instances of disclosure of their medical information with certain exceptions such as disclosures made to persons involved in the patient's medical care or ones made for national security reasons. As of this writing, details of what can be disclosed and to whom disclosures can be made are substantial and appear to be changing as a result of recent federal action. Medical office managers are strongly advised to undertake a more detailed study of these rules as found under the HITECH Act portion of ARRA.

- Patients are to be given the opportunity to request that PHI communications be forwarded to an alternative location or by another method where the request is reasonable and where the patient states that the disclosure may constitute a safety risk.

- The patient may request that the medical provider restrict the use or disclosure of PHI for carrying out medical treatment, payment purposes, or health care operations. This has historically been a tricky situation where the rights of the patient can conflict with the legal obligations of the medical provider (e.g., payment transactions and disclosures required by law). Here again, due to rapid changes as a result of recent federal action such as the implementation of portions of the HITECH Act, the patient's rights have been expanded and the medical office manager is advised to seek legal counsel on these matters.

- The medical provider must allow the patient to submit a complaint about their policies and procedures or the noncompliance with the Privacy Rule. The patient must be notified as to the process for filing such a complaint with the Office of Civil Rights (OCR), Department of Health and Human Services.

One of the key issues with regard to the relationship between the medical office manager and the Privacy Rule is the establishment within the medical practice of an effective means of notification of patients of their rights under HIPAA. The medical office manager should supervise the creation and dissemination of such a notice which should contain, at a minimum, the following points:

- A description of the uses and disclosures of health information that are routinely made by the medical practice, along with examples

- A statement about whether the organization uses patient information to issue appointment reminders, to support marketing and fundraising efforts, and/or to report information to the sponsors of the individual's health plan.

- A statement of the rights of individual patients

- A description of the mechanism for making complaints about violations of the medical practice's stated privacy policies

- Any other information about the medical practice's use and disclosure of patient information[1]

HIPAA Privacy Rule and the Doctor and the Hospital

The HIPAA Privacy Rule is not intended to impede the provision of comprehensive medical services to the patient. These services may occasionally involve inpatient stays at hospitals and similar facilities that could require the transmission and use of PHI that is protected under the Privacy Rule. The vast majority of physicians maintain an affiliation with an inpatient facility/hospital. Thus, privacy issues concerning the flow of PHI, both to an affiliated inpatient facility from the medical practice and from the affiliated medical facility to the medical practice, are at issue.

One issue is the exchange of treatment, payment, and operations information (TPO). Whereas the Privacy Rule generally requires patient authorization for release and use of a patient's PHI, the rule carves out an exception when that information is used for treatment purposes. However, even though patient PHI may be so exchanged

Office of Civil Rights (OCR): A subagency of the U.S. Department of Education that is primarily focused on protecting civil rights in federally assisted education programs and prohibiting discrimination on the basis of race, color, national origin, sex, handicap, age, or membership in patriotic youth organizations.

Treatment, Payment, and Operations Information (TPO): Those areas defined in the HIPAA Privacy Rule under which a covered entity is prohibited from using or disclosing protected health information (PHI). The core health care activities of "treatment," "payment," and "health care operations" are defined in the Privacy Rule at 45 CFR 164.501.

Minimum Necessary: A provision under HIPAA that specifies that when using, disclosing, or obtaining from others, protected health information, all effort should be made to only use, disclose, or request the minimum information absolutely needed to satisfy the intention of that use, disclosure, or request.

without violating the Privacy Rule, the medical office manager should strongly consider implementing a comprehensive patient authorization policy to forestall any question of liability.

A corresponding issue deals with a provision in the Privacy Rule that otherwise requires any patient PHI disclosed to be only the "minimum necessary" to accomplish the legitimate task related to the disclosure. For example, only information related to the patient's current diagnosis (the minimum necessary) should be considered for release to an insurance company to justify payment of a claim. However, much more information may be needed by either the physician or the inpatient facility to facilitate treatment. And patient PHI may be released for treatment purposes to both affiliated and nonaffiliated facilities and practices where such information is deemed medically necessary.

Organized Health Care Arrangement: An arrangement of covered clinically integrated providers where individuals typically receive care from more than one provider and who present themselves as such and who must have joint utilization review or quality assurance and share financial risk.

Some legal relationships between the office of a medical provider and an inpatient facility may also create some circumstances where the patient PHI confidentiality under the Privacy Rule may be waived. The medical office manager should be informed whether the practice is legally "affiliated" with or in an "organized health care arrangement" with another health care organization by common ownership or control. If this is the case, authorization requirements under the HIPAA Privacy Rule are waived. Again, the medical office manager is urged to seek competent legal counsel in these situations.

The Privacy Rule may also be waived in the event of a disaster such as public health emergencies. Under these conditions, the medical office manager should contact authorities such as the Veterans Administration, Office of Civil Right of the Department of Health and Human Services, or state and local emergency management staff or competent legal counsel.

HIPAA Security Rules

HIPAA is made up of seven titles covering such areas as health care access, portability and renewability, tax-related health provisions, and group health plan requirements. As we have seen, the Privacy Rule deals with just that—the privacy to which the patient is entitled vis-à-vis his or her own medical record. With the advent of the electronic medical record, it was shown that safekeeping of the record was subject to severe and frequent compromise with little chance of preemptive solution—it was harder to trap and bring back a wayward electronic medical file than to try to do the same with a simple file folder! The HIPAA Security Rules expand the Privacy Rule protecting the medical record from tampering which may cause misrepresentation of the medical record.

Electronic Patient-Protected Health Information (ePHI): Provision under HIPAA defining any information in electronic format about health status, provision of health care, or payment for health care that can be linked to a specific individual including any part of a patient's medical record or payment history.

Of the four provisions of HIPAA that protect individually identifiable health information, the Security Rules focus on the record that is transmitted by or maintained electronically, otherwise referred to as electronic patient-protected health information (ePHI). In contrast, the HIPAA Privacy Rule covers all forms of a patient's PHI including written and oral communication. The Security Rules expand the security of patient PHI significantly over the Privacy Rule, and thus its provisions should be carefully explored and understood by the medical office manager.

The Security Rules apply to the same medical health organizations or covered entities (CEs) as the Privacy Rule. While the Office of Civil Rights within the Department of Health and Human Services is tasked with oversight and enforcement of the HIPAA Privacy Rule, the CMS is similarly tasked with oversight and enforcement of the Security Rules. The Security Rules deal only with health information and not materials that deal with other business activities such as marketing unless these contain patient-identifiable factors.

Additionally, the medical office manager should not forget that although the Security Rules do not apply to any format other than electronic information, if those electronic medical records are printed on paper for storage for example, then these paper records WOULD BE subject to the Security Rules.

Covered Entities (CEs): Under HIPAA, any entity defined in the rule as covered must comply with the HIPAA Privacy Rule. Originally, health care payers, health care providers, and medical claims clearinghouses were covered entities but under the Health Care Reform Act of 2009, the list was expanded to include business associates and also to increase the penalties for violation.

Compliance with HIPAA Security Rules

The scope of the Security Rules is broad and detailed and the CMS is trying hard to assist the medical office manager to implement policies and procedures to ensure compliance.

The medical office manager will play a fundamental role in the development and implementation of compliance policy. The CMS has recommended that the development process might include

1. Assessing the current level of security, risks, and problems in the office
2. Developing a viable implementation plan
3. Implementing solutions to challenges
4. Documenting procedural and policy decisions
5. Conducting periodic reassessment and implementing adjustments based thereon[2]

The HIPAA Security Rules apply only to patient's ePHI including those originally produced electronically and subsequently printed on paper but not records originally produced on paper or orally. The medical office manager must consider the production and or acquisition of ePHI data and its handling and storage as well as the distribution and/or transmission to proper parties and even its eventual destruction. Protections are called for that address physical, technical, and administrative issues of the ePHI.

Physical/Technical Safeguards

Of primary concern should be access control—who has the ability to access the ePHI and how is that access effectively limited but not to the point of crippling operations. The compliance policy should include details regarding the process of authorization and modification and termination thereof. Delineation of chain of command (who may issue or rescind authorization) and the authentication of users should be addressed (Fig. 9.3).

All office work areas where ePHI might be handled should be carefully checked for potential lapses in the safety and security of the record.

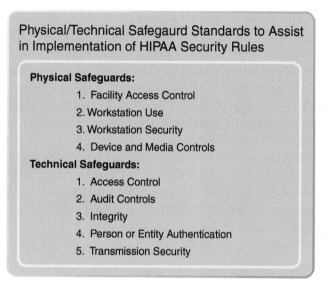

Figure 9.3 Physical/technical safeguard standards to assist in implementation of HIPAA security rules.

A specific part of the access control policy should be developed and promulgated among the staff detailing how every electronic record is received, what records are kept regarding transmittal of any part of the record, and who is responsible for what areas of the ePHI. Limitation of access to the ePHI should be strong and deep, being careful to control how access will be protected, allowing limited right of entry to identified individuals, and providing those individuals with assurances of both quick and accurate admittance to the medical record as well as ensuring privacy and security.

So, too, should the maintenance and upgrading of the compliance system as a whole and the electronic access subsystem thereto be subject to detailed scheduled review. Provision should be made for regular audits of the security system incorporating technological updates in both hardware and software. The medical office manager should consider bringing in a reliable, bonded software inspection team to sweep the system for malware, bugs, spyware, and any kinks in the system that might allow unauthorized access to the medical records. Of course, these procedures should be documented in the access control policy.

In designing the medical records security system, consideration should be given to including an alarm system to immediately notify the proper authority when an illegal entry has been made or attempted or when the system has crashed. The medical office manager should also try to influence the design to include some sort of authentication mechanism to confirm that the person trying to access the system is who they say they are (this could include an automatic fingerprint identification system [AFIS] or a magnetic stripe security badge).

What would happen if the lights went out—for an hour, a day, or a week or more? The medical office manager should include contingency plans for just such an event and the myriad other challenges that could be filed under "What if...?" The ePHI is relatively easy to backup and provision should be made for regular backups of the record. The

Automatic Fingerprint Identification System (AFIS): A national automated fingerprint identification and criminal history system maintained by the Federal Bureau of Investigation (FBI). AFIS allows search, exchange, and storage capabilities.

Magnetic Stripe Security Badge: A type of authentication verification in which a magnetic stripe containing data about the authorized badge owner to ensure the person has legal rights to access PHI. It works like the magnetic stripe on a debit card.

contingency plan should include the frequency of the backup process, the extent of the backup, the person or persons responsible for it, and the location of the stored files.

Updates should be built into the plan both for contact for professional data recovery service should this become necessary and for regular audits of the system to upgrade hardware and software. Included in this should be a provision for training—but remember, training should be done ONLY on dedicated test data and never on live data!

This type of comprehensive contingency plan for the medical record of the practice will basically kill two birds with one stone: An excellent contingency plan will ensure continuity of patient services at least on a limited scale and such a plan should fulfill the HIPAA Security Rules as well.

Administrative Safeguards

While almost every office staff structure is unique, all are comprised of certain general positions. The HIPAA Security Rules require the medical office manager to consider staffing a new position: information security officer. The information security officer is tasked with the development and implementation of the information security policy of the compliance plan for the medical practice (Fig. 9.4). This includes

Information Security Officer: An identified officer tasked with the development and implementation of the information security policy of the compliance plan for the medical practice.

- Design and implementation of a risk analysis to determine areas that present security challenges
- Implementation of policy to address these risks (risk management)
- Development and implementation of penalties against security violations
- Design and configuration of the system as a whole

For this position, the medical practice's hiring team should look for a capable, technically competent individual who understands the way information is acquired and used in the practice and the need for security. But of equal concern should be a demonstrated appreciation of the state and federal regulations that are unique to medical practices in

> **Administrative Safegaurd Standards to Assist in Implementation of HIPAA Security Rules**
>
> 1. Security Management Process
> 2. Assigned Security Responsibility
> 3. Workforce Security
> 4. Information Access Management
> 5. Security Awareness Training
> 6. Security Incident Reporting
> 7. Contingency Plan
> 8. Evaluation
> 9. Business Associate Contracts and Other Arrangements

Figure 9.4 Administrative safeguard standards to assist in implementation of HIPAA security rules.

general and to the integrity and accreditation of the practice and of the medical office management in particular.

COMPLIANCE WITH FRAUD AND ABUSE REGULATIONS

The American Health Information Management Association defines fraud as

> A false representation of fact or a failure to disclose a fact that is material (relevant) to a healthcare transaction that results in damage to another part that reasonably relies on the misrepresentation or failure to disclose.[3]

Further, the AHIMA defines abuse as

> Provider, supplier or practitioner practices that are inconsistent with accepted sound fiscal, business or medical practices, which directly or indirectly may result in unnecessary costs to the program, improper payment, services that fail to need professionally recognized standards of care or are medically unnecessary, or services that directly or indirectly result in adverse patient outcomes or delays in appropriate diagnosis or treatment.[3]

The financial loss due to health care fraud is estimated to be between $70 billion to an astounding $234 billion a year.[4] Every provider, every patient, and every third-party payer should concern themselves ipso facto with this egregious abuse of the greatest health care system in human history but such is not the case. Instead, vast public energy and resources are spent on remedying these often criminal activities. Indeed, such is the state of the misconduct in the health care system that it has been found necessary to craft broad yet detailed regulations designed to curb abuses by requiring compliance with federal and state laws and rules prohibiting fraudulent activity and to certify proper reimbursement for services rendered.

Moreover, the risks to patients due to fraudulent and abusive activity are substantial. For example, a bogus diagnosis entered into a patient's medical record in order to submit a fraudulent claim for reimbursement becomes part of the permanent medical record and can affect future treatment and insurability. Some patients have lifetime caps on health insurance coverage and a fraudulent claim can significantly diminish or even wipe out this coverage. Patients can even be at risk of physical hazard if a fraudulent misdiagnosis subjects the individual to unnecessary or dangerous medical procedures.

According to the National Health Care Anti-Fraud Association, the most common types of fraud committed by dishonest providers include

- Billing for services that were never rendered—either by using genuine patient information, sometimes obtained through identity theft, to fabricate entire claims or by padding claims with charges for procedures or services that did not take place.

- Billing for more expensive services or procedures than were actually provided or performed, commonly known as "upcoding," that is, falsely billing for a higher-priced treatment than was actually provided (which often requires the accompanying "inflation" of the patient's diagnosis code to a more serious condition consistent with the false procedure code).

- Performing medically unnecessary services solely for the purpose of generating insurance payments—seen very often in diagnostic-testing schemes.

- Misrepresenting noncovered treatments as medically necessary covered treatments for purposes of obtaining insurance payments—widely seen in cosmetic-surgery schemes, in which noncovered cosmetic procedures such as "nose jobs" are billed to patients' insurers as deviated-septum repairs.

- Falsifying a patient's diagnosis to justify tests, surgeries, or other procedures that aren't medically necessary.

- Unbundling—billing each step of a procedure as if it were a separate procedure

- Billing a patient more than the co-pay amount for services that were prepaid or paid in full by the benefit plan under the terms of a managed care contract.

- Accepting kickbacks for patient referrals

- Waiving patient co-pays or deductibles and overbilling the insurance carrier or benefit plan[4]

There are both state and federal weapons available to fight fraud and abuse including the False Claims Act (FCA), 31 USC 3729 (1986), which allows people to file actions against federal contractors for knowingly submitting fraudulent claims against the government (such as a medical practice submitting claims for reimbursement under Medicare and Medicaid). The act of filing such actions is informally called "whistle-blowing." Persons filing under the act stand to receive a portion (usually about 15% to 25%) of any recovered damages. Any practice found liable under the federal False Claims Act can be fined up to three times the amount in question in addition to fines of up to $11,000 per claim.

Under the Federal Anti-Kickback Statute (42 USC 1320a-7b[b]), anyone who knowingly and willfully receives or pays anything of value to influence the referral of federal health care program business, including Medicare and Medicaid, can be held accountable for a felony punishable by a fine up to $25,000 per occurrence or imprisonment for up to 5 years or both. The Federal Anti-Kickback Statute is very broadly worded and consequently Congress has carved out many exceptions to these directives, some of which deal with discounts which are otherwise properly disclosed and reflected in the costs claimed by the provider and payments made by a provider to group purchasing arrangements. In addition, there are many so-called safe harbor activities which are designations to protect deals between and among providers which are for fair market value and are considered "commercially reasonable" such as deals for space and equipment rental and sale of practices by one practitioner to another. While she or he does not normally come into contact with these types of arrangements, the

False Claims Act (FCA): A federal law that imposes penalties, such as fines and imprisonment on persons or companies who defraud any governmental program (e.g., Medicare or Medicaid).

Whistle-Blowing: The reporting to the public or someone in authority about alleged dishonest or illegal activities or misconduct occurring in government, public or private organizations, or companies.

Federal Antikickback Statute: A statute that specifies anyone who knowingly and willfully receives or pays anything of value to influence the referral of federal health care program business, including Medicare and Medicaid, can be held accountable for a felony punishable by a fine up to $25,000 per occurrence or imprisonment for up to 5 years or both.

Safe Harbor: Legal provisions that immunize certain payment and business practices that are implicated by the antikickback statute from criminal and civil prosecution under the statute.

Civil Monetary Penalty Act (CMP): An act authorizing the Office of Inspector General to assess and seek civil monetary and other penalties (i.e., exclusion from participation in Medicare) against people who commit health care fraud, violate the antikickback statute, or commit any other abuse of federal health care funds.

Stark Law: Regulates physician self-referral for Medicare and Medicaid patients.

medical office manager who demonstrates a true appreciation of these regulations is most valuable not only to the medical practice but to the patients whom it serves.

Both of the above-referenced laws plus the federal Civil Monetary Penalty Act (CMP) section of the Social Security Act (42 USC 1320a-7a) have combined to provide potent weapons in the fight against medical information fraud and abuse. Fines and penalties that can be assessed under the CMP have been enhanced under HIPAA and now reflect amounts of up to $10,000 per occurrence in a broad spectrum of federal programs (including Veterans Affairs and the Public Health Service) for infractions such as incorrect coding or provision of medically unnecessary services or persuading a patient to order products or services from a particular provider by offering a bribe.

Filing false claims usually involves improper coding and attempts to gain reimbursement for medically unnecessary services which makes this a violation of HIPAA and thus a federal offense. The Federal Bureau of Investigation (FBI) is charged with investigation of these offenses.

Finally, physicians are prohibited from referring patients to other medical providers with whom the originating physician has a financial relationship. Known as the "Stark law," these rules originally affected the ordering of clinical lab services but have since been expanded to include a series of "designated health services" including physical therapy services, durable medical equipment, and outpatient prescription drug provision among other areas. Again, serious monetary penalties can greatly enhance the obedience of these rules.

A number of government agencies, including the Office of Inspector General (OIG) and the FBI, are charged with investigating fraud and abuse of activities within the health care industry. The OIG investigates fraud and abuse cases via audits and inspections. The rules for compliance are very detailed and the medical office manager is advised to undertake further study to become familiar with them as appropriate. The most common violation is under the False Claims Act, which deals with claims for services that either were not performed or resulted in misleading process or costs.

The idea of developing compliance programs and policies to address fraud and abuse gained momentum as a result of federal sentencing guidelines adopted in 1991 that allowed corporations who were found to have dealt fraudulently with the government to avoid catastrophic fines and penalties by showing that they had substantially complied with the laws in place at the time. The falloff of these programs—that organizations used these mandatory programs and procedures to identify problems and improve operations—made the concept of regulatory compliance programs even more attractive to the health care industry which had a significant component related to governmental reimbursement.

The medical office manager will be involved in the planning, development, and execution of a program designed to ensure compliance. The OIG has issued specific compliance guidance to designated individual and small group physician practices to assist in crafting a program specific to the needs of the individual organization:

From AHIMA: Content for compliance education and training activities

- Medicare Billing Rules: emphasis on areas that have been problematic, e.g. billing of consultants, billing of annual exams, billing of services "incident to," appropriate assignment of Diagnosis Related Groups (DRG's), and billing for consolidated services in skilled nursing facilities.

- Documentation Guidelines and Accessing Personal Health Information: including required elements of the patient record accessing patient information and record maintenance and retention of patient records, and release of information. Included in this section would be what is expected to be documented in the medical record (e.g. who can make entries, how entries may be revised, who should authenticate, etc.).

- Medicare Bulletins, Seminars, Other Related Compliance Resources: on-going and yearly updates, revisions and new resources related to compliance that should be shared throughout the organization.

- Coding, Billing and Claim Submission: yearly updates on ICD-9 and CPT changes with emphasis on appropriate use of modifiers, global surgery package rules, add-on codes, E&M coding and documentation, and coding conventions in general.

Figure 9.5 From AHIMA: Content for compliance education and training activities.

1. Conducting internal monitoring and auditing through the performance of periodic audits

2. Implementing compliance and practice standards through the development of written standards and procedures

3. Designating a compliance officer or contact(s) to monitor compliance efforts and enforce practice standards

4. Conducting appropriate training and education on practice standards and procedures

5. Responding appropriately to detected violations through the investigation of allegations and the disclosure of incidents to appropriate government entities

6. Developing open lines of communication, such as (1) discussions at staff meetings regarding how to avoid erroneous or fraudulent conduct and (2) community bulletin boards to keep practice employees updated regarding compliance activities

7. Enforcing disciplinary standards through well-publicized guidelines[5]

See Figure 9.5 for an example of content for compliance education and training activities.[6]

Quality improvement organizations (QIOs) and recovery audit contractors (RACs) are private contractors with arrangements with CMS to independently audit claims. The 3-year demonstration project ended in March 2008 and identified $992.7 million in overpayments and $37.8 million in underpayments via Medicare. Based on these results, permanent RAC programs are now in place in four regions in the United States.

The types of audits utilized by government and private companies include

- Random one-record prepayment audits—conducted for simple one-patient visits

Quality Improvement Organizations (QIOs): Private contractor extensions of the federal government that work under the auspices of the U.S. Centers for Medicare and Medicaid Services (CMS) to monitor the appropriateness, effectiveness, and quality of care provided to Medicare beneficiaries.

Recovery Audit Contractors (RACs): Program was created through the Medicare Modernization Act of 2003 (MMA) to identify and recover improper Medicare payments paid to health care providers under fee-for-service Medicare plans (FFS plans).

- Electronic claims submission audits—the most common type of audit; these can pertain to one-patient visits or multiple visits/procedures on the same or different patients
- Focused health record reviews—where the provider is identified as having provided a service that falls outside the norm for similar providers
- Comprehensive health record reviews—where the providers' charges for 6 months are audited as a whole

Provider Self-Disclosure Protocol (SDP): Provisions for voluntary disclosure by health care providers of self-discovered evidence of potential fraud to the U.S. Department of Health and Human Services Office of the Inspector General.

In addition to audits, the OIG has introduced what it hopes will be a streamlining of the process by allowing providers to participate in the provider self-disclosure protocol (SDP). Not meant for simple billing errors or overpayments, the SDP guides providers to self-disclose violations involving the anti-kickback laws and the physician self-referral or Stark law. Medical practices can help avoid sanctions by establishing their own compliance programs that enable them to self-regulate their efforts in appropriate billing and development of policies and procedures that protect patient information while continuing to operate at the highest possible level of service.

A significant resource for designing and implementing compliance programs is the American Health Information Management Association (AHIMA).[7] AHIMA has indicated that compliance programs should include at least seven major elements:

1. Oversight—designating who is responsible for corporate compliance (single individual or team); involving all staff members from the beginning; involving legal counsel
2. Policies and procedures—stating the compliance mission of the practice; establishing written policies and procedures tailored to the individual practice while addressing each and every appropriate compliance issue
3. Training and education—instilling continuing training in compliance issues as part of the culture of the practice; focus especially on staff involved with billing and coding
4. Communication method and tools—addressing issues such as existence and efficacy of the internal and external communication mechanisms of the practice; who, what, when, where, how, and why does the practice talk with patients, staff, and the community
5. Internal audit and controls—OIG recommends combining internal with external audits; establish the scope of audits; review audits should be conducted regularly
6. Enforcement and follow-up—detailing who has responsibility for what measures of enforcement; provide adequate notice of consequences of noncompliance
7. Problem resolution and corrective action—dealing with corrective action on a multidisciplinary team level; using the skills of health information management professionals

All levels of human resources activity should be aware of compliance issues. The medical office manager is tasked with introducing the benefits and responsibilities of following compliance policies to new employees and to design regular continuing education programs that effectively address compliance issues in all areas of the practice including wages and benefits, discrimination, OSHA requirements, social security and retirement issues, and immigration law.

MEDICAL IDENTITY THEFT—THE RED FLAGS RULE

The problem of identity theft in America is serious and growing. Estimates are that as many as nine million Americans have elements of their identities stolen each year causing each victim untold embarrassment and misery, hours of lost time to try to identify and correct problems, and potentially devastating damage. Much of the problem is directly attributable to the proliferation of electronic data processing that has infused itself into almost every aspect of modern life. The medical office is, of course, a prime example, for with the great advancements offered by the emergence of the electronic medical records system there came equally great perils.

The theft of medical identity information can have particularly severe consequences: thieves may use the information to procure medical services or goods without the permission of the victim's knowledge or consent or unscrupulous providers may file false claims for medical services. These practices can cost medical providers and insurers millions of dollars in damages each year and erode confidence and trust in the health care system. But the more sinister result of medical identity theft is the possibility of falsification, alteration, or intentional misuse of a patient's own medical health record, potentially jeopardizing both the financial as well as the physical health of the patient.

If this were a problem that could be limited to one office or one town or even one region, localized procedures could be put in place to minimize the spread of medical identity theft, just like offices implement infection control procedures. But the unique design of electronic data processing that fostered the creation of the Internet makes the problem of medical identity theft a worldwide phenomenon. So broad are the possible pitfalls that the U.S. Congress has passed national legislation designed to reduce the occurrence of offenses and diminish any resulting damages. Although these rules were successfully challenged as not being enforceable with regard to medical practices in December 2010, many practices have determined that the Red Flags Rule is worthwhile to enforce.

Pursuant to this directive, the Federal Trade Commission (FTC) has identified five warning categories or "Red Flags" that would raise suspicion of possible identity theft:

- Alerts, notification, or warnings from a consumer reporting agency
- Suspicious documents
- Suspicious personally identifying information, such as a suspicious address
- Unusual use of or suspicious activity relating to a covered account

Red Flags Rule: Policy created by the Federal Trade Commission; sets out how certain businesses and organizations must develop, implement, and administer their identity theft prevention programs.

- Notices from customers, victims of identity theft, law enforcement authorities, or other businesses about possible identity theft in connection with covered accounts

The FTC called for certain entities that regularly extend or renew credit or allow deferred payments to design, implement, and administer identity theft prevention programs. Because they routinely perform a service, then receive payment once the work is complete, most medical practices will fall under this category. Further, because of the limited nature of most medical practices, a program appropriate to the size and complexity of the practice can be straightforwardly designed to accomplish the goal. Each program must include four basic elements:

1. Identify relevant Red Flags
   Identify the Red Flags of medical identity theft the practice is likely to encounter
2. Detect Red Flags
   Set up procedures to detect Red Flags in day-to-day operations
3. Prevent and mitigate identity theft
   Take action to prevent theft of medical information and reduce damages
4. Update your program
   Evaluate your program regularly and train staff to spot changes and meet new threats

While your practice can comply with the requirements of the Red Flags Rule by retaining professional help to design, implement, and administer the program for a fee, many practices can create their own program using the template provided by the FTC at http://www.ftc.gov/bcp/edu/microsites/redflagsrule/RedFlags_forLowRiskBusinesses.pdf. The template is for small, very low–risk practices, thus its applicability should be judged accordingly. Whichever method of design is chosen, the program must be approved by the board of directors or senior management of the practice. Senior management must also be designated to oversee the implementation, administration, and regular evaluation of the program.

While there are no criminal sanctions imposed for failure to comply with the Red Flags Rule, a practice risks civil liability with the possibility of enhanced damages for failure to have an identity theft prevention program in place even thought the law requiring these rules was successfully challenged making medical practices exempt. More information about the Red Flags Rule can be found at http://www.ftc.gov/bcp/edu/pubs/business/idtheft/bus23.pdf.

In the spirit of building patient loyalty, see Figure 9.6 for Medical Identity Theft and Abuse guidelines for providers and patients which a savvy practice manager will implement and make available to each patient.

PARTIES	ACTION ITEM
Provider	1. Identify areas of potential abuse or misuse of medical identity information in the office setting. a. Note "icebergs" or key problem points related to electronic medical records
	2. Develop effective medical identity information theft prevention programs based on best practices/risk-assessment values a. Use approach similar to that used to respond to financial identity theft b. Address prevention, identification and incident response issues. b. Include mechanisms for sharing information with health care payers c. Ensure cross-communication among different departments/areas to share information regarding possible medical record identity theft
	3. Develop appropriate educational programs about medical information identity theft for training of staff and service providers a. Include thorough, clear/concise/accurate discussion of HIPAA Privacy Rule and HIPAA Security Rules including directions to resources b. Ensure adequate initial training for all team members and providers c. Evaluate effects of training on medical record security as well as patient satisfaction d. Conduct regular systematic updates to accommodate changes e. Consider development of controlled tests of identification and incident response procedures
	4. Include information on medical identity theft in patient education materials
	5. Conduct regular systematic audits of medical identity theft prevention program and make appropriate adjustments
	6. Develop relationship with local law enforcement a. Provide appropriate educational materials to local law enforcement agencies regarding medical identity information theft
	7. Consider development of and/or participation in local or regional incident response systems
Patient	1. Become proactive in your own security. b. Familiarize yourself with tools you can use in case you are victimized. i. Stolen Social Security number stolen? Contact the Social Security Administration at 1-800-269-0271 ii. Stolen mail? Contact your local Post Office or 1-800-275-8777 iii. Stolen checks or credit cards? Contact your bank or credit card issuer immediately – DO NOT WAIT! iv. Upon suspicion of any misuse or abuse of medical identity information, START TAKING NOTES IMMEDIATELY! Document all correspondence, telephone calls, E-mails with the date and time and the party who you correspond with. v. Make copies of everything related to the complaint and keep in a separate file. vi. Consider filing a complaint with the Identity Theft Data Clearinghouse run by the Federal Trade Commission at http://www.ftc.gov/bcp/edu/microsites/idtheft/
	2. Your medical provider is the immediate point of entry for victim report of potential abuses of medical information a. CONTACT THE PROVIDER WHERE THE SUSPECTED MEDICAL IDENTITY THEFT OCCURRED IMMEDIATELY! i. Establish a single point of contact if possible; one person with whom you can deal regarding your complaint ii. STOP the flow of information immediately! iii. Try to establish the extent of the abuse; what was stolen or determined to be inaccurately recorded and to whom this information was sent. b. All potential abuses will be thoroughly investigated and forwarded to law enforcement where appropriate.
	3. If you would like more information or guidance on actions you can take after speaking to your provider: a. You may file a report with Office of Civil Rights at the Department of Health and Human Services at 1-800-368-1019 or go online: i. For HIPAA complaints, go to http://www.hhs.gov/ocr/privacy/hipaa/complaints/index.html ii. For Patient Safety and Quality Improvement Act complaints, go to http://www.hhs.gov/ocr/privacy/psa/complaint/index.html b. You may report the case to local law enforcement, the local district attorney, the state attorney general, the state office of consumer protection or other bureau specifically designated for medical identity information theft protection c. To report fraud in Medicare, Medicaid and Children's Health Insurance Program (CHIP) go to http://www.healthcare.gov/news/factsheets/tools_to_fight_fraud.html

Figure 9.6 AMA medical identity theft response checklist for consumers at http://library.ahima.org/xpedio/groups/public/documents/ahima/bok1_039114.pdf.

Box 9.1

Opportunity to Enhance Customer Loyalty

The perceptive medical office manager will realize that compliance with the Red Flags Rule assures patients that your practice is doing its part to protect them from the scourge of medical identity theft.

Case Study

NANCIE JONES AND LEGAL ASPECTS OF HEALTH INFORMATION

Nancie Jones has been hired as the practice administrator. Her predecessor left without notice due to a conflict with the managing physician. On her first day of employment, she has been given access codes to the electronic medical record file by the receptionist of the practice. She notes that the system was installed 24 months prior to her hiring and has not been updated since that time. During an orientation meeting with staff, a clerk comes to Nancie with a report that one day before she left, Nancie's predecessor responded to a call for assistance from the clerk who complained that the system continually froze up on her and that Nancie's predecessor apparently fixed the problem by inserting a flash drive into the staffers computer and typing some commands. The next day, Nancie is inundated with calls: one from a patient who was referred to psychotherapy who complains he has been denied access to his medical record, another from a patient whose insurance indicated a bill for a procedure the patient claims never took place, another is a report that a scheduled surgery of a patient has to be cancelled due to conflicting information on the patient's medical history, and another patient reports experiencing harassing phone calls from durable medical equipment providers regarding sexual dysfunction therapy. The final call of the day is from an attorney who demands any and every piece of data ever produced, kept, archived, or sent for destruction concerning his client, a former patient.

What would you do?

Nancie has seemingly walked into the proverbial hornet's nest! A good way for her to get started on solving these crises would be to remember the cardinal rule of the practice—to provide excellent medical care to the patient. Thus, the initial effort would be to secure the urgent safety and health of patient in need of surgery. Then she might evaluate each of these issues in terms of their effect on the legal liability to the practice and the possible prosecution of parties for criminal or civil violations or potential civil rights violations. At the same time, she should be evaluating the existing policies of the practice with a view toward implementing immediate and short- and long-term changes to prevent future occurrences.

THE LEGALLY SOUND MEDICAL RECORD

Patient health records are maintained by a variety of health-related organizations as a means of providing proof of service and care furnished to the patient. Records can vary in content and format but are all maintained to meet patient care needs and to comply with legal requirements. Defining the legal medical record requires us to balance the service-oriented clinical purposes of record-keeping with the more esoteric reasons demanded by the legal system.

Whether that record is maintained on paper, in an electronic health record (EHR) or some combination of both formats, the medical office manager will face challenges in designing and implementing a system that protects the confidentiality, security, and privacy of the patient record. Physician practices must adhere to state and federal laws and accrediting and licensing provisions protecting the patient record and guiding their use. Determining what constitutes a legally sound medical record and the procedures governing its use are essential issues to both protect a medical practice and to help it flourish.

Patient health records serve several important purposes:

- The chief purpose of the medical record is to document patient contact and care.
- The medical record may be shared by physicians making clinical decisions.
- The record can offer information about the effectiveness of care provided.
- Data contained in the medical record is vital to ongoing research and continuing education.
- Continuing evaluation of the record can support the overall operation of the practice.
- Reimbursement and support for legal challenges require accurate medical record-keeping.

While the principles outlined above remain unchanged, the composition of the legal health record (LHR) becomes problematic when contemplating the migration to the EHR. See Figure 9.7 for the legal EHR basics. Redefining what makes up the LHR/EHR is affected by legislation as well as by continuing advancements in technology both in terms of patient care as well as improvements in records generation and retention. And because various pieces of patient health care data can come in various forms (paper records, transcripts, prescription records, films, and test results are just a few examples), defining what is and is not a necessary part of the LHR/EHR can be tricky.

Because the scope of such a project is broad and highly subjective to individual medical practice (not to mention full of legal pitfalls), medical office managers should consider advising that the practice retain expert assistance when developing a new LHR or transitioning to an LHR/EHR. Knowledge of key areas of consideration to assist in the determination of what to include in the LHR/EHR, however, is important to the process. There are eight generally recognized areas of consideration:

Legal Health Record (LHR): A medical record that is in full compliance with all rules, regulations, and laws governing how the record is created, updated, maintained, stored, accessed, transmitted to another party, and amended.

The Legal Electronic Medical Record

HiMSS

Healthcare providers across the country recognize the benefits of electronic medical records (EMRs) to improve care, reduce costs and improve efficiency. But as medical professionals, we know the challenges of keeping up with technology. The Healthcare Information and Management Systems Society (HIMSS) has developed some suggestions for you as you plan EMR implementation for your practice. This brochure discusses the EMR as a legal record.

WHAT IS THE LEGAL ELECTRONIC MEDICAL RECORD (EMR)?

- The medical record is a healthcare organization's most important business and legal record.
- Legal requirements, well defined for maintaining paper medical records, are additionally complex for electronic records.
- Medical records must be maintained in a way that is legally sound or they risk being challenged as invalid.

EMR selection criteria must include ensuring that a given EMR is appropriately designed and can be appropriately used to ensure adherence to federal and state rules, as well as institutional requirements and additional certification standards that may apply to their organization.

WHY DOES THE EMR NEED TO BE A LEGAL RECORD?

Simply, a healthcare organization must have a medical record. Its "medical record" must, by definition, meet all statutory, regulatory, and professional requirements for clinical purposes as well as for business purposes. If the record does not qualify as a legal record, it becomes hearsay and therefore is much less legally valid for business or for medical-legal purposes. Unless the practice intends to maintain separate paper records that comply with legal requirements, its EMR, to be a legal record, must conform to the same requirements as medical records in general and for business records on computers more specifically.

WHAT IF MY EMR DOES NOT MEET THE REQUIREMENTS FOR A LEGAL RECORD?

- As an invalid business record, a problematic EMR can be challenged by payors for billing or Pay for Performance (P4P).
- With an invalid medical-legal record, risk of adverse litigation outcomes and costs rise.

> *Regardless of format, whether paper, hybrid, or electronic, the medical record must meet the requirements of the legal and business record for the organization.*

LEGAL EMR BASICS

Don't assume that a given EMR will meet your requirements for a legal record. As the EMR marketplace increases awareness of these matters, products will continue to improve. Here are four areas to look at:

How is documentation created?

- Is the author of each element of documentation accurately recorded, including vitals, chief complaint, history of present illness, orders, plans, and prescriptions?
- How are different, successive versions of the encounter (before signature) treated?
- Do signature procedures and tools meet your state's and your organization's requirements?

How is documentation managed and preserved over time?

- After signature, if a correction, clarification, or amendment is added, is it clear what is original and what is not and can all original documentation be recovered if needed?
- How is documentation protected from being altered, in all parts of the system including the underlying database?
- How are new templates, guidelines, forms, etc., created, preserved, retired?
- Are all clinical messages and clinical behaviors (prompts, etc.) reproducible and recoverable?
- Do other periodic and necessary tasks, such as report-creation and auditing, also expose documentation to additional security risks?
- Are critical support functions, such as auditing, always operable and reasonably accesible or do they require vendor supports or other extra costs?

How does documentation interact with billing?

- Does the system prompt users to add documentation for "improved revenue"?
- Does the system allow the sending of billing information without completion of documentation?
- Does the system send billing information for tests without means to ensure the tests were actually done?

How is documentation presented?

- When asked to produce a view or a printout of an encounter, does the system offer a view that conforms to your organization's definition of its legal record?
- If documentation has been amended or otherwise altered, is that clearly identified in the viewed and printed version?

Figure 9.7 Legal EHR basics. (Source: from HIMSS The Legal Electronic Record http://www.himss.org/content/files/LegalEMR_Flyer3.pdf)

1. **Sources and secondary data:** If more than one location holds the LHR/EHR, the practice must determine which source is the "source of truth."

2. **Detail vs. summary data:** Practice must decide whether to include detail and summary forms of findings of diagnostic studies.

3. **Paper vs. images:** Local laws may allow, require, or be ambivalent toward keeping both paper and other images of the same data.

4. **Data not to include:** Documents that do not meet Business Records Hearsay Exception (e.g., incident reports, insurance forms, psychotherapy reports, e-mails between patient and provider, and data imported from patients to other providers into provider-hosted Web-based portals and patient-created personal health records [PHRs])

5. **Decision support:** Alerts, pop-up notices and reminders of tests and procedures that affect treatment decisions that ultimately impact a patient's care should probably be included.

6. **Sources of communication:** Voice mails, e-mails, and other Web-based communications that provide documentation of the patient's care, treatment, or diagnosis should be included.

7. **Personal health records:** Because these would likely not qualify as a business record, patient-produced PHRs should probably not be included in the LHR/EHR.

8. **Sharing of data between providers:** If the data shared between providers is used in the patient's care, treatment, or diagnosis, it should be kept—the receiving provider should make this decision.[8]

In the event of a legal challenge in a practice, it is likely that records will be sought by both sides first as a means of determining the credibility of a case and then as evidence should the case be prosecuted. This process is called "discovery." With the explosive proliferation of information technology, the tendency to archive increasing amounts of data related to the care, treatment, and diagnosis of a patient has become a tidal force. There is danger that information legally discoverable under the Federal Rules of Evidence can become intermingled with otherwise non-discoverable data irrelevant to a legal issue. Overbroad records can subject the practice to unnecessary legal maneuvering and harassment. On the other hand, an LHR/EHR that is incomplete does not serve the cause of justice in legitimate questions of legal liability and could subject the practice and various entities therein to legal sanctions, licensing questions, and continued practice.

Although training as a legal professional is certainly not a prerequisite for a successful medical office manager, she or he should be experienced and comfortable with the unique rules for the legal discovery of the LHR/EHR which, in the case of electronic records, is referred to as "e-discovery." Medical office managers and associated HIM professionals should carefully distinguish between the medical practice's LHR/EHR and patient's DRS as provided for by the HIPAA Privacy Rule. While the DRS has been referenced earlier, at this point, a full understanding of the concept is called for. According to AHIMA, a DRS is

> A group of records maintained by or for a covered entity encompassing medical records and billing records about enrollment, payment, claims, adjudication, and case or management record systems maintained by or

Business Records Hearsay Exception: Records are considered hearsay (they record what others said and did and are maintained by other than those directly involved in litigation) and are not usually admissible in court. Medical records are the business records of health care and are an exception to the hearsay rule as long as they meet certain criteria such as being maintained in the course of business and recorded at or very near the time of the event by someone who has personal knowledge of the event, that is, a practitioner.

Personal Health Records (PHRs): A health record where health data is maintained and controlled by individual users themselves.

Discovery: Part of the pretrial litigation process during which each party requests relevant information and documents from the other side in an attempt to discover facts pertinent to the case and includes depositions, interrogatories, requests for admissions, document production requests, and requests for inspection.

E-Discovery: The collection, preparation, review, and production of electronic documents in litigation discovery. This includes e-mail, attachments, and other data stored on a computer, network, backup, or other storage media.

for a health plan, used in whole or in part, by or for the covered entity to make decisions about individuals.[6]

Patients have the right to inspect and obtain a copy and request amendment of medical and billing information used to make decisions about their care under HIPAA standards and the DRS is used to accomplish this. Generally, because it is not used as an official business record for legal purposes, the information included in the DRS is far more broad and inclusive than that required for the LHR/EHR. Thus, the medical office manager should firmly advise the practice that these two data sets should be separately maintained and only correlate where necessary.

In the design and implementation of the LHR/EHR, consideration should also be given to the issues of retention and destruction of records. Various rules and laws dictate how long any given piece of data must be kept for any of a variety of purposes, both business and legal. Here again, given the vast increase in the amount of data being created in the practice of modern medicine, the medical office manager has the daunting task of determining what to keep and what to throw away! A cardinal rule of e-discovery with respect to retention and destruction of records is that the course of action that governs these procedures in any medical practice MUST BE FULLY DOCUMENTED IN THE COMPREHENSIVE COMPLIANCE PROGRAM OR POLICY OF THE PRACTICE! The same admonition applies to "spoliation of records," which is "the intentional destruction, alteration or concealment of relevant data: records should be kept and policy in place to prevent the destruction, tampering, alteration or concealment of electronic records."[8]

Spoliation of Records: The alteration or destruction of medical records.

SUMMARY

The medical office manager plays a key role in directing compliance with all rules and regulation regarding the HIPAA Privacy Rule and Security Regulation, fraud and abuse regulations, protection from identity theft, and maintenance of the legally sound medical record. Complete understanding of these rules will assist in the production of policy and procedure protecting the various interests of the responsible medical practice. She or he may be ably assisted in this task by a variety of resources including various federal and state Web sites and agencies, the AHIMA, and public and private organizations as well as regular contact with outside legal counsel.

CHAPTER REVIEW QUESTIONS

1. What are the seven major elements recommended by AHIMA for the development of a compliance manual addressing the medical-legal aspects of health information management?

_____

_____

_____

2. How can the medical office manager demonstrate the ability to ensure the HIPAA compliance procedures are communicated to all team members and maintained to accommodate changes?

_____

_____

3. What is the difference between fraud and abuse and what measures have been put in place by the government to eliminate fraud and abuse?

_____

_____

_____

4. What is the Red Flags Rule and give an example of how an office complies with this rule?

_____

_____

_____

5. Give an example of federal requirements governing medical records documentation.

_____

_____

_____

6. Give an example of a recommended medical record practice in the absence of a more stringent state rule.

_____

_____

_____

7. Give an example of a common type of fraud committed by dishonest providers.

_____

_____

_____

8. Recall the important distinctions between legal discovery and e-discovery particularly with respect to the LHR/EHR and the DRS.

_____

_____

_____

REFERENCES

1. Rinehart-Thompson L. A. JD, RHIA, CHP. Chapter 9. Risk Management and Liability (Figure 9.13 p.282 "Inclusions for the Notice of Privacy Practices"). In Fahrenholz, C. G. (2011). *Documentation for Medical Practices*. Chicago, IL: AHIMA.
2. Centers for Medicare and Medicaid Services. 2004. (November) HIPAA Security Series: Security 101 for Covered Entities. Volume 2, paper 1. Available at: http://www.cms.hhs.gov/EducationalMaterials/Downloads.Security101forCovered-Entities.pdf
3. Brodnik M, et al. *Fundamentals of Law for Health Informatics and Information Management*. Chicago, IL: AHIMA; 2009.
4. Combating Health Care Fraud in a Post-Reform World: Seven Guiding Principles for Policymakers. 2010. National Health Care Anti-Fraud Association White Paper http://www.nhcaa.org/eweb/docs/nhcaa/PDFs/Member%20Services/WhitePaper_Oct10.pdf
5. Department of Health and Human Services. Office of Inspector General. OIG Compliance Program for Individual and Small Group Physician Practices. September 27, 2000. http://oig.hhs.gov/authorities/docs/physician.pdf
6. Brodnik M, et al. *Fundamentals of Law for Health Informatics and Information Management*. Chicago, IL: AHIMA; 2009:332.
7. AHIMA Compliance Taskforce. Practice brief: seven steps to corporate compliance: the HIM role. *J AHIMA* 1999;70(9):84A–84F.
8. Servais C. *The Legal Health Record*. Chicago, IL: AHIMA; 2008.

Workbook for
Chapter 9

Workbook:
Chapter 9 Managing the Legal Aspects of Health Information

9.A: YOUR TURN: WRITE AN ANTIFRAUD POLICY AND PROCEDURE

Review the National Healthcare Anti-Fraud Association's list of most common types of fraud committed by dishonest providers. Select any one of these and write an office policy and procedure to demonstrate an attempt to prevent this problem.

9.B: TEAM PROJECT: COMPLETE A COMPLIANCE CHECKLIST

Access the template provided by the FTC to help smaller practice implement a compliance policy to help prevent identity theft. Complete the checklist for a fictional practice. Then brainstorm with teammates on ideas for ways to effectively disseminate this information to patients.

9.C: ILLUSTRATION: RANK SECURITY REGULATIONS IN ORDER OF IMPORTANCE

Using Figure 9.4 regarding Administrative Safeguard Standards to Assist in Implementation of HIPAA Security Regulations, rank the standards according to your perception of most important to least important and briefly explain your ranking rationale.

9.D: YOUR TURN: DESIGN A POSTER

Design a poster for a medical practice that will remind employees about the importance of medical records information safety and safe practices.

9.E: EXPERT PANEL

Recall the case scenario in this chapter.

Nancie Jones has been hired as the practice administrator. Her predecessor left without notice due to a conflict with the managing physician. On her first day of employment, she has been given access codes to the electronic medical record file by the receptionist of the practice. She notes that the system was installed 24 months prior to her hiring and has not been updated since that time. During an orientation meeting with staff, a clerk comes to Nancie with a report that one day before she left, Nancie's predecessor responded to a call for assistance from the clerk who complained that the system continually froze up on her and that Nancie's predecessor apparently fixed the problem by inserting a flash drive into the staffers computer and typing some commands. The next day, Nancie is inundated with calls: one from a patient who was referred to psychotherapy who complains he has been denied access to his medical record, another from a patient whose insurance indicated a bill for a procedure the patient claims never took place, another is a report that a scheduled surgery of a patient has to be cancelled due to conflicting information on the patient's medical history, and another patient reports experiencing harassing phone calls from durable medical equipment providers regarding sexual dysfunction therapy. The final call of the day is from an attorney who demands any and every piece of data ever produced, kept, archived, or sent for destruction concerning his client, a former patient.

Nancie has identified many issues that should be addressed. Your assignment is to ascertain as many potential privacy, security, identity theft, or other legal issues as you can and then identify what steps the administrator should take to respond to one of these issues. You will most likely need to research your solution using one of the resources mentioned in this chapter. Your instructor may have you break into teams or respond as an individual expert. Each team or individual needs to document the steps in the solution to the issue chosen.

10

Managing Health Information Technology

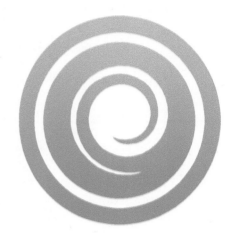

Upon completion of this chapter, the student should...

- Define and differentiate between electronic health records (EHRs), electronic medical records (EMRs), and patient health records (PHRs)
- Describe the limitations of paper-based health records and why EHRs are important
- List the key components of an EHR
- Describe the 2009 Medicare and Medicaid reimbursement for EHRs
- List the key functions of a practice management (PM) system.
- Identify the key advantages and obstacles in converting from paper records and a stand-alone PM system to an integrated or interfaced EHR with PM software
- Document strategies for evaluating, selecting, purchasing, and implementing the best EHR/PM system for a practice's size, specialty, and culture
- Document the workflow in a medical office that utilizes a PM system integrated or interfaced with an EHR
- Discuss how health information is exchanged between medical offices and other entities
- Discuss the advantages of patient portals and describe how they are used in medical practices

Center for Information Technology Leadership (CITL)

Certification Commission for Healthcare Information Technology (CCHIT)

Claim

Electronic Health Record (EHR)

Electronic Medical Record (EMR)

Personal Health Record (PHR)

Health Information Exchange (HIE)

Health Information Organization (HIO)

Interoperability

Modular

Nationwide Health Information Network (NHIN)

ONC-Authorized Testing and Certification Bodies (ONC-ATCBs)

Patient Portals

Regional Extension Centers (RECs)

Regional Health Information Organization (RHIO)

Request for Information (RFI)

Request for Proposal (RFP)

Secure Messaging

⊗ OVERVIEW

Leading people through change is one of the most challenging aspects of being a practice administrator. Health information technology changes at such a rapid pace that a successful administrator must constantly balance the processing of new information with the most effective way of communicating and implementing change to the team—in a manner that promotes trust and enthusiasm. The purpose of this chapter is to provide a foundation of general knowledge regarding the importance of health information technology, what is currently available, and how to move a practice forward toward optimizing technology.

⊗ ELECTRONIC HEALTH RECORDS

Electronic health records (EHRs) have been central to the discussion of health care reform in the United States. EHRs have been touted to improve patient safety, productivity, and the quality of medical care.[1,2] Furthermore, electronic patient data produced by EHRs can be used for multiple purposes: disease management, pay for performance, coordination of care, and research. EHRs have the potential to generate volumes of important patient data that can be mined and used for improving the practice of medicine. That is why the federal government chose to reimburse clinicians and hospitals in the stimulus package for the use of EHRs, which we discuss in another section.

The history of EHRs in the United States is relatively short, occurring over the past three decades. In 1991, the Institute of Medicine (IOM) recommended EHRs as a solution for many of the problems facing modern medicine, but since then little progress has been made for multiple reasons.[3]

We only discuss outpatient (ambulatory) EHRs in this chapter. Inpatient EHRs share many similarities to ambulatory EHRs, but the scope, price, and complexity are different. In this section, we discuss the EHR adoption rate, important definitions, the importance and obstacles of EHRs, key EHR components, the EHR spectrum, stimulus package reimbursement, and an overview of how to purchase and implement an ambulatory EHR.

Ambulatory EHR Adoption

In 2008, a study reported on the adoption rate of outpatient EHRs in the United States. Osteopaths, residents, and federal physicians were excluded from this survey so the overall U.S. adoption rate is probably higher. The most significant finding was that only 4% of respondents reported using a comprehensive EHR (order entry capability and clinical decision support), whereas 13% reported using a basic EHR system. This study, along with others, reported that the adoption rate was much higher for large medical groups or medical centers. Importantly, physicians who responded to this survey did report multiple beneficial effects of using EHRs.[4]

Definitions

In 2008, the National Alliance for Health Information Technology (NAHIT) released the following definitions in an effort to standardize terms used in HIT. For consistency, we have adopted these definitions:

Electronic medical record (EMR): "An electronic record of health-related information on an individual that can be created, gathered, managed and consulted by authorized clinicians and staff within one healthcare organization."

Electronic health record (EHR): "An electronic record of health-related information on an individual that conforms to nationally recognized interoperability standards and that can be created, managed and consulted by authorized clinicians and staff across more than one healthcare organization."

Personal health record (PHR): "An electronic record of health-related information on an individual that conforms to nationally recognized interoperability standards and that can be drawn from multiple sources while being managed, shared and controlled by the individual."[5]

Why are EHRs important?

The Paper Record Is Severely Limited

Much of what can be said about the limitations of handwritten prescriptions can also be said about handwritten office notes. Shortcomings of paper include illegibility; expensive to copy, transport, and store; easy to destroy; difficult to analyze and determine who has seen it; and the negative impact on the environment. Electronic records represent a quantum leap forward in legibility and speed to retrieve information.

It is much easier to retrieve and track patient data using EHRs and patient registries than to use labor intensive paper chart reviews (Fig. 10.1). EHRs are much better organized than paper charts and much of patient data is computable, thus allowing data mining. Studies show that paper charts are missing 25% of the time and even when present, missing information is noted 14% of the time.[6,7] According to the President's Information Technology Advisory Committee, 20% of laboratory tests are reordered because previous studies are not accessible.[8]

Electronic Medical Record (EMR): An electronic record of health-related information on an individual that can be created, gathered, managed, and consulted by authorized clinicians and staff within one health care organization.

Electronic Health Records: An electronic record of health-related information on an individual that conforms to nationally recognized interoperability standards and that can be created, managed, and consulted by authorized clinicians and staff across more than on health care organization.

Personal Health Records (PHRs): A health record where health data is maintained and controlled by individual users themselves.

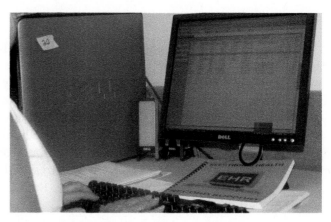

Figure 10.1 EHR screen on computer.

The Need for Improved Efficiency and Productivity

The goal is to have patient information available to anyone who needs it, when they need it, and where they need it. With an EHR, lab results can be retrieved much more rapidly, thus saving time and money. EHRs are more efficient because they reduce redundant paperwork, faxing, and have the capability of interfacing with practice management (PM) systems that submit claims electronically. EHRs can help with productivity if templates are used judiciously. Templates allow for point and click histories and physical exams, thus saving time. Several EHR companies also offer a centralized area for all physician approvals and signatures of lab work, prescriptions, etc. This improves workflow by avoiding the need to pull multiple charts or enter multiple EHR modules.

The Need for Improved Quality of Care and Patient Safety

EHRs improve medical quality and patient safety through many mechanisms: (1) improved legibility of clinical notes; (2) improved access anytime and anywhere; (3) reminders that tests or preventive services are overdue; (4) clinical decision support that reminds clinicians of patient allergies, correct drug dosages, etc.; (5) electronic problem summary lists provide diagnoses, allergies, and surgeries at a glance; and (6) disease registries that organize all patients with a specific disease such as diabetes. Health care organizations have been able to manage large groups or entire populations with these electronic tools. As an example, Kaiser Permanente used EHR data and determined that the drug Vioxx had an increased risk of cardiovascular events before that information was published.[9] Similarly, within 90 minutes of learning of the withdrawal of Vioxx from the market, the Cleveland Clinic queried its EHR to see which patients were on the drug. Within 7 hours, they deactivated prescriptions and notified clinicians via e-mail.[10]

EHRs can include clinical practice guidelines that are embedded or linked, to provide clinicians with treatment and prevention guidance, at the point of care.

Financial Savings

The Center for Information Technology Leadership (CITL) has suggested that ambulatory EHRs would save $44 billion yearly and eliminate more than $10 in rejected claims per patient per outpatient visit. CITL concludes that not only would there be savings from eliminated chart rooms and record clerks, there would be a reduction in the need for transcription. There would also be fewer callbacks from pharmacists with electronic prescribing. It has been shown that copying and labor costs would be reduced with EHRs. More rapid retrieval of lab and x-ray reports results in time saving as does the use of templates. More efficient patient encounters mean more patients could be seen each day. Improved savings from medication management is possible with reminders to use the "drug of choice" and generics.[11] Furthermore, it is believed that EHRs improve the level of coding. Templates may help remind clinicians to add more history or details of the physical exam, thus justifying a higher level of coding.

It is not known if EHR adoption will decrease malpractice, hence saving physician and hospital costs. A 2007 survey by the Medical Records Institute of 115 practices involving specialties showed that 20% of malpractice carriers offered a discount for having an EHR in place. Of those physicians who had a malpractice case in which documentation was based on an EHR, 55% said the EHR was helpful.[12]

Improved Patient Care Coordination

According to a Gallup poll, it is extremely common for older patients to have multiple physicians, thus mandating good communication between primary care physicians, specialists, and patients.[13] This becomes even more of an issue when different health care systems are involved. A survey of patients with chronic conditions showed that 18% of the population received duplicate tests or procedures, 17% received conflicting information from other clinicians, and 14% received different diagnoses from different physicians.[14] In the future, EHRs will be integrated with health information exchanges, so that inpatient and outpatient information can be shared, therefore improving care coordination. Home monitoring (telehomecare) can transmit patient data from home to an office EHR, also assisting in the coordination of care.

EHR Obstacles

Financial Barriers

Although there is evidence that ambulatory EHRs can save money, the reality is they are expensive. Multiple studies report that lack of funding is the number one barrier to EHR adoption.[15] In a 2005 study published in *Health Affairs*, initial EHR costs averaged $44 K (range $14 to $63,000) per FTE (full time equivalent) and ongoing costs of $8.5 K per FTE. These costs included the purchase of new hardware, etc. Financial benefits averaged about $33,000 per FTE provider per year due to improved efficiencies and more than half the benefit was from improved coding. This study looked at 14 primary care practices using two well-known EHRs. The average practice showed a return on investment (ROI) in only 2.5 years.[16]

Center for Information Technology Leadership (CITL): An academic research organization founded in 2002 and focused on assessing the impacts and costs of health information technologies.

Physician Resistance

Another leading obstacle for EHR adoption is physician resistance. Clinicians have to be shown a new technology makes money, saves time, or is good for their patients. None of these can be proven for certain for every practice. EHR adoption will reduce productivity in the office for 3 to 12 months, which is difficult for clinicians, even though their productivity will likely improve above baseline in the future. There are many legitimate concerns by clinicians such as workflow interference, security, ease of use, concerns about ROI, and future modifications. We now know that some practices have opted to change or discontinue their use of an EHR. A 2007 survey demonstrated that fewer than 20% of respondents had uninstalled their EHR in an effort to step down to a less expensive alternative and 8% had returned to paper.[17]

Lack of Data Standards

One can assume that an EHR purchased today will not communicate with other EHRs, although vendors are being pressured to make their products interoperable. The Certification Commission for Healthcare Information Technology (CCHIT) was established with the goal of certifying technologies, such as EHRs, to include interoperability standards.[18]

Loss of Productivity

Most physicians will have to work at reduced capacity for several months with gradual improvement depending on training, aptitude, etc. This is a period when physician champions can help maintain momentum with a positive attitude.

Separating Fact from Fiction

It is important to critically evaluate EHRs and avoid hyperbole. Clinical decision support systems (CDSS), such as alerts and reminders are relatively new and have not been adequately studied.[19] Moreover, reports from medical centers that have used homegrown systems for many years cannot be compared to the average medical office or hospital. Also, there have been several studies that have shown increased errors as a result of implementing computerized order entry.[20,21]

EHR Key Components

The IOM set forth eight EHR core functions[22] they felt were transformational:

- Health information and data: lists diagnoses, medications, allergies, patient demographics, encounters, and lab results
- Result management: the ability to rapidly retrieve results, consultations, x-rays (images), etc.

- Order management: the ability to electronically order medications, labs, images, etc.
- Decision support: includes reminders for tests such as mammograms and alerts about drug allergies, drug–drug interactions, etc.
- Electronic communication and connectivity: the ability to communicate electronically with other clinicians as well as secure e-mail and electronic interfaces with disparate systems. Interoperability is discussed in another section.
- Patient support: patient education can be generated from the EHR and home monitoring (blood sugars, blood pressures, etc.) can be inputted into some EHRs
- Administrative processes: includes scheduling, eligibility, billing, and claims management
- Reporting and population health: includes internal and external quality reports, disease management, biosurveillance, etc.

In order to carry out the eight functions above as well as a few additional ones, the following components are desirable in any EHR:

- Computerized physician order entry (CPOE) used for inpatient and outpatient ordering of labs, x-rays, medications, consults, etc.
- CDSS to include alerts, reminders, and clinical practice guidelines. CDSS is associated with CPOE.
- Secure messaging (e-mail) for communication between patients and office staff and among office staff. Telephone triage capability is important.
- An interface with PM software, scheduling software, and patient portal (if present). This feature will handle billing and benefits determination.
- Managed care module for physician and site profiling. This includes the ability to track Health Plan Employer Data and Information Set or similar measurements and basic cost analyses.
- Referral management feature
- Retrieval of lab and x-ray reports electronically
- Retrieval of prior encounters and medication histories
- Electronic patient encounters
- Multiple ways to input information into the encounter: free text (typing), dictation, voice recognition, and templates
- The ability to input or access information via a PDA, smartphone, or tablet PC
- Remote access from the office or home
- Electronic prescribing
- Integration with a picture archiving and communication system
- Knowledge resources for physician and patient, embedded or linked
- Public health reporting and tracking
- Ability to generate quality reports for reimbursement

- Problem summary list that is customizable and includes the major aspects of care: diagnoses, allergies, surgeries, and medications. Also, the ability to label the problems as acute or chronic, active or inactive.
- Ability to scan in text or use optical character recognition
- Ability to perform evaluation and management (E&M) determination for billing
- Ability to create graphs or flow sheets of lab results or vital signs
- Ability to create electronic patient lists or disease registries
- Preventive medicine tracking that links to clinical practice guidelines
- Security compliant with HIPAA standards
- Backup systems in place
- Ability to generate an interoperable patient summary document known as a continuity of care document or continuity of care report
- Client-server or application service provider (ASP) options: a standard client-server EHR package, which means having the software on your own computers and servers. The other choice is an ASP that uses a remote server that hosts the EHR software and your patient data. Each has its merits and shortcomings. Features of an ASP model:
  - Vendor charges monthly fees to provide access to patient data on a remote server. Fees will usually include maintenance, software upgrades, data backups, and help desk support.
  - Pros: Lower start-up costs; ASP maintains and updates software; requires very little local tech support, thus saves money. Often a better choice for small practices with less IT support. Enables remote log-ons, for example, from home, hospital, or satellite offices.
  - Cons: If your ISP is not working, you aren't either; concerns about security and HIPAA; concerns about who owns the data and cost of monthly cable fees. Speed may be a little slower compared to the client-server model. Must have fast Internet connection; should be cable modem, DSL, or T1 line.[23]

EHR Systems Available

If a medical practice desires Medicaid or Medicare reimbursement from the stimulus package, they will have to select EHRs that are certified and meet "meaningful use" criteria (next section). At the time of publication, there was no final definition of meaningful use and there may be several certifying organizations, in addition to CCHIT. There are over 300 EHR vendors with prices ranging from free such as Practice Fusion[24] to approximately $50,000 per clinician for initial purchase. Furthermore, there are an increasing number of open source EHRs that are unassociated with a licensing fee but generally require contractor support for installation, maintenance, and customization.[25] At least one survey would suggest that there is no clear correlation between the price of the EHR and user satisfaction.[26] Purchasing a top of the line EHR, particularly a client-server model, may mandate in-house tech staff. For smaller clinics and those with little technology expertise, the ASP model

Table 10.1	Medicare reimbursement for EHRs						
Adoption Y	Y 1	Y 2	Y 3	Y 4	Y 5	Total	Penalty
2011 or 2012	$18,000	$12,000	$8,000	$4,000	$2,000	$44,000	0
2013	$15,000	$12,000	$8,000	$4,000	0	$39,000	0
2014	$15,000	$12,000	$8,000	0	0	$35,000	0
2015	0	0	0	0	0		1%
2016	0	0	0	0	0		2%
2017	0	0	0	0	0		3%
2018	0	0	0	0	0		3%–4%
2019 +	0	0	0	0	0		3%–5%

is strongly recommended. Be aware that the majority of EHR vendors do not list charges on their Web site and they expect to negotiate the price. Exceptions to this rule are SOAPware[27] and eClinical[28] works that post their charges clearly on their Web sites.

EHRs and the American Recovery and Reinvestment Act of 2009

Tables 10.1 and 10.2 cover American Recovery and Reinvestment Act (ARRA)-based Medicare and Medicaid reimbursement for EHR adoption. At the time of publication it was clear that EHRs would have to be certified and meet meaningful use criteria, defined broadly as the requirements of electronic order entry, interoperability, quality report generation, and electronic prescribing. The final definition of meaningful use was not available until the spring of 2010. Reimbursement is for nonhospital-based physicians and they cannot be reimbursed by both Medicare and Medicaid. For Medicaid reimbursement, clinicians must have 30% Medicaid volume (20% for pediatricians).[29]

Beginning in 2010, the ONC created ONC-Authorized Testing and Certification Bodies (ONC-ATCBs) as follows from the Official Government Health IT Web site (http://healthit.hhs.gov/portal/server.pt/community/healthit_hhs_gov__home/1204):

ONC-Authorized Testing and Certification Bodies (ONC-ATCBs): Authorized by the Office of the National Coordinator for Health Information Technology, ONC-ATCBs are required to test and certify that certain types of EHR technology (complete EHRs and EHR modules) are compliant with the standards, implementation specifications, and certification criteria adopted by the HHS secretary and meet the definition of certified EHR technology.

Table 10.2	Medicaid Reimbursement for EHRs						
Clinician	Y 1	Y 2	Y 3	Y 4	Y 5	Y 6	Total
Physician	$21,250	$8,500	$8,500	$8,500	$8,500	$8,500	$63,750
Certified nurse midwife	$21,250	$8,500	$8,500	$8,500	$8,500	$8,500	$63,750
Dentist	$21,250	$8,500	$8,500	$8,500	$8,500	$8,500	$63,750
Nurse practitioner	$21,250	$8,500	$8,500	$8,500	$8,500	$8,500	$63,750
Physician assistant	$21,250	$8,500	$8,500	$8,500	$8,500	$8,500	$63,750

ONC-ATCBs

The following organizations have been selected as ONC-ATCBs:
Certified Health IT Product List

The online list of certified EHR technology is updated as ONC-Authorized Testing and Certification Bodies certify new products.

- Surescripts LLC —Arlington, VA
  Date of authorization: December 23, 2010.
  Scope of authorization: EHR Modules: E-Prescribing, Privacy and Security.

- ICSA Labs —Mechanicsburg, PA
  Date of authorization: December 10, 2010.
  Scope of authorization: Complete EHR and EHR Modules.

- SLI Global Solutions —Denver, CO
  Date of authorization: December 10, 2010.
  Scope of authorization: Complete EHR and EHR Modules.

- InfoGard Laboratories, Inc. —San Luis Obispo, CA
  Date of authorization: September 24, 2010.
  Scope of authorization: Complete EHR and EHR Modules.

- Certification Commission for Health Information Technology (CCHIT)—Chicago, IL
  Date of authorization: September 3, 2010.
  Scope of authorization: Complete EHR and EHR Modules.

- Drummond Group, Inc. (DGI)—Austin, TX
  Date of authorization: September 3, 2010.
  Scope of authorization: Complete EHR and EHR Modules.

The organizations listed above have been authorized to perform Complete EHR and/or EHR Module testing and certification. These ONC-ATCBs are required to test and certify EHRs to the applicable certification criteria adopted by the secretary under subpart C of Part 170 Part II and Part III as stipulated in the Standards and Certification Criteria Final Rule.

Certification by an ATCB will signify to eligible professionals, hospitals, and critical access hospitals that an EHR technology has the capabilities necessary to support their efforts to meet the goals and objectives of meaningful use.

Check this Web site for updates at the time a practice is interested in selecting an EHR that meets the meaningful use criteria.

INTEGRATED PRACTICE MANAGEMENT SYSTEMS

Overview of Practice Management Systems

Most medical offices have had computerized practice management systems (PMS) for many years, regardless of whether that office maintains paper medical records, EHRs, or records that are a hybrid of these two.

As we will point out, there are many reasons why PM systems have become so prevalent but one of the main reasons is for more rapid claims submission and adjudication. Without an electronic system, time and money would be lost on faxes, phone calls, and snail mail. The American Medical Association estimated that inefficient claims submission systems lead to about $210 billion annually in unnecessary costs.[30] A PM system is designed to capture all of the data from a patient encounter necessary to obtain reimbursement for the services provided. This data is then used to

Claim: A standardized document–CMS 1500 in the case of health care practitioners containing all necessary information and submitted to a third-party payer in order for the practitioner to be reimbursed for eligible services provided to a patient who has health insurance.

- Generate claims to seek reimbursement from health care payers
- Apply payments and denials
- Generate patient statements for any balance that is the patient's responsibility
- Generate business correspondence
- Build databases for practice and referring physicians, payers, patient demographics, and encounter transaction (i.e., date, diagnosis codes, procedure codes, amount charged, amount paid, date paid, billing messages, place and type of service codes, etc.)

Additionally, a PM system provides routine and ad hoc reports so that an administrator can analyze the trends for a given practice and implement performance improvement strategies based on the findings. For example, a medical office administrator is able to use the PM system to compare and contrast different payers with regard to the amount reimbursed for each given service or the turnaround time between claims submission and payment. The results lead to deciding which managed care plans the practice will participate in versus those plans that the practice may want to consider not accepting in the future. Another example is to analyze all payers for a given service performed in the practice to determine if that service is a good use of the practice's clinical time. This analysis provides one aspect of whether the practice should consider continuing to offer a certain service such as case management of a patient who is receiving a home health service. Of course, the administrator has to weigh services that aren't profitable against any negative impact on overall patient loyalty, but the PM system provides a means of analyzing payment performance.

Most PM systems also offer patient scheduling software that further increases the efficiency of the business aspects of a medical practice. Finally, some PM systems offer an encoder to assist the coder in selecting and sequencing the correct diagnosis (International Classification of Diseases, current revision, clinically modified for use in the US or ICD-X-CM) and procedure (Current Procedural Terminology, fourth edition or CPT-4 and Healthcare Common Procedure Coding System or HCPCS) codes. Even when a physician determines the appropriate codes using a "superbill," a list of the common codes used in that practice along with the amount charged for each procedure, there are times when a diagnosis or procedure isn't listed on the superbill and an encoder makes it efficient to do a search based on the main terms and select the best code. Furthermore, some encoders are packaged with tools such as a subscription to the American Medical Association's "CPT Assistant" that help the practice comply with correct coding initiatives, which in turn optimize the reimbursement to which the practice is legally and ethically entitled and avoids fraud or abuse fines for improper coding.

Clinical and Administrative Workflow in an Electronic Medical Office

The practice administrator must be aware of workflow regardless of the status of paper versus EHRs. It is of special importance to the success of implementing an EHR system integrated with PM software to analyze where any inefficiencies in current workflow may be found to avoid just moving an inefficiency over from a manual to an electronic process. Recall from Chapter 1, several steps are common to almost any medical practice with regard to treating patients and getting reimbursed properly for the services provided. The first step is to get the patient registered. In a fully electronic medical office, this can be accomplished via a practice Web site or by secure messaging, which is discussed in more detail later in this chapter. For each step of the typical office workflow, there are functions available using an integrated PM system with a robust EHR that increase the efficiency and accuracy of each step of the patient encounter process.

Patient Registration and Scheduling

If a practice offers Web-based patient registration, there are some choices ranging from designing the Web site and all applicable online forms internally to contracting with a forms services company. Based on the amount of money the practice is willing to spend, a forms company offers basic forms design for use on the practice's own Web site. Alternately, they can subcontract to use the company's server and Web site for forms design, updating, processing, and transmitting information to the practice's EHR or PM system. See Medical Web Office services[30] for a sample range of forms and communications services available for medical practices.

Patient Check-In

Scanning patient demographic information is an option with an EHR. Most practices that have a PM system that is integrated with an EHR can scan the documents (including bubble sheets completed by the patient at time of registration) into the system once and the information is posted to the appropriate places in both the EHR and the PM system. Sometimes the data that is used by both the EHR and the PM software, such as patient name, is saved to a common database in an integrated system. Other times, however, the shared data is communicated electronically between the EHR and the PM system even though the databases are separate. It is important to know that when the systems have a shared database, this database only contains the part of the clinical record that is used to obtain reimbursement such as the patient demographics, diagnoses and procedures, and dates of service. However, the purely financial information is only found in the PM system—such as amount billed and amount paid or information about health plans.

This is because it is not advisable to combine the business aspects of health information with clinical aspects. What procedure is done on a given date and the diagnosis that justifies the medical necessity of a procedure is both clinical and financial, but how much the procedure costs, how much the patient paid out of pocket, etc., is purely financial.

Clinical Encounter

In an EHR system, clinicians have several options for inputting patient information into the clinical record. They can use voice recognition software, standard dictation, or templates. This can be accomplished on a PC or in a wireless mode with a tablet PC or PDA. For example, an EHR is formatted with physician workflow in mind and then customizable by each individual physician to optimize efficiency based on specialty and personal preferences. The customization "initially takes time and patience but is well worth the effort in a practice that sees a lot of patients daily with the same symptoms such as an ear infection for a pediatrician."[32] Therefore, when the physician is face to face with the patient, the EHR would have already been started for that encounter by a nurse or other physician extender who would have entered the patient's chief complaint, vital signs, and possibly any updates to the patient's subjective history. Clinical notes are compiled in what is known as SOAP order. This acronym represents the *s*ubjective and *o*bjective findings, *a*ssessment, and *p*lan for each patient. Therefore, the patient's description of the chief complaint and responses to questions about body systems (review of systems) is the subjective portion of SOAP notes. The physician will continue building the encounter notes by using a series of drop-down menus to indicate body systems examined, tests performed, tests or prescriptions ordered (the objective portion of the SOAP notes), the assessment, and the plan. Each selection made by the physician adds to the clinical notes. If free text is required to further clarify a selection, there are options based on the type of information so the free text is displayed in the proper location in the encounter notes. If a physician prefers not to use the free text option, naturally speaking software is available in many EHRs to electronically transcribe the dictation and place it appropriately in the notes. An alternative to naturally speaking software that many physicians prefer is to hire a medical scribe. A scribe is trained to follow the physician throughout the patient encounter in order to capture all pertinent dialogue for live input directly into the EHR, via a wireless device. Another option is to dictate the encounter and have a transcriptionist manually update the record using a combination of drop-down options and free text. The disadvantage is that the note isn't ready to print out for the patient at the end of the visit and the physician has to double-check the notes at a later date, when his or her memory is not as fresh, in order to electronically sign the note.

Clinical notes are a good example of data that is maintained in the EHR but not shared with a PM system. However, EHRs that use computer-assisted coding technology can convert the standardized notes into codes and the codes are used by both the EHR and the PM system. For example, many EHRs can run the office notes through logic to assign CPT evaluation and management (E&M) codes based on either the 1995 or 1997 guidelines. The EHR system can pass these codes plus many ICD-9-CM/ICD-10-CM codes over to integrated (same vendor) or interfaced (different vendors) PM system when the systems are compatible. However, a person responsible for correct coding and billing must still verify that all applicable codes were brought over to the PM system, add any codes that the system did not assign automatically since it does not completely code all diagnoses and procedures for every encounter, and scrub the codes, which means to link the diagnoses to the correct procedures to justify medical necessity and check for obvious errors in order to get them ready to submit as claims to payers. The physician then discharges the patient with any applicable drug samples and patient education literature. Any lab samples are sent to the lab and, if the patient needs a prescription and the practice uses e-prescribing, a prescription is sent from the EHR to the pharmacy electronically or via Fax.

Patient Checkout

The EHR can interface with the PM system scheduler so the physician can schedule a follow-up visit and the patient can take home a printout of the office notes, any education material, date and time of the next appointment, information on any scheduled lab or imaging center appointments ordered electronically by the practitioner, and any prescriptions ordered through electronic prescribing.

Charge Entry and Claim Generation/Submission

In an integrated PM with EHR system, the information needed is sent directly from the EHR to the PM system and a claim is built as described above. Once the claim is built in an electronic system, the claims are sent, usually to a clearinghouse for editing, and then out to the appropriate payers for processing.

Receipt of Remittance Advice and Explanation of Benefits

In electronic processing, a deposit is made electronically directly into the practice's bank account by the payer and the practice receives a notice of the amount deposited and the details of which payments were made on which line of service within each claim processed on that particular remittance advice.

Payment Posting

Electric remittance advices automatically update the PMS but, depending on the system, there is a varying degree of work required by the billing specialist in order to ensure every service is updated appropriately and any outstanding balances that aren't written off are in a status to be sent in the next cycle to either a secondary payer or the patient.

Reporting

Integrated EHR with PM systems are capable of producing standard and customized reports. These reports can help analyze virtually any business aspect of the practice as well as researching patient clinical trends and other clinical reports for analysis.

Telephone calls in a medical office

As discussed earlier, telephone calls to a practice are extremely varied in nature and must be handled in a manner that ensures patient safety first with customer service always being an important aspect of building patient loyalty. Many EHR systems enable the message taker to electronically route the call directly to the intended recipient instead of having to take a paper message. In this case, protocols exist in which the person answering the phone can take certain actions or make some decisions. For example, the receptionist may be able to determine if outside lab results have been received by the practice or not. If they have, the receptionist can route a message directly to the appropriate clinician requesting the patient be called regarding the results. In more urgent cases, a patient may have a nonemergency, but urgent condition and request to be seen that day. The receptionist may be able to schedule that person and tell them when to arrive. If the receptionist is uncertain, he or she may route an urgent message to the most appropriate clinician for a decision about whether the patient can be seen that day. The messages go directly to the recipient's attention and may be color coded to highlight urgent versus nonurgent.[33,34]

Practice Management Systems and EHRs

When the administrators of a medical practice commit to the conversion of paper-based or hybrid records to an EHR system, they should strongly consider converting their existing PMS to one that is integrated with the EHR they chose. Although this strategy means a higher initial investment of both time and money, many practices report that part of their overall success with implementing an EHR with a PM system is due to the increased efficiency and accuracy of the billing process when the systems are integrated. One alternative to discontinuing an existing PM system—especially one that works very well and that everyone in the office who uses it is comfortable with—is to find a reputable EHR vendor that offers interface capabilities with your existing PM system vendor. For example, Eclipsys has a list of PM systems with which their EHR interfaces. One potential setback is anytime a vendor upgrades its software, the interfaces have to be tested and both vendors may need to get involved.

As mentioned earlier in this chapter, formal studies of ROI for an EHR in medical practices are very limited at this time and although some of these studies mention how many of the practices surveyed implemented an EHR in conjunction with an integrated PMS, they don't differentiate the results as to the impact on ROI of an integrated EHR/PM system versus a stand-alone EHR project.

There are some testimonials and customer information pages available on many of the vendor Web sites that discuss success stories of EHR implementation in which some of the cost savings were realized by the integration of the EHR with a PM system. Some of these Web sites also list the ROI based on an integrated EHR/PM system.[35,36]

For example, e-MDs, inc., has an ROI page on their Web site under the topic of education. "Six Ways to Return On Investment: Using an electronic medical record integrated with a robust practice management application can generate real cost savings as well as enhanced revenue. The scope of improved efficiency varies with degree of implementation, and includes reduced labor costs, improved cash flow, streamlined clinical and financial management workflow, increased reimbursement, and detailed financial reporting. All these factors can contribute to making a healthcare delivery system of any size more profitable... In a best case scenario, assuming you expense all costs up front, the combination of better billing and reduced costs results in an estimated increase in income of $118,000 per physician in the first year. After the first year, the increase in income from pre-EMR deployment can be as high as $158,500 annually. It can be expected that offices which do not operate at peak efficiency, or avail themselves of all of the EMR time-saving features, should be roughly 50% of these numbers."

Another example is a quote from a single physician practice manager who implemented an integrated EHR/PM System from e-ClinicalWorks. "Every day before I leave the office, all claims are posted, audited and electronically sent out. Filing claims is simple and it's now done every day. With our last system, Medical Manager, we filed once a week because of the cumbersome nature of the software. Therefore, we have much less insurance outstanding in the older categories. We can work the claims more quickly bringing in money more quickly. Your dollar is worth much more when you bring it in sooner rather than later. Or, if there is a claim rejected, we can fix the problem with the push of a button and resubmit a corrected claim much earlier in the process—again making A/R in better shape."

In March 2008, the Medical Society of New York reported on the experience of a solo, internal medicine practice in identifying, purchasing, implementing, and maintaining an EHR with a PM system. Some of the highlights from this article include

- Choosing an in-office server over ASP because it was more affordable since the practice already had old computers that could be used as workstations and they did not already have business-grade broadband Internet service provider necessary for an ASP arrangement
- Choosing to pay a monthly subscription fee to use the EHR/PM software because it was less expensive than purchasing software and hardware required. Lease agreement was approximately $400 per month for software and off-site HIT support.
- HIT vendor providing most of the on-site technical support during the first three months
- Choosing the EHR from same vendor as PM, because "to run an efficient office, the two systems should be totally compatible and ideally share the same database."
- The criteria most important to Dr. Volpe included performing the same functions as a paper record only better affordability and navigability for all users between both the EHR and the PM systems;

adaptability—the records and templates for information were easily modified and customized as patient information and practice needs changed; track record of vendor, ease of data entry, tight security, and CCHIT certification

- The transition from paper was easy (by comparison) for the doctor and his staff because they had already used an e-prescribing system and a patient Web portal. They transitioned from the old billing system to the new PM system gradually over 30 to 90 days by using the old system for any patient billing that was in process or occurred before the staff training was complete and then used the new system for all encounters occurring after the staff was trained.

- The overall assessment considering the improvement in efficiency, improved patient care, and improved claims coding and submission is "within one year, Dr. Volpe had paid off the cost of his new hardware, his office had returned to full productivity, and he was earning over $30,000 more than he had the year before, due primarily to reduced overhead costs (space for paper records has been converted to an additional exam room, for example). He, his family, his staff and his patients all love the new system."[37]

According to a recent newsletter offered by the Health Information Management Systems Society (HIMSS), "A tool was recently launched to measure the healthcare industry's move from paper-based processes to electronic business applications. Called the US Healthcare Efficiency Index, this tool is intended to raise awareness about the cost savings that can be achieved by increasing the adoption of electronic business processes. One third of respondents believed that the largest cost savings would come in the area of claims submission. Nearly half of respondents that work for a healthcare provider organization reported that they submitted claims payments electronically. A similar percent also reported that their organization submitted claims eligibility and claim remittance advice transactions electronically. Another potential area of cost savings would be to have claims payments issued via direct deposit."[38]

Steps to Purchase an EHR Integrated or Interfaced with a PM system

The following are phases and steps to purchase and implement an EHR. These phases are based on the model of choosing to implement an integrated EHR with PM system but the steps are similar for implementing a stand-alone EHR or one that will be interfaced with an existing system.

Phase I: Planning

1. Develop an office strategy. It is the practice administrator's responsibility to coordinate with the physicians and list priorities for the practice. Now is the time to study workflow and see how it will change your practice. This is when frequent conferences with your front office staff will be critical to get their input about the processes that need to improve. This collaboration with staff will increase morale, decrease anxiety, and generally result in a team effort.

> **TIP**
>
> The amount of effective planning is directly related to the success of implementing a new system.

While working with staff in the planning and analysis of current processes stage, the administrator should also look for at least one physician champion, meaning a physician that will assist in getting the other physicians and clinical staff to overcome resistance to change. Keep your staff well—informed, involved, and onboard. Factor in future requirements: more partners, offices, or specialties? Plan for initial decreased productivity. Use a checklist to stay organized.[39] Begin the educational process by reading one of several helpful books on EHRs and informatics or taking a course.

2. List the EHR features you need (known as functional requirements). Review the key components section. Choose the method of inputting: keyboard, mouse, stylus, touch screen, or voice recognition? Determine if any of the physicians will prefer to use a medical scribe either initially or long term but discourage traditional transcription since scanned documents, unlike data keyed directly into the EHR templates, are not able to be analyzed.

3. Decide on client-server versus the ASP option.

4. Decide early on if you plan to purchase a combined EHR and PMS or do you need an interface to be created with your existing PM system?

5. Survey hardware and network needs. How many more computers will you need to buy? Do you need to hard-wire a network and/or are you going wireless? Are you going to need an in-house server with its dedicated closet, air conditioning, and backup? Do you need a network switch and commercial-grade firewall? You will need backup and a disaster plan. Plan for a commercial-grade uninterruptible power supply. Also, plan for a service-level agreement if you opt for the ASP model.

6. What interfaces do you need? Will you need interfaces to external laboratory, pharmacy, and radiology services or is that part of the package purchased?

7. Do you need third-party software? As an example: patient education material, ICD-9 codes, CPT codes, HCPCS database, SNOMED, drug database, voice recognition, etc. Ask if that is part of the purchased package. Also be sure to ask if the contract will cover upgrades to accommodate conversion from ICD-9-CM to ICD-10.

8. Address financing. Many offices will evaluate if they qualify for stimulus package reimbursement, covered in another section.

9. Although paper chart conversion is covered in phase III, discussion should start early.

Phase II: EHR Selection

1. Develop your vendor strategy. Write a simple "request for proposal" (RFP) or "request for information" (RFI). This will cause you to put on paper all of your requirements. Each vendor will need to respond in writing how they plan to address them. Exact pricing should be part of the RFP. Sample RFPs are available on the Web.[40] There is a Web-based search engine that will search 324 EHR vendors with the filters for practice specialty, practice size, ASP versus client server, EHR or EHR plus PMS, and whether the

Request for Proposal (RFP): A process at the beginning of a project whereby an invitation is presented for suppliers, often through a bidding process, to submit a proposal on a specific commodity or service.

Request for Information (RFI): A business process whose purpose is to collect written information about the capabilities of various suppliers, normally following a format that can be used for comparative purposes and often used in combination with the request for proposal (RFP), request for tender (RFT), and request for quotation (RFQ).

EHR is CCHIT certified.[41] After the RFPs/RFIs return, narrow the field down to no more than three to five potential choices.

2. Obtain several references from each vendor and visit each practice if possible. Be sure to select similar practices to yours. The following excellent reference provides an EHR demonstration rating form, questions to ask vendors, forms, EHR references, and a vendor rating tool.[42] Create a scoring matrix to compare vendors. There are also several fee-based sites to compare EHR products, such as KLAS.[43] Obtain in writing commitments for implementation and technical support, including data conversion from paper records, interfacing with PM software, and exact schedule and time line for training.

3. Select a vendor and have a contract drawn up and reviewed by legal counsel.

Phase III: Training and Implementation

1. Begin in-person or online training. With comprehensive client-server software, in-person training is strongly recommended.

2. Implement decision made during planning regarding whether you want implementation to be modular or all at once ("big bang")

3. Implement decision made during planning regarding whether to scan and upload all paper charts or active patients only or input key components such as problem summary lists, allergies, and medications. Do you want an outside nurse to key in information into the EHR and/or hire an outside scanning operation to do the work?[44] Remember that scanned-in information become images that are difficult to search versus keyed-in information that can be searched.

4. Be prepared for reduced productivity. Have frequent staff meetings to work out the kinks.

Practice Management System Examples

There are more than 200 PMSs on the market with a variety of PM features to include integration with an EHR and the availability as both a client-server model and/or an ASP model. In Table 10.3, we have included a list of the better-known vendors who offer a combined EHR-PM that is CCHIT certified and available in the ASP model. In the resource section, we direct you to methods to search all available PM systems.

Resources

Although there is very little written about the merits and limitations of PMSs, we can direct you to several helpful resources. A 2009 monograph by the California HealthCare Foundation "Practice Management Systems for Safety-Net Clinics and Small Group Practices: A Primer"[45] discusses how important PM systems are for safety net clinics but also provides an excellent overview on the subject.

> **TIP**
>
> In hind sight, many managers have realized that training is as crucial as planning with regard to successful implementation of a new system.

Modular: An electronic health record system implementation strategy whereby functional modules, such as e-prescribing, are implemented in a planned manner versus implementing the full EHR at one time.

Table 10.3	EHR-PM Integrated Systems that are Certified Under One of the New ONC-ATCBs	
EHR-PM System	**Web site**	**Features**
ABELMed v11	HYPERLINK "http://www.abelsoft.com/" www.abelsoft.com	ASP available
Allscripts MyWay PM Allscripts Professional PM	HYPERLINK "http://www.allscripts.com/" www.allscripts.com	ASP available. Small-medium practices
Athena Clinicals	HYPERLINK "http://www.athenahealth.com/" www.athenahealth.com	Only ASP. Can outsource the billing service
Cerner PowerWorks	HYPERLINK "http://www.cerner.com/" www.cerner.com	ASP available. Small-large practices
e-MDs Solution Series 7.0	HYPERLINK "http://www.e-mds.com/" www.e-mds.com	ASP available
eClinicalWorks	HYPERLINK "http://www.eclinicalworks.com/" www.eclinicalworks.com	ASP available. Small-large practices
GE Centricity Practice Solution	HYPERLINK "http://www.gehealth.com/" www.gehealth.com	ASP available. Medium-large practices
Medical and Practice Management Magic 5.64	www.lssdata.com	ASP available
NextGen Healthcare	HYPERLINK "http://www.nextgen.com/" www.nextgen.com	ASP available.
Perfect Care	www.ncgmedical.com	ASP available
Sage Intergy Meaningful Use Version	HYPERLINK "http://www.sagehealth.com/" www.sagehealth.com	ASP available
Waiting Room Solutions v4	HYPERLINK "http://www.waitingroomsolutions.com/" www.waitingroomsolutions.com	ASP available. Covers 26 specialties

See the Health IT Web site at healthit.hhs.gov for the most updated and complete list of certified EHRs and modules, with or without integrated PMs.

For prospective purchasers of PM systems and/or EHR systems, several resources are worth mentioning:

- Capterra is a Web site that includes a search engine with filters for operating systems (platform), number of users, PM features, inclusion with EHRs, location (e.g., the Unites States), and annual revenue. Over 200 products are included with hyperlinks to the individual Web sites, demos, and tours.[46]

- "Selecting a Practice Management System" is a monograph by the American College of Physicians.[47] Members can access this resource that focuses how to go about selecting a PM system, in terms of the steps that are necessary prior to purchase.

- "Medical Practice Management Buyer's Guide" is a May 2008 Web-based resource that includes pricing and tips before purchase.[48]

- The Online Consultant is a fee-based generator of "requests for proposal" (RFP).[49] In the case of PM systems, they generate detailed questions about price and functional requirements. Once the RFP is complete, they offer the ability to graph and create comparison reports between vendors. Charge is $695 for PM RFP.

⊘ INTEROPERABILITY: HEALTH INFORMATION ORGANIZATIONS AND THE NATIONWIDE HEALTH INFORMATION NETWORK

Health information technology (HIT) interoperability means that electronic applications, devices, systems, or networks are able to share health-related information. Interoperability is a critical element in the exchange of information at the local, regional, and national level. As an example, patient data within an EHR is interoperable if it can be shared with other computers or networks. In order to accomplish this, data standards such as HL7, LOINC, and DICOM are required but will not be covered in this chapter. Practically speaking, interoperability is important in several common settings:

1. EHRs need to interface with PMSs, as already discussed. Most experts recommend purchasing an EHR and PMS from the same vendor so they interface without difficulty.

2. Other EHR interfaces: it would not be unusual to have to pay for the creation of EHR interfaces, so that orders for lab and imaging will be transmitted to local hospitals, commercial labs, etc., and reports returned to the EHR. Depending on complexity, interfaces cost between \$3,000 and \$15,000 and may need to be modified whenever there is a software upgrade. A new open source data integration engine, known as Mirth, has made the process easier and less expensive.[50]

3. Exchange of health information locally, statewide, or nationwide between clinicians and health care organizations. Several definitions are important:

   a. Health information exchange (HIE)—the electronic movement of health-related information among organizations according to nationally recognized standards

   b. Health information organization (HIO)—an organization that oversees and governs the exchange of health-related information among organizations according to nationally recognized standards

   c. Regional health information organization (RHIO)—a health information organization that brings together health care stakeholders within a defined geographic area and governs health information exchange among them for the purpose of improving health and care in that community[51]

Interoperability is important to all health care organizations, but particularly for federal agencies. The federal government determined that the exchange of health information was essential to improve the disability process, continuity of medical care issues, biosurveillance, research, and natural disaster responses. Electronic exchange of data should result in faster and less expensive transactions when compared to standard mail and faxes. In order to accomplish this goal, multiple partners would need to communicate using data standards. The end result has been that the federal government has been a major promoter of HIT interoperability.[52] Toward that goal, in 2004 President Bush signed

Interoperability: The ability for health information systems, using approved standards, to exchange health care data and information in a meaningful manner between disparate systems and organizations.

Health Information Exchange (HIE): The electronic movement of health-related information among organizations according to nationally recognized standards.

Health Information Organization (HIO): An organization that oversees and governs the exchange of health-related information among organizations according to nationally recognized standards.

Regional Health Information Organization (RHIO): A group of organizations within a specific geographical area that share health care–related information electronically according to national standards.

Nationalwide Health Information
Network (NHIN):   A network that
will provide a secure, nationwide,
interoperable health information
infrastructure that will connect providers, consumers, and others involved
in health care. Once in place, it will
enable health information to follow
the consumer, be available for clinical
decision making, and support appropriate use of health care information
beyond direct patient care so as to
improve health.

Executive Order 13335 creating the Office of the National Coordinator for Health Information Technology (ONC) and at the same time calling for interoperable EHRs within the next decade.[53]

To promote interoperability, the federal government, with civilian input, decided that there was a need for a national interoperable network, now known as the Nationwide Health Information Network (NHIN). It would be created and based on a decentralized "network of networks" that also meant that there would not be a centralized data repository of all patient information as illustrated in Figure 10.2. In order for the NHIN to be successful, it would need to connect to hundreds of HIOs, created by localities, regions, and states. The vision is for physicians to adopt EHRs that would generate digital patient data that would be shared with HIOs that in turn could be shared with other health care organizations and federal agencies by connecting to the NHIN.

The Social Security Administration was the first federal agency in 2009 to use the NHIN to connect to the MedVirginia HIO in order to request patient information for disability determinations. The time to retrieve the necessary information has been less than one minute, in most cases, a huge improvement over prior paper-based average of 65 days to process a claim. Given the fact that the majority of veterans and active duty service members receive medical care outside their respective systems, it is likely there will be additional trials, with new partners in the near future.[54]

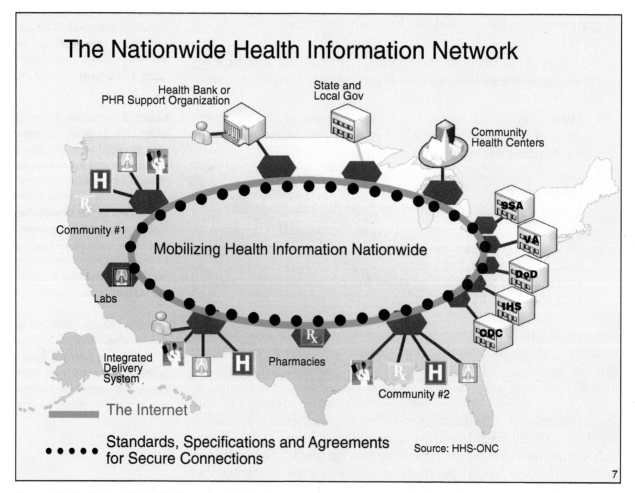

Figure 10.2 The Nationwide Health Information Network

HIOs require cooperation among multiple disparate partners, governance, and a long-term business plan. The technology used is based on service-oriented architecture to deliver Web services. Most HIOs begin with simple processes such as test results retrieval, electronic claims submission, secure messaging, e-prescribing, simple order entry, and, much later, EHRs. Downstream HIOs may be able to amass data to look at quality of care, patient safety, and biosurveillance (public health). Patient information can be based on actual results or claims data. Ideally, participating clinicians will order and retrieve information using EHRs but in the absence of EHRs results can be delivered to a Web-based electronic inbox. HIOs can help satisfy the "meaningful use" criterion of exchanging information "among providers of care." The planning phase of a HIO generally takes several years, requires a great deal of cooperation among disparate partners, and usually necessitates initial grant support.

The expectation is that HIOs will save money by reducing office inefficiencies (routine mail, faxing, etc.) and duplication of orders. It is clear that one of the benefits of HIOs is more cost-effective electronic claims submission.

According to a report published in 2009, there are about 40 HIOs actually exchanging clinical information and about 200 in the formative stages.[54]

Funding from the 2009 HITECH Act established regional extension centers (RECs) throughout the United States to help as many eligible providers as possible attain meaningful use criteria by implementing interoperable EHRs that have been certified under one of the approved ONC agencies. The latest information on RECs can be located at the Web site www.regionalextensioncenters.com.

Regional Extension Centers (RECs): An extension program authorized by the HITECH Act, RECs support and serve health care providers to help them quickly become adept and meaningful users of electronic health records (EHRs).

SECURE MESSAGING IN A MEDICAL OFFICE

Secure messaging is a communication mode used to communicate internally with office staff in a medical practice or externally with patients. Secure messaging can be part of an EHR or a patient portal (covered in next section). It is not recommended that medical offices use standard e-mail to communicate with patients, as that mode is not secure. Instead, it is recommended that electronic communication includes usernames, passwords, and encryption. Figures 10.3, 10.4, and 10.5 are screen prints of a secure messaging system. Secure messaging in an office setting has many advantages:

Secure Messaging: Technology for protecting sensitive data when sent beyond the corporate borders and providing compliance with industry regulations such as HIPAA.

- It is asynchronous, so office nurses, staff, and physicians can respond to issues when time allows and thus avoid "telephone tag."
- It is self-documenting as seen in the figure below. An audit trail is created so future reference is possible.
- The process can lead to virtual or electronic visits (e-visits) down the road, if reimbursement is available.
- Patients appreciate an alternative method to contact the office. Increasingly, new methods to contact patients are appearing: text messages, e-mail reminders, etc.

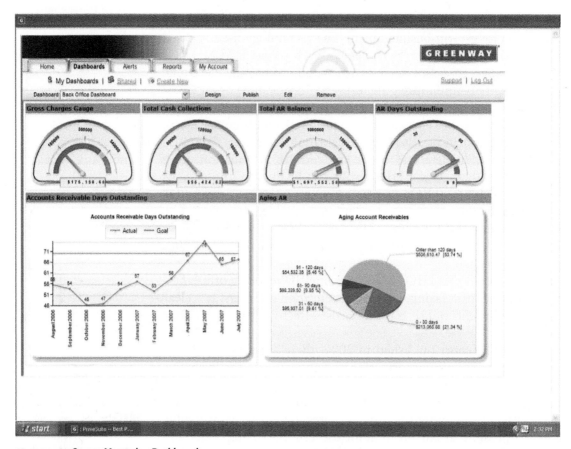

Figure 10.3 **Secure Messaging Dashboard**

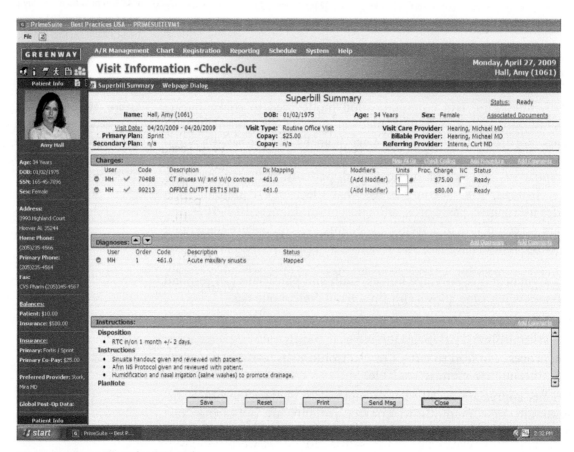

Figure 10.4 **Secure Messaging Scorecards**

Collection Scorecard

KPI	Actual	Target	% Goal	% Goal MTD	Trend
Total Cash Collections	$87,847.52	$55,000.00	159.36%	196.86%	
Total Accounts Receivable Balance	$3,259,599.06	$2,500,000.00	76.69%	77.91%	
Primary Cash Collections Percentage	95.89%	90.00%	106.55%	131.62%	
Patient Cash Collections %	2.31%	2.00%	115.66%	142.87%	
Average Days to Pay	112	110	101.52%	125.41%	
Accounts Receivable Days Outstanding	177	150	117.94%	145.69%	

Billing Scorecard

KPI	Actual	Target	% Goal	% Goal MTD	Trend
Primary Billings Percentage	68.97%	60.00%	114.94%	141.99%	
Secondary Billings Percentage	10.73%	15.00%	71.52%	88.35%	
Patient Billings Percentage	20.31%	25.00%	81.23%	100.34%	
Number of Claims Billed	261	250	104.40%	128.96%	
Gross Charges	$318,322.91	$200,000.00	159.16%	196.61%	
Average Days Unbilled		200	0.00%	0.00%	
Average Days To Bill	20	20	98.79%	122.04%	
Average Daily Billings	$18,425.45	$20,000.00	92.13%	113.80%	

Frontdesk Scorecard

KPI	Actual	Target	% Goal	% Goal MTD	Trend
Point of Service Cash Collected	$2,027.47	$2,500.00	81.10%	100.18%	
Number of Patients Seen	160	180	88.89%	109.80%	
New Patients Percentage	108.13%	80.00%	135.16%	166.96%	

Figure 10.5 Secure Messaging: Patient Encounter Documentation Screen

PATIENT PORTALS

Patient portals are Web-based programs that patients can access for health-related services. A Web portal can be a stand-alone program or it can be integrated with an EHR. Patient portals began as a Web-based entrance into a health care system for the purpose of learning about a hospital, health care system, or physician's practice. They were clearly a marketing ploy to attract patients who were Internet savvy. Currently, patient portals offer multiple features and functions as summarized in Table 10.4.

A minority of Web portals actually integrate with an EHR, which means that most patient data has to be manually inputted. As EHRs become more widespread, selected patient lab results will automatically upload to the patient portal, thus saving time and money. Patients will also be able to access parts of their EHR.

Patient portals are moderately popular with patients but little has been written about the objective benefits for the average consumer. Group Health Cooperative, a large mixed-model health care organization, studied the effect of integrating its new comprehensive patient portal MyGroupHealth with its Epic EHR. As of December 2005, the highest monthly user rates per 1,000 adult members were for test results, med refills, after-visit summaries, and patient-provider messaging. A patient survey revealed that the satisfaction rates were 94% were

Patient Portals: Health care-related online applications that allow patients to interact and communicate with their health care providers, such as physicians and hospitals.

Table 10.4 Web Portal Features and Functions

Feature	Function
Online registration	Allows patients to complete information before a visit or hospitalization
Medication refills	Secure message can be left for physician to refill or renew medications, instead of telephone calls
Laboratory results	Patients can find results on recent tests as well as an explanation
Electronic visits	Portals exist that facilitate e-visits and the payment process
Patient education	Links to common educational sites
PHRs	Allows patients and their families to create and update their PHR
Online appointments	Allows patients to see what appointments are available and when
Referrals	Patients can request referrals to specialists, e.g., OB-GYN
Secure messaging	More convenient than playing phone tag
Bill paying	Online payment using credit card is faster than snail mail
Document uploading	Several portals allow uploading of medical records to their site
Tracking function	Portal allows patients to upload diet, blood sugars, blood pressures, etc.

satisfaction overall, 96% for med refills, 93% for patient-provider messaging, and 86% for test results. Although early use of the Web portal was low, there was a steady increase over time. Attrition rates were not reported.[56,57] Many excellent patient portals exist but we will only discuss one, RelayHealth,[58] a product line of McKesson Corporation. They have been very successful in getting insurance companies such as Aetna, Cigna, and Blue Cross/BlueShield to utilize their platform. Their business model is to charge physicians a monthly fee. They offer the following standard features:

- E-visits are part of the portal and the vendor handles eligibility, claims and collections.
- 100 interactive structured interviews to keep the e-visit focused and fact based
- PHRs
- Access to lab results
- E-prescribing and refills
- Online appointments
- Preregistration
- Phone message routing
- Ability to create a practice Web site
- Colleague to colleague secure messaging
- Interoperability tool kit to link to EHRs (McKesson, GE Centricity, NextGen, Epic, Cerner, AllScripts Touchworks, A4 HealthMatics, and Practice Partner)
- Electronic data exchange (Results Distribution Service) to transmit lab, x-ray, discharge summaries, etc., to physician offices or to the EHR. Results can then be forwarded to patients or other clinicians.
- The ability to store portal information on Microsoft's HealthVault

SUMMARY

Regardless of where in the United States a medical practice administrator works and what size of practice is being managed, there will be a demand for the ability to understand and use health information technology. Leadership of people is crucial during all phases of adapting new technology or upgrading existing systems in a medical office. The successful administrator will plan well, choose the most effective system available to meet the unique aspects of the practice, obtain staff input and collaboration, communicate consistently, train well, and stay current on all relevant regulations, trends, and technology in a rapidly changing environment.

CHAPTER REVIEW QUESTIONS

1. What is the main difference between an EMR and an EHR?

_____

_____

_____

2. What is the main difference between a client-server and an ASP agreement for using an EHR?

_____

_____

_____

3. List three uses of the data that is collected by a PMS.

_____

_____

_____

4. What does the acronym SOAP represent? What is an example of data that would be collected under the "O" part of SOAP notes?

_____

_____

_____

5. What does a medical scribe do?

_____

_____

_____

6. What are the three phases of purchasing and implementing a new EHR with PM system?

_____

_____

_____

7. What is interoperability and why is it important in health care?

_____

_____

_____

8. List five of the features of a patient portal.

_____

_____

_____

REFERENCES

1. Hillstead R, Bigelow J, Bower A, et al. Can electronic medical record systems transform healthcare? Potential health benefits, savings and cost. *Health Aff.* 2005;24(5):103–117.
2. Institute of Medicine Reports. Key Capabilities of an Electronic Health Record System. Institute of Medicine Web site. 2003. Available at: http://www.iom.edu/en/Reports/2003/Key-Capabilities-of-an-Electronic-Health-Record-System.aspx. Accessed October 4, 2009.
3. Dick RS, Steen EB, Detmer DE, eds. *The Computer-Based Patient Record: An Essential Technology for Healthcare.* Washington, DC: National Academy Press; 1997.
4. DesRoches CM. Electronic health records in ambulatory care—a national survey of physicians. *N Engl J Med.* 2008;359:50–60.
5. National Alliance for Health Information Technology. 2008 Available at: www.nahit.org. Accessed May 20, 2008.
6. Tang P. Measuring the effects of reminders for outpatient influenza immunizations at the point of clinical opportunity. *J Am Med Informatic Assoc.* 1999;6:115–121.
7. Smith P. Missing clinical information during primary care visits. *J Am Med Assoc.* 2005;293:565–571.
8. Presidents Information Technology Advisory Committee. 2006; Available at: http://www.nitrd.gov/pubs/pitac. Accessed January 28, 2006.
9. *US FDA.* 200; Available at: http://www.fda.gov/ola/2004/vioxx1118.html. Accessed August 15, 2006.

10. Badgett R, Murlow C. Using information technology to transfer knowledge: a medical institution steps up to the plate. *Annal Intern Med.* 2005;142:220–221.

11. CPOE in Ambulatory Care. CITL Web site. 2005. Available at http://www.citl.org/research/ACPOE.asp. Accessed December 22, 2009.

12. New Survey Addresses Relationship of EMRs to Malpractice Risk. *Medical Records Institute.* 2007; Available at http://www.medrecinst.com/MRI/emrsurvey.html. Accessed December 4, 2007.

13. Jacobe D. *Gallup Poll.* 2002. Available at: http://poll.gallup.com/content/default.aspx?ci=6325&pg=1. Accessed January 29, 2006.

14. *National Public Engagement Campaign on Chronic Illness-Physician Survey.* Princeton, NJ: Mathematica Policy Research Inc.; 2001.

15. Wang SJ. A cost-benefit analysis of electronic medical records in primary care. *Am J Med.* 2003;114:397–403.

16. Miller RH, West CE. The value of electronic health records in solo or small group practices. *Health Aff.* 2005;24:1127–1137.

17. Ninth Annual Survey of Electronic Medical Records Trends and Usage. Medical Records Institute Web site. 2007. Available online at www.medrecinst.com/MRI/emrsurvey.html. Accessed December 4, 2007.

18. Certification Commission for Health Information Technology. 2009; Available at http://www.cchit.org. Accessed October 20, 2009.

19. Hunt DL et al. Effects of Computer-Based Clinical Decision Support Systems on Physician Performance and Patient Outcomes: A systematic review. *JAMA.* 1998; 280(15);1339-1346.

20. Han YY. Unexpected increased mortality after implementation of a commercially sold computerized physician order entry system. *Pediatrics* 2005;116:1506–1512.

21. Bates DW. Computerized physician order entry and medication errors: finding a balance. *J Bioinformatic.* 2005;38:259–261.

22. Dick RS, Steen EB, Detmer DE, eds. *The Computer-Based Patient Record: An Essential Technology for Healthcare.* Washington, DC: National Academy Press; 1997.

23. Carter J. Selecting an electronic medical records system. American College of Physicians, Practice Management Center. 2008. Available at: www.acponline.org/pmc. Accessed December 22, 2009.

24. Practice Fusion. 2009. Avaiable at: http://www.practicefusion.com. Accessed October 15, 2009.

25. Faus SA, Sujansky W. California Healthcare Foundation. 2008. Available at http://www.chcf.org/documents/chronicdisease/OpenSourceEHRSystemsExecSummary.pdf. Accessed August 12, 2008.

26. Edsall RL, Adler KG. American academy of family physicians. family practice management. 2008. Available at: http://www.aafp.org/fpm/20080200/contents.html. Accessed November 1, 2009.

27. SOAPware. 2009. Available at: http://www.soapware.com. Accessed November 2, 2009.

28. eClinicalWorks. 2009. Available at: http://www.eclinicalworks.com. Accessed November 3, 2009.

29. Public Law 111–5. American Recovery and Reinvestment Act of 2009. 2009. Available at http://www.gpo.gov/fdsys/pkg/PLAW-111pub15/content-detail.html. Accessed August 13th, 2009.

30. Pulley J. The claims scrubbers. *Government Health IT.* 2008;10–14.

31. Medical Web Office. Available at: http://www.medical weboffice.com. Accessed December 18, 2009.

32. Gartee R. *Electronic Health Records: Understanding and Using Computerized Medical Records.* Upper Saddle River, NJ: Pearson/Prentice Hall; 2007.

33. Gartee R. *Electronic Health Records: Understanding and Using Computerized Medical Records.* Upper Saddle River, NJ: Pearson/Prentice Hall; 2007.

34. Torpey D. Physician office workflows. Lecture. *UWF.* 2009.

35. E-MDs, Inc. Available at: http:www.e-mds.com/education/articles/roi.html. Accessed December 18, 2009.

36. EClinicalWorks. Available at: http://www.eclinicalworks.com/casestudy6.php. Accessed December, 18, 2009.

37. HIT Taken to the Next Level: NYS Practices that have Successfully Adopted EMR & PMS. *Medical Society of the State of New York.* March 2008: pp. 5–6.

38. Electronic Claims. *Health Information Management Systems Society: Vantage Point.* February 2009.

39. Sample EHR implementation plan, 2009.

40. Health Resources and Services Administration. 2009. Available at http://www.hrsa.gov/healthit/ehrguidelines.htm. Accessed July 20, 2009.

41. EHR Scope. 2009. Available at: http://www.ehrscope.com/emr-comparison/. Accessed September 11, 2009.

42. Adler KG. How to Select an Electronic Health Record System. American Academy of Family Practice: Family Practice Management. 2005. Available at: http://www.aafp.org/fpm. Accessed September 19, 2009.

43. KLAS. 2009. Available at: http://www.klasresearch.com. Accessed August 12, 2009.

44. Adler KG. How to Sucessfully Navigate Your EHR implementation. American Academy of Family Practice: Family Practice Management. 2007. Available at: http://www.aafp.org/fpm. Accessed August 12, 2009.

45. Sujansky W, Sterling R, Swafford R. Practice management systems for safety-net clinics and small group practices: a primer. Available at: www.chcf.org. Accessed December 18, 2009.

46. Medical Practice Management Software. Capterra Web site. Available at: http://www.capterra.com/medical-practice-management-software. Accessed December 18, 2009.

47. Selecting a Practice Management System. ACP Online. 2007. Available at: http://www.acponline.org/running_practice/technology/pms. Accessed December 18, 2009.

48. Medical Practice Management Buyer's Guide. Buyer Zone. May 2008. Available at: http://www.buyerzone.com/software/mpm/buyers_guide1.html. Accessed December 18, 2009.

49. Selecting a New Physician Practice System? Online Consultant. Available at: http://olcsoft.com/physician_practice_management_software_requirements.htm. Accessed December 18, 2009.

50. Mirth. 2009. Available at: http://www.mirthcorp.com. Accessed October 19, 2009.

51. National Alliance for Health Information Technology. 2008. Available at: http://www.nahit.org. Accessed May 20, 2008.

52. Commonweath Fund. 2003. Available at: http://www.cmwf.org/surveys/surveys_show.htm?doc_id=278869. Accessed December 4, 2004.

53. Executive Order: Incentives for the Use of Health Information Technology and Establishing the Position of the National HIT Coordinator. 2004. Available at: http://www.whitehouse.gov/news/releases/2004/04/20040427-4.html. Accessed February 18, 2006.

54. National Health Information Exchange Begins First Exchange. iHealthBeat Web site. March 2, 2009. Available at: www.ihealthbeat.org. Accessed December 22, 2009.

55. Adler-Milstein J, McAfee AP, Bates DW, et al. The State of Regional Health Information Organizations: Current Activities and Financing.

56. Group Health Patient Portal. Group Health Cooperative Web site. Available at: http://www.ghc.org/mygrouphealthpromos/onlinesvcs.jhtml. Accessed December 22, 2009.

57. Ralston JD, Carell D, Reid R, et al. Patient Web services integrated with a shared medical record: patient use and satisfaction. *JAMA* 2007;14:798–806.

58. Relay Health. Relay Health Web site. Available at: https://www.relayhealth.com/. Accessed December 22, 2009.

Workbook for
Chapter 10

Workbook:
Chapter 10 Managing Health Information Technology

10-A: ILLUSTRATION AND INTERNET ACTIVITY—EHR AND PM DEMOS

Using Table 10.3 and any other EHR with PM systems with Web sites listed in the references for this chapter, access the Web sites and look for a demo. Watch the demo and then rate your impression of each in order. Explain what features or other information on the Web site led you to your preferred ranking order.

10-B: INTERVIEW: E-PRESCRIBING

Interview one pharmacist or pharmacy technician and one physician or staff member from a physicians practice near you and ask each the following questions: (1) Do you use e-prescribing? (2) If not, do you plan to start using it in the near future? (3) If not, what are all of the reasons you've chosen not to transition to e-prescribing. (4) If you are using e-prescribing currently, what are all of the things you like about the process and what obstacles or disadvantages have you encountered? (5) Approximately, what percentage of your prescriptions are electronic versus manual or fax? (6) Physicians only: Does your EHR support e-prescribing and do you have alerts built into this system?

10-C: OPTUM ACTIVITY—EHR AND PM

(Please access the companion website on thePoint for these activities)

10-D: INTERNET SCAVENGER HUNT: EPOCRATES

Go to http://www.epocrates.com and create a free account. Look up five diseases that interest you and find out which drug or drugs are used to treat that disease. Turn in a table with the following columns: disease, drug(s), contraindications, or cautions. Then, list the five diseases in the first column and complete the other categories of information for each.

10-E: INTERNET SCAVENGER HUNT: HEALTH INFORMATION EXCHANGE AND NATIONAL INITIATIVES

Go to http://www.healthit.hhs.gov/portal/server.pt.

Click on the tab to the left for National Health Information Network (NHIN). What is the NHIN? What is Connect? What were the original core set of capabilities desired of the NHIN? What are the key priorities of the NHIN? What is the current status?

11

Managing the Physicians and Keeping Up with Emerging Trends

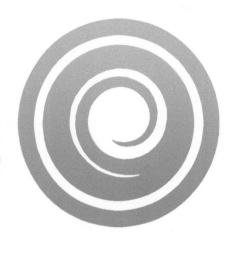

LEARNING OUTCOMES

Upon completion of this chapter, the student should...

- Explain what information is typically required for physician credentialing and how to obtain that information
- Complete a credentialing application packet
- Complete an itinerary and check list of all of the things a manager must do to help a physician schedule attending an out-of-town conference
- Delineate between the various types of medical facilities—both physician based and hospital based
- Understand the concept of physician office laboratories along with the requirements and exceptions under the Clinical Laboratory Improvement Act (CLIA) from both a management perspective and from the interaction between a regular physician practice and either a physician office laboratory or other laboratory facilities
- Understand how to interact with any type of health care facility in which patients may receive services not available in many physician practices and also be able to explain management considerations in other physician-based facilities
- Describe the main differences between ICD-9-CM and ICD-10-CM
- Discuss implementation strategies for HIPAA Transaction Updates (5010) and ICD-10 code sets

OVERVIEW

There are a number of nonroutine tasks that administrators do to help "manage the physicians." The best manager is one who anticipates the needs of the physicians and meets those needs while concurrently keeping the rest of the team motivated by ensuring each individual's needs are also met.

One nonroutine but somewhat common task a manager performs is completing paperwork for physicians to get credentialed or reappointed for approval to serve on the medical staff organization at a hospital or to be authorized to get reimbursed through a third-party payer such as Medicare or a managed care organization. Although physician credentialing from a "hospital privileges" and liability perspective was briefly discussed earlier under the risk management and under legal considerations, the credentialing process must be completed not only for each hospital where a physician has privileges but also for every third-party payer for whom the physicians in the practice desire to participate. This chapter explains how the manager assists the physicians in completing the credentialing process for each of these entities. Also, the most recent CMS Provider Enrollment, Chain and Ownership System (PECOS) changes are discussed.

Other nonroutine activities that are common for the manager to oversee include completing the planning and paperwork for a physician to attend or to speak at an event. The upcoming implementation of HIPAA final rules governing updates to HIPAA transactions and code sets is discussed as an example of how a proactive manager handles significant changes in rules, regulations, or laws governing the revenue cycle and other aspects of medical practice.

Finally, the savvy manager needs to be aware of how to best interact with other health care facilities in which patients may receive tests or treatment including those where the physician may treat the patient such as ambulatory surgery centers (ASCs) and also unique management considerations for the office manager who is employed by a physician-based laboratory or other specialty facility.

Physician Credentialing: The process of gathering information and presenting it for review regarding a physician's qualifications for appointment or reappointment to either have privileges at a hospital or to participate with a managed care organization.

PHYSICIAN CREDENTIALING

For the purposes of obtaining hospital privileges, physician credentialing is the process of gathering information regarding a physician's

Sunshine Managed Care Corporation
Application for Credentialing a Physician with Sunshine Managed Care Corporation
(Please note that this application may be submitted via email as an attachment along with the
required attachments noted in the application form itself to ProviderInfo@SunshineMCO.org)

Section 1: Physician Personal Information
Physician Name: (Last)_____(First)_____ (MI)___
Prior Legal Names:_____
_____
SSN: _____ DOB:_____
Applying as: ___Primary Care Physician
___Specialist with a specialty in _____
___Hospitalist
___Allied Health Practitioner (NP, PA, Midwife, Nurse Anesthesist)

Section 2: Practice Information
Applying as a ___Member of Physician Group   ____Solo Practitioner/Clinician
Name of Practice:_____
Address of Practice: _____
_____
Primary Telephone Number:_____Fax:_____
Email:_____
Office Days and Hours of Operation:_____
Available on call to Established Patients: ____Yes ____No
Primary Contact Name for Credentialing Questions:_____

Figure 11.1 Sample first page provider application for credentialing form.

qualifications for appointment to the medical staff or reappointment every 2 years. A subset of credentialing for hospital privileges is delineation of privileges which entails the hospital specifying which services or specific procedures a physician is authorized to provide at the given hospital. Each member of the medical staff must be subject to periodic review as part of the performance improvement activities of the organization.

Third-party payer provider credentialing is required for the same basic reasons as hospitals credential physicians before granting privileges—ensuring quality of care. See Figure 11.1 for a sample of the type of information gathered on the first page of what is typically a 10-to-15-page form. Hospitals and third-party payer Web sites generally have a link to their application form for the provider credentialing process. For example, access the following AvMed Web site for a typical application form: http://www.avmed.org/pdf/unsecure/Forms/Providers/Credentialing%20application.pdf

Note that there are 12 pages and that it is very important to address every field even by indicating that particular data is not applicable in this case. The forms also indicate attachments that are required as part of the submission process. Some of these applications can be done exclusively online, while others need to be mailed with the required attachments. Typically, these applications require the following attachments, at a minimum:

- Proof of current malpractice insurance with effective dates of coverage
- Curricula vitae (CV) with current work history by date with gaps explained
- Proof of any recent Continuing Medical Education units (CMEs) earned (especially general practitioners)
- Documentation for any positive responses to questions on the application form such as questions regarding litigation over medical malpractice

Continuing Medical Education (CME): Continuing medical education consists of educational activities which serve to maintain, develop, or increase the knowledge, skills, and performance of a physician and are required for maintenance of credentials.

If a physician attends an event that qualifies for CMEs, the manager is often responsible for ensuring those CMEs are reported in the next credentialing cycle. For example, a hospital will typically grant privileges to a physician for 2 years and then require the physician to apply for reappointment by submitting proof of CMEs and other required maintenance of licensure and, as applicable, board certification as well as proof that no negative activity has been taken against the physician such as a suit for malpractice or suspension of license.

CMS PROVIDER ENROLLMENT, CHAIN AND OWNERSHIP SYSTEM

CMS requires a slightly different method of credentialing physicians who bill services for Medicare or Medicaid. In addition to ensuring quality care, CMS is also trying to eliminate payments to nonexistent or unqualified providers. CMS has historically paid out billions of dollars in fraudulent claims—many from phony physician practices or medical suppliers. CMS is continually making changes to its strategies to recover money already paid out for claims that fall under fraud or abuse in addition to preventing future fraudulent payments.

Provider Enrollment, Chain and Ownership System (PECOS): Supports the Medicare provider and supplier enrollment process by managing, tracking, and validating enrollment data collected in both paper form and electronically via the Internet.

In an effort to support the goals of eliminating fraudulent payments, CMS insists that every provider who receives money for services under Medicare, had to enroll or reenroll if they enrolled prior to the changes made to the Provider Enrollment, Chain and Ownership System (PECOS). As of January 3, 2011, claims from providers who had not registered under PECOS were held until physicians could retroactively enroll. Figure 11.2 is a copy of the PECOS enrollment welcome screen. From that site, the manager, as an authorized user, can navigate through the screens to enroll a physician or update physician information for the practice.

The following Web site is an excellent overall resource for practice managers and specifically includes extensive resources to help individual physicians and group practices comply with all PECOS requirements so no claims are suspended or denied due to noncompliance with timeliness and other requirements: http://www.managemypractice.com/attention-

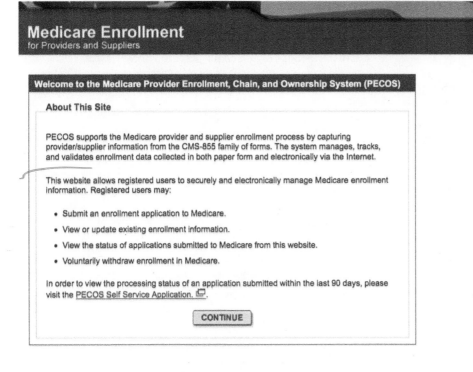

Medicare Enrollment
for Providers and Suppliers

Welcome to the Medicare Provider Enrollment, Chain, and Ownership System (PECOS)

About This Site

PECOS supports the Medicare provider and supplier enrollment process by capturing provider/supplier information from the CMS-855 family of forms. The system manages, tracks, and validates enrollment data collected in both paper form and electronically via the Internet.

This website allows registered users to securely and electronically manage Medicare enrollment information. Registered users may:

- Submit an enrollment application to Medicare.
- View or update existing enrollment information.
- View the status of applications submitted to Medicare from this website.
- Voluntarily withdraw enrollment in Medicare.

In order to view the processing status of an application submitted within the last 90 days, please visit the PECOS Self Service Application.

CONTINUE

Web Policies & Important Links | Department of Health & Human Services | CMS.gov | PECOS FAQs | Accessibility

CENTERS FOR MEDICARE & MEDICAID SERVICES, 7500 SECURITY BOULEVARD, BALTIMORE, MD 21244

CMS/

Figure 11.2 PECOS welcome screen: https://pecos.cms.hhs.gov/pecos/login.do.

medical-practice-staff-medicare-changes-the-rules-for-credentialing-and-retro-billing/

PHYSICIAN SCHEDULES AND EVENTS

Managers typically assist physicians with planning, travel arrangements, itineraries, and making sure the physician has coverage for any hospital rounds or emergency admission of a patient to the hospital during his or her absence. A travel planning and procedures checklist will make each time a physician or other member of the team, including a manager, has to travel for business, a more efficient process. As shown in Figure 11.3, a generic planning and procedures checklist allows flexibility for type of travel (rental car, personal car, or air travel), whether or not certain meals are provided as part of the registration fee and other items that may vary from trip to trip. An Internet search provides the ability to select dates and times for air travel and then will display the fares and airlines in price order. For major conferences, a discount arrangement for attendees with the hotel in which the conference is being held is generally available on the registration brochure, as also, which meals are provided and which ones have to be purchased by the attendee(s).

Travel Planning Checklist Travel Dates: From_____ to _____ Name of Traveler_____ Purpose of Travel_____ Department Cost Center_____		Check when Complete or N/A
Block out dates on practice management scheduler and reschedule any appointments that may already be on the calendar for those dates	Must be completed as soon as dates for travel are known	
Arrange for a physician to be on call for emergencies while the traveler is away	Must be completed as soon as dates for travel are known	
Contact hospital(s) where traveler has rounds and let them know the dates the traveler will be unavailable and who is taking emergency calls for the physician	Must be completed as soon as the physician who agrees to be on time is confirmed	
If conference or convention, complete application form, note what is included in the price, and use the appropriate credit card for the physician's department to pay the conference fees. Reserve hotel room where the conference is being held (unless physician requests you search for less expensive accommodations within a given distance (perhaps walking distance). Either way, reserve room.	Confirmation number (Conference) _____Charges_____ Confirmation number (Hotel) _____Charges_____	
AIR TRAVEL: Research online for best airfare. If there is more than a couple of weeks, see which of the lower priced flights still have room. If there are a lot of seats, request an alert if price drops. If no alert within a few days, reserve air travel.	Confirmation number, (Airfare) _____Charges_____	
Car Travel: Rental – if trip by rental car or if traveler needs a rental car at destination airport, reserve car. If frequent travel, try to get a corporate discount with a reliable rental company.	Confirmation number, (Rental Car) _____Charges_____	
Does traveler need transportation to airport from office and back on return? If so, reserve shuttle. If not, does driver intend to park at airport while traveling? If so, check rates off site.	Confirmation number, (Shuttle) _____Charges_____ Confirmation, (offsite parking)_____ Charges_____	
Make sure traveler has a corporate credit card and/or cash advance depending on policy	Signature/Date Manager Signature/Date Traveler	

Figure 11.3 Travel planning procedures and checklist.

If a physician is going to speak at an event, the organization that invites the physician will often apply to the appropriate agency so attendees earn continuing medical education (CME) hours (Fig 11.4). This process means the host will need the physician to submit an outline of the presentation with samples of any handouts and PowerPoint slides as well as a CV demonstrating the physician's expertise on the topic, as early as possible because the CME-approval process may take several weeks. This information is used secondarily to provide the sponsor with enough details to market the event, prepare an introduction of the speaker, and determine the best time slot for the speaker. Although many physicians put together their own presentations, the manager should be able to help with editing, formatting, Internet research, documenting references and other assistance as requested.

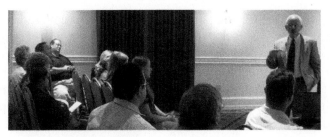

Figure 11.4 Physician speaker.

MANAGEMENT AND COMMUNICATIONS CONSIDERATIONS FOR DEALING WITH HEALTH CARE FACILITIES OTHER THAN A PHYSICIAN PRACTICE

As mentioned previously, a practice manager interacts with representatives in other health care facilities from various perspectives which include the following:

- Patient referrals and follow-up
- Reimbursement considerations
- Management of unique aspects of these facilities

The most common types of health care facilities other than physician practices that a practice manager should be familiar with include

- Hospitals (inpatient and outpatient or ambulatory services)
- Stand-alone imaging centers
- Stand-alone laboratories
- Physician office laboratories
- Stand-alone ASCs—usually physician owned

Patient Referrals and Customer Service

From a patient referral and customer service perspective, it is common to refer patients for various services not available at the initiating physician's practice. Common examples include referring patients to

- Specialists outside of the initiating practice's expertise
- Stand-alone or hospital-based diagnostic tests (laboratory tests, imaging, stress tests, etc.)
- Stand-alone or hospital-based surgeries or therapies (physical, speech, occupational, etc.)
- Inpatient hospital treatment or services that can't be done on an outpatient basis

In each case, if at all possible, the office of the primary care physician should ensure that a valid diagnosis code justifying the medical necessity of the service is provided to the place to which the patient is referred along with verification that the patient's insurance will cover the referred service (or the patient is aware it is not covered and willing to sign a waiver), assist the patient with obtaining any required prior authorization from the patient's insurer, scheduling, and, follow-up after the scheduled services to make sure the primary care physician updates the patient's medical record with any relevant information. If the facility is contacted by anyone in the office, the facility representative should be treated with respect and courtesy so they will be more likely to comply with any requests and therefore treat the patient in the same customer-focused manner as the staff in the primary care office.

Reimbursement Considerations

It is common for primary care physicians or specialists to provide services or procedures to patients in almost any clinical department of the hospital (Emergency department, outpatient surgery department, or inpatient units such as intensive care, coronary care, medical–Surgical, etc.) as well as in nonhospital-based ASCs, acute care nursing facilities, and other locations.

In this case, it is common for the medical office staff to have a process in place to be sure the services rendered outside of the practice's office are billed properly to any third-party payer or to the patient as applicable. The office manager needs to determine how they are going to obtain any medical record documentation required for reimbursement including any financial information that the patient provides to the facility so that the office has the most current information. Also, the manager needs to establish a collaborative relationship with an appropriate hospital representative—usually in health information management—in case there are any issues with consistency between the codes and dates the hospital submits for the facility to get reimbursed and the codes and dates the physician's office submits to get the physician reimbursed. With increased use of interoperable electronic health records, it is becoming more common for the physician's office staff to have online access to the patient's medical record for services provided at a hospital or other facility. The same philosophy applies to any other facility in which a physician or other practitioner provides services or procedures. At the time any physician is credentialed to provide services at another facility, the practice manager or appropriate staff member should discuss procedures for obtaining facility records such as accessing a Web-based electronic health record or requesting paper copies of medical reports dictated by the physician but transcribed by a transcriptionist with the facility.

The medical staff organization and the required medical staff credentialing process for a physician to gain privileges at that hospital were discussed previously in both the quality management chapter and in the legal chapter. However, in general, a practice manager should be aware of different types of hospitals and typical departments found in an acute care hospital.

Regardless of ownership (privately owned which is also called proprietary or for-profit, government owned such as a VA hospital, or owned by private, not-for-profit entities such as churches or a club like the

Rotary), there are various types of hospitals with which a physician may provide services. The more common types include

- Teaching hospitals that train medical students and other students such as nurses or technologists and other allied health students
- Hospitals that are accredited by the American Osteopathic Association (AOA) and provide an environment for Doctors of Osteopathic Medicine (D.O.s) a facility that is modeled after the D.O.'s philosophy, even though as physicians, D.O. are licensed to practice at any facility
- Specialty hospitals such as behavioral health hospitals, children's hospitals, and rehabilitation hospitals
- General hospitals

Hospitals always have a medical staff. The medical staff is comprised of any licensed practitioner including physician extenders discussed earlier in this book. The medical staff organization is required to have bylaws, rules, and regulations dictating how the hospital complies with all clinical licensure and accreditation requirements including the content, format, and timeliness of completing medical records and also ensuring quality oversight of all hospital services to minimize adverse drug reactions, adverse blood transfusion reactions, medical and surgical errors, hospital-acquired infections, etc. Medical staff may be employed by the hospital or may be independent but have privileges at the hospital.

Hospitals also have clinical departments responsible for both inpatient and outpatient services and procedures such as nursing, medicine, surgery, pathology, radiology, therapy departments, and emergency medicine. Nonclinical departments are those that don't treat the patient but perform support functions such as patient financial services, human resources, and health information management (responsible for all medical records, indexes, registries, transcription, coding, etc.).

Management Considerations

A medical office manager may be responsible for the management of other than a traditional medical practice. Two examples include a physician office laboratory (POL), which was initiated as a cost-savings because it is less expensive than using a hospital-based laboratory for tests that are generally required before a patient is admitted to the hospital for inpatient or outpatient surgery or other treatment, and a physician-owned Ambulatory Surgery Center (ASC).

Physician Office Laboratories

The principles of leadership and management are the same for any environment; however, what a manager must know about the function being managed varies greatly. So far, this book has explained the knowledge a medical practice manager must have to be effective. If the manager specializes in other than a regular physician practice or clinic, however, there are some additional things he or she must be aware of regarding specific tasks performed in specialized offices.

Physician Office Laboratory (POL): A laboratory within the medical practice so that patients or samples don't have to be referred to an outside laboratory for those tests the lab is certified to perform.

Clinical Laboratory Improvement Act (CLIA): An act passed in 1988 delineating the conditions a laboratory must meet in order to be certified and therefore to receive any reimbursement under CMS.

For the physician office laboratory (POL), which means a physician's office has its own laboratory, a manager needs to be aware of the Clinical Laboratory Improvement Act (CLIA) of 1988 and its amendments of 1997 in addition to knowing about a Certificate of Waiver (COW) and certain specialized lab functions.

CLIA regulations require that any practice that performs tests for the purpose of diagnosing and treating patient signs, symptoms, and diseases must perform the tests in a defined manner and maintain all pertinent medical record and general documentation. A registered POL can perform screening tests, preadmission tests, emergency tests (e.g., a patient in the office who is displaying symptoms of severe electrolyte imbalance should be tested as quickly as possible to determine if the patient needs to be transported to an emergency department or if the planned service can still be rendered without endangering the patient), tests that confirm a preliminary diagnosis, and tests to monitor patients during treatment such as an infusion to ensure the patient is not getting too much of the substance or having a reaction. All tests are categorized by the government as waived, low complexity, moderate complexity, and high complexity to guide the POL staff in compliance.

POLs are able to apply for a COW for tests that meet certain criteria under CLIA regulations such as they can be administered in the home environment or they are deemed safe enough to pose little or no risk to the patient including any unintended results of a misread test result (e.g., urine tests using a dipstick, blood sugar levels using an approved device or blood stick, and pregnancy tests). The COW still requires POLs to obtain a certificate of registration that attests to the fact that the POL will follow the most current testing instructions by the manufacturer; follow the calibration instructions; use reagents in the proper form; follow all storage and handling instructions; not use any expired reagents; maintain documentation of any training or proof of competency of any person with lab-related responsibilities; and follow all OSHA rules.

POLs may also obtain a special certificate to use a microscope during a patient encounter when the specimen being examined cannot be transported easily. This certificate is called a Provider Performed Microscopy (PPM) certificate.

Managers of POLs must always be prepared for the possibility of a CLIA inspection. The documentation that is required for compliance and therefore available for inspection includes all human resources files documenting the licensure, training, and competency of any employee who performs any part of a lab test in a POL: the policy and procedures manual for the POL; the logs documenting maintenance of equipment, temperature, calibration, and quality control; patient test management documentation and patient medical records for lab procedures. All documentation must be signed and dated as applicable.

POLs should run internal inspections periodically to verify they are in compliance with all CLIA regulations based on the types of tests they perform (waived, etc.).

The inspectors have the right to verify any aspect of compliance including having personnel run sample tests or perform other lab procedures. The following Web sites are helpful in setting up and managing a POL:

- Commission on Laboratory Accreditation (COLA): www.cola.org/pol
- CLIA section of CMS Web site, http://www.cms.gov/clia/, which includes all rules and regulations, lists of criteria, lists of waived tests, and the PPM procedures listing
- The Federal Drug Administration listing of test complexity: www.access.data.fda.gov/scripts/cdrh/cfdocs/cfCLIA/search.cfm
- Centers for Disease Control CLIA requirements: www.phppo.cdc.gov/clia/regs/toc.aspx

Ambulatory Surgery Centers

Sometimes ambulatory care is used interchangeably with the term outpatient care. It's most accurate to say that ambulatory services encompass any service or procedure delivered on an outpatient basis, in other words, any service that is provided to a patient who has not been admitted as an inpatient to a hospital or other health care facility. Ambulatory care locations include, but are not limited to, physician offices, clinics, outpatient departments of hospitals, laboratories, imaging centers, and ambulatory surgery centers (ASCs).

ASCs are facilities that are typically owned by either physicians or a combination of physicians and development companies for the primary purpose of providing nonemergency surgical procedures that do not usually require overnight hospitalization but are more complex than can routinely be performed in a physician office setting. A common example is an endoscopic procedure such as upper or lower gastrointestinal endoscopies or procedures involving endoscopic repair of joints (arthroscopic procedures, e.g., repair of a shoulder joint tear).

CMS certification of ASCs requires the ASC to be a distinct entity. Therefore,

> The regulatory definition of an ASC does not allow the ASC and another entity, such as an adjacent physician's office, to mix functions and operations in a common space during concurrent or overlapping hours of operations. CMS does permit two different Medicare-participating ASCs to use the same physical space, so long as they are temporally separated. That is, the two facilities must have entirely separate operations, records, etc., and may not be open at the same time. However, ASCs are not permitted to share space, even when temporally separated, with a hospital, e.g., a hospital outpatient surgery department....[1]

Managers of an ASC need to fully understand the CMS requirements for certification, maintenance, reimbursement of services (including medical record documentation content), and other considerations such as the federal program to reduce health care acquired infections in hospitals and ASCs. State licensure requirements are also critical to know.

The following Web sites are useful to assist any ASC manager:

The Ambulatory Surgery Center Association: http://ascassociation.org

Center for Medicare and Medicaid Services (CMS) ASC homepage including free training modules: http://www.cms.gov/center/asc.asp

Ambulatory Surgery Centers (ASC): A distinct entity with the primary purpose of providing nonemergency surgical procedures that do not usually require overnight hospitalization but are more complex than can routinely be performed in a physician's office setting.

The American Associations for Accreditation of ASCs: http://www. aaaasf.org/

IMPLEMENTING HIPAA TRANSACTION UPDATES (5010) AND ICD-10

In January 2009, the Department of Health and Human Services published two final rules to adopt updated HIPAA standards and code sets. This means that a proactive manager would have known about the proposed changes during the "public comment" period that precedes every major change and is available through the daily Federal Register. Once the public comment period is over and the final version of the rule is announced, the rule becomes enforceable as law to anyone receiving payment for medical care from any federal third-party payer such as Medicare or Medicaid. These changes, announced in 2009, are being discussed now because of the future implementation dates but also as excellent examples of how a manager deals with major changes to minimize cost and disruption to the practice. The significance of the date the final rules were announced is the fact that they are closely tied to the overhaul of health care delivery in the United States that relate to the American Recovery and Reinvestment Act (ARRA) of 2009, specifically the Health Information Technology for Economic and Clinical Health (HITECH) Act, a subact of ARRA.

HIPAA Transaction Standards

One rule is commonly referred to as Version 5010 because it pertains to the newest version of the transaction standards required for HIPAA compliance in transmitting health information electronically. This rule also includes an update to Medicaid pharmacy transactions. The implementation date is January 1, 2012, for all covered entities except small health plans, which will have until January 1, 2013, to comply. The implementation date is designed to allow the industry time to upgrade and test all impacted systems, including the exchange of health information between various agencies. It also allows time between implementation of these transactions and the subsequent adoption of the second

---

Box 11.1

Proactive leadership

Many practices implement required changes inefficiently causing much more disruption and possible issues with compliance largely due to not being aware of the requirement until a tight deadline is approaching. A proactive leader will network with other practice managers, check official state and federal Web sites routinely, subscribe to practice management newsletters and other related strategies to identify pending changes early, communicate pending changes with the team members, and plan for smooth, efficient implementation of any changes.

rule, the adoption of the International Classification of Diseases, 10th Revision, Clinical Modification (ICD-10-CM) for all diagnoses reporting (and ICD10-Procedural Coding System [PCS]—for coding inpatient hospital procedures).

Version 5010 of the first rule accommodates the ICD-10 code sets and will be implemented earlier to provide adequate test time between the two new substantial rule updates.

Compliant vendors will be instrumental in the technical aspects of implementing and testing these changes but a significant amount of planning and training is required of all management in health care to ensure the team members are properly trained and ready to implement the changes with minimal disruption to the flow of patient care, HIPAA compliance and revenue cycle processes.

ICD-10-CM and ICD-10-PCS

These new code sets replace the current ICD-9-CM volumes 1 and 2 for diagnostic coding which also justifies medical necessity to support reimbursement of services and procedures performed, and Volume 3 for inpatient procedure coding. Remember from earlier chapters, ICD-9-CM volumes 1 and 2 justify the medical necessity of Volume 3 procedures for hospital reimbursement and CPT-4 codes for outpatient hospital reimbursement as well as all physician services and procedures for which the provider is seeking reimbursement. HCPCS Level II Codes are used for services, drugs, and supplies for which the CMS does not find CPT-4 specific enough to fully describe. The implementation date for ALL covered entities (any entity receiving funds from the federal government) is proposed for October 1, 2015.

Unfortunately, there are a lot of rumors in the media regarding the expense and interruption to medical practice of converting from ICD-9-CM diagnostic coding to ICD-10-CM diagnostic coding.

The American Health Information Management Association (AHIMA) and its coding professionals believe that one person in the office needs to spend some time understanding the benefits of ICD-10 and learning how the coding system works so they can get one or more clinician champions in the practice to make the transition a positive, efficient process. Physicians will most likely only need about 4 hours of training to convert from ICD-9 to ICD-10 diagnostic coding. This training may be available free to many physicians through the hospitals where they have privileges. Improved documentation will promote optimal use of ICD-10. Hospitals may ask surgeons to increase their documentation on operative reports pertaining to inpatients because the new ICD-10-PCS system is significantly different from Volume 3 of ICD-9-CM and requires the hospital coders to build codes from tables. This transition should have little to no impact on the practice itself or managing the practice.

Certified coders must complete CEUs in coding anyway so the additional hours required should not be a burden to the practice. Some managers and physicians are concerned that the sheer substantial

Conventions: Conventions are a tool used in medical coding to alert the coding professional that there is something unique about a code. For example, the code is new this year or the coder has to add another code to the one being considered in a specific sequence, etc.

increase in the number of codes in ICD-10 versus ICD-9 will automatically pose training issues. In reality, diagnostic coding under ICD-10 will be more efficient because the increased specificity makes code choices less ambiguous and often creates a combination code in situations that require two codes in ICD-9.

Many of the ICD-10 conventions are the same as those in ICD-9. For example, the coder will first look in the alpha index and then go to the appropriate tabular section to select the most appropriate code. Another similarity is that a code can be as short as three characters in both coding systems. On the other hand, ICD-9 has a maximum of five characters, while ICD-10 has a maximum of seven characters. Also, all but V and E codes begin with a numeric digit in ICD-9, while all ICD-10 codes begin with an alpha character.

SUMMARY

A practice manager is responsible for day-to-day operations of a practice as well as handling nonroutine tasks and responsibilities. The manager should be able to balance the needs of the physicians with the needs of the other members of the team in order to ensure all team members can focus on the patients without worrying about their individual needs. There are three fairly common nonroutine tasks a typical manager will encounter occasionally. These are physician credentialing, planning for physician travel when the physician is going to either speak or earn CMEs, and implementing changes to practice procedures that result from external entities such as CMS or other third-party payers.

CHAPTER REVIEW QUESTIONS

1. What is credentialing for hospital privileges?

_____

_____

_____

2. What is delineation of privileges for a physician at a hospital?

_____

_____

_____

3. List the typical attachments that are required to be submitted with an application for physician credentialing.

_____

_____

_____

4. How often does a physician have to renew hospital privileges?

_____

_____

_____

5. What does the acronym PECOS represent and what are the two main reasons for this process?

_____

_____

_____

6. What 2009 Act and subsection call for a major overhaul to health care in the United States?

_____

_____

_____

7. What code set replaces ICD-9-CM?

_____

_____

_____

8. What code set replaces Volume 3 of ICD-9 and what purpose does it serve?

_____

_____

_____

REFERENCE

1. Centers for Medicare and Medicaid Services (CMS), Ambulatory surgery centers at http://www.cms.gov/CertificationandComplianc/02_ASCs.asp. Accessed July 1, 2011.

Workbook for
Chapter 11

Workbook:
Chapter 11 Managing the Physicians and Keeping Up with Emerging Trends

11.A: INTERNET ACTIVITY: CONDUCT A SEARCH ON THE STATUS OF ICD-10-CM IMPLEMENTATION

Access www.**cms.gov**/ICD10 for the official CMS ICD-10-CM/PCS Web site. Then do a search of other Web sites to determine the current status of ICD-10-CM implementation. Write a summary of the current status and list any issues practices are having along with any advice you find on how to resolve the issues.

11.B: INTERNET ACTIVITY: CONDUCT A SEARCH FOR A SAMPLE ICD-10-CM SUPERBILL

Find a sample superbill for a medical practice—general practice or any specialty. Print out that superbill. Then, go to http://www.cms.gov/ICD10/Downloads/GEMs-CrosswalksTechnicalFAQ.pdf and look up the crosswalk code for any of the diagnoses listed on the superbill. List the ICD-9-CM code or codes that would be used to submit a claim for a date of service prior to 10-1-2013 for any of the ICD-10-CM codes on the superbill. Note the crosswalks will be available, both directions (ICD-9 to 10 and ICD-10 to 9), for at least 3 years but also note that there is not an exact match so sometimes it takes more than one ICD 10 code to describe what was a single ICD-9 code and vice versa.

11.C: INTERVIEW A PRACTICE MANAGER REGARDING ICD-10 TRAINING AND IMPLEMENTATION

Prepare a list of questions to ask a practice manager regarding how that manager is preparing for the training and implementation for ICD-10-CM coding. Call practices that are conveniently located, identify yourself as a student in whichever program (e.g., administrative medical assisting, health information technology, and medical office administration), and the name of your college or technical institution. Ask if you may schedule a brief appointment as a required assignment to determine how he or she is preparing for ICD-10 implementation. Then, dress professionally for the interview, arrive a few minutes early, and bring a notepad and a prepared list of questions. Be efficient in jotting down notes because if you try to write down every word, the manager will become impatient. Just jot down the key words that will refresh your memory and then complete the assignment later that same day while the interview is fresh on your mind. You may ask initially if it's ok to record the interview but that does make some people uncomfortable, so efficient notetaking is preferable.

11.D: ILLUSTRATION: PREPARE A PHYSICIAN CREDENTIALING APPLICATION PACKET

Using Figure 11.1 from your textbook, complete that application form using a physician you make up (or look at some physician profiles on any practice Web site). Also, be sure to create your own information for the attachments so that there is a complete "mock" package ready to submit to your instructor. If you use templates from various Web sites, be sure to make all of the dates and names consistent. Indicate on a cover sheet who you would mail the application to and the address to be used.

11.E: ILLUSTRATION: CREATE AN ITINERARY FOR A PHYSICIAN'S OUT-OF-TOWN CONFERENCE

Using Figure 11.3 from your textbook, find any upcoming conference on the Internet that would be appropriate for a physician to attend. Using the illustration as a guide, follow each step and then document an itinerary. For example, if your practice is in Florida, and the American Medical Association's annual conference is going to be in Chicago this year, you would create an itinerary that includes flying in the day before the first day of the conference and flying home either late the night it ends or the next morning. Complete the checklist as you complete the itinerary including name of hospital notified for coverage, airlines, times, transportation to and from airports, etc. Use the conference brochure to guide you regarding hotel information and which meals are provided as part of the conference.

Appendix
Common Forms Used by Medical Office Managers

Provider Enrollment, Chain and Ownership System (PECOS) -Tips

Provider Enrollment, Chain and Ownership System (PECOS) Enrollment Form

Application to become a Participating Physician with Medicare

Application to become an AvMed Credentialed Provider

Application to Certify a Laboratory Under the Clinical Laboratory
Improvement Act (CLIA)

Tips to Facilitate the Medicare Enrollment Process

To ensure that your Medicare enrollment application is processed timely, you should:

1. **Consider using Internet-based Provider Enrollment, Chain and Ownership System (PECOS) to enroll or make a change in your Medicare enrollment if it is available for your provider or supplier type.**

   The Internet-based PECOS allows physicians and non-physician practitioners to enroll, make a change in their Medicare enrollment, or view their Medicare enrollment information on file with Medicare.

   Internet-based PECOS is a scenario-driven application process with front-end editing capabilities and built-in help screens. The scenario-driven application process will ensure that physicians and non-physician practitioners complete and submit only the information necessary to enroll or make a change in their Medicare enrollment record.

   All information for Internet- based PECOS can be found by logging on to the Medicare Provider and Supplier Enrollment webpage (www.cms.gov/MedicareProviderSupEnroll) and clicking on the *Internet-based PECOS* link located on navigation menu.

2. **Submit the current version of the Medicare enrollment application (CMS-855).**

   The Centers for Medicare & Medicaid Services (CMS) revised the Medicare enrollment application (i.e., CMS-855A, CMS-855I, CMS-855B, and CMS-855R) in February 2008. CMS revised the DMEPOS supplier enrollment application (i.e., CMS-855S) in March 2009.

   While Medicare contractors will continue to accept the 02/2008 version of the Medicare enrollment application (CMS-855I and CMS-855B) through November 2009, physicians, non-physician practitioners, and other suppliers should begin to use the new Medicare enrollment applications (i.e., "(02/2008) (EF 07/2009)" immediately.

   A copy of the Medicare enrollment application can be found at: http://www.cms.hhs.gov/CMSForms/CMSForms/list.asp

3. **Submit the correct application for your provider or supplier type to the Medicare fee-for-service contractor servicing your State or location.**

   The Medicare contractor that serves your State or practice location is responsible for processing your enrollment application.   Applicants must submit their application(s) to the appropriate Medicare fee-for-service contractor.   A list of the Medicare fee-for-service contractors by State can be found in the download section of www.cms.hhs.gov/MedicareProviderSupEnroll.

4. **Submit a complete application.**

   If you are enrolled in Medicare, but have not submitted the CMS-855 since November 2003, you are required to submit a complete application.   Providers and suppliers should follow the instructions for completing an initial enrollment application.

When completing a CMS-855 for the first time for any reason, each section of an application must be completed.   When reporting a change to your enrollment information, complete each section listed in Section 1B of the CMS-855.

5. **Request and obtain your National Provider Identifier (NPI) number before enrolling or making a change in your Medicare enrollment information.**

   CMS requires that providers and suppliers obtain their National Provider Identifier (NPI) prior to enrolling or updating their enrollment record with Medicare.

   If you do not have an NPI, please contact the NPI Enumerator at https://nppes.cms.hhs.gov or call the Enumerator at 1-800-465-3203 or TTY 1-800-692-2326.

6. **Submit the Electronic Funds Transfer Authorization Agreement (CMS-588) with your enrollment application, if applicable.**

   CMS requires that providers and suppliers, who are enrolling in the Medicare program or making achange in their enrollment data, receive payments via electronic funds transfer. Reminder: when completing the CMS-588 complete each section.

   The CMS-588 must be signed by the authorized official that signed the Medicare enrollment application.

   Note: If a provider or supplier already receives payments electronically and is not making a change to his/her banking information, the CMS-588 is not required.

   If you are a supplier who is reassigning all of your benefits to a group, neither you   nor the group is required to receive payments via electronic funds transfer.

7. **Submit all supporting documentation.**

   In addition to a complete application, each provider or supplier is required to submit all applicable supporting documentation at the time of filing. Supporting documentation includes, if applicable, an authorization agreement for Electronic Funds Transfer Authorization Agreement (CMS-588).

   Note: Only durable medical equipment, prosthetics, orthotics, and supplies (DMEPOS) suppliers are required to submit the National Provider Identifier notification received from the National Plan and Provider Enumeration System.

   See Section 17 of the CMS-855 for additional information regarding the applicable documentation requirements.

8. **Sign and date the application.**

   Applications must be signed and dated by the appropriate individuals.   Signatures must be original and in ink (blue preferable). Copied or stamped signatures will not be accepted.

9. **Respond to fee-for-service contractor requests promptly and fully.**

   To facilitate your enrollment into the Medicare program, respond promptly and fully to any request for additional or clarifying information from the fee-for-service contractor.

Please check one. Directions for completing this form begin on page 3.

☐ New Application
☐ Change Request
☐ Voluntary Termination

DEPARTMENT OF HEALTH AND HUMAN SERVICES
CENTERS FOR MEDICARE & MEDICAID SERVICES

Form Approved
OMB No. 0938-0929

SECTION 1011 PROVIDER ENROLLMENT APPLICATION

1. Applicant's Legal Business Name as Reported to the IRS and Individual Physician Name when applicant is Physician in Box 9

2. Doing Business AS (DBA) Name (if applicable)

3. Physical Address

4. Name, telephone number, and address of person to be contacted on matters involving the application.

5. County	6. E-mail address of person to be contacted on matters involving the application.

7. State of Service (Note: A separate application must be submitted for each State of Service)	8. Current Medicare Fiscal Intermediary or Carrier

9. Type of Applicant (Check one)
☐ Hospital
☐ Physician
☐ Physician Group (must complete attachments 1 and 2)
☐ Ambulance

10. Applicant's Medicare Identification Number, NPI and SSN

Hospital_____ (Medicare #/CCN and NPI)

Physician_____ (NPI and UPIN or PTAN)

Physician_____ (SSN (voluntary))

Physician Group _____ (NPI and UPIN or PTAN)

Ambulance _____ (NPI and UPIN or PTAN)

11. Hospital Election (Hospital only)
☐ Payment for hospital and physician services
(Note: Hospitals electing to receive payment for both hospital and physician services must complete Attachment 1.)

☐ Payment for hospital and a portion of on-call payments made by the hospital for physician services.
(Note: If a hospital elects this option, physicians will separately bill for section 1011 services.)

12. Physician Privileges (Note: If a physician has privileges at multiple hospitals, the physician must complete Attachment 2)

Hospital Name: _____ Medicare Number: _____ NPI Number: _____

☐ Physician Group Privileges (Note: If enrolling a group, the group must complete Attachments 1 and 2)

13. Applicant's Federal Tax Identification Number	14. Applicant's Routing Transit Number, Deposit Account Number
	Routing Transit # _____ ☐ Checking
	Account # _____ ☐ Savings

Form CMS-10115 (04/12)

1

ALL PROVIDERS

In order to receive payment under section 1011 of the Medicare Modernization Act of 2003, the provider submitting this enrollment application agrees to collection requirements approved under the Paperwork Reduction Act. This agreement, upon submission by the provider of services and acceptance by the Secretary of Health and Human Services, shall be binding on the provider of services and the Secretary.

The hospital, physician, ambulance provider, or any other person or entity receiving section 1011 payments (hereinafter "payee") acknowledges that those payments may be retroactively adjusted at the end of each fiscal year in accordance with subsection (c)(2) of section 1011. If CMS determines that payments must be retroactively adjusted, the payee agrees that it will promptly remit the full amount of the reduction to CMS in accordance with instructions provided with the notice of retroactive adjustment. Payee acknowledges that there will be no appeal or review of the determination of retroactive adjustment. Any payment owed to CMS must be remitted promptly, but in no event later than 30 days after notice.

HOSPITALS ONLY

I agree to provide patient eligibility information to physicians and ambulance providers within 120 days of the date of service. I agree to notify the physicians within my hospital about my payment election (see item 10 above.) I further agree to reimburse physicians in a prompt manner after receiving section 1011 reimbursement and agree not to charge an administrative or other fee with respect to transferring reimbursement to a physician.

ATTENTION: READ THE FOLLOWING PROVISION OF FEDERAL LAW CAREFULLY BEFORE SIGNING.

Whoever, in any matter within the jurisdiction of any department or agency of the United States knowingly and willfully falsifies, conceals or covers up by any trick, scheme or device a material fact, or makes any false, fictitious or fraudulent statement or representation, or makes or uses any false writing or document knowing the same to contain any false, fictitious or fraudulent statement or entry, shall be fined not more than $10,000, imprisoned not more than 5 years, or both (18 U.S.C. section 1001).

To the best of my knowledge and belief, all data in this application are true and correct, and the governing body of the applicant has duly authorized the document.

15. Write Name and Title of Authorized Official	16. Telephone Number (including area code)
17. Signature of Authorized Official	18. Date

APPLICATION DEFINITIONS AND INSTRUCTIONS
Section 1011 Provider Enrollment Application—Form CMS-10115

The purpose of collecting the information on the section 1011 Enrollment Application is to determine or verify the eligibility of individuals or organizations enrolling in the section 1011 program as providers. This information will also be used to ensure that payments are made to eligible providers as described in section 1011(e)(4) of the Medicare Prescription Drug, Improvement, and Modernization Act of 2003. All information on this form is required for new applications to be processed. Applications not properly or fully completed are denied and returned as incomplete.

APPLICATION DEFINITIONS

CMS Form 10115
This application allows eligible providers to apply for payment of some or all of their unreimbursed costs of providing services required by Section 1867 of the Social Security Act and related hospital inpatient, outpatient, and ambulance services furnished to undocumented aliens, aliens paroled into the United States at a U.S. port of entry for the purpose of receiving such services, and Mexican citizens permitted temporary entry to the U.S. with a laser visa.

Application Submission
To enroll in this program, a provider must **MAIL** an original **APPLICATION** with an original signature to the following address. An original or copy of the Medicare 855i or your Medicare confirmation letter must be included. Applicable attachments must be included with the application as well as an Electric Funds Transfer (EFT) Agreement, (FORM CMS-588) and an Electronic Remittance Advice (ERA) Request Application. Applications missing any information, attachments or EFT Agreement and ERA application will be denied and returned to the provider.

> **Novitas Solutions, Inc.**
> **Attn: Section 1011**
> **P.O. Box 890121**
> **Camp Hill, PA 17089-0121**

Change Requests
Once a section 1011 Provider Identification Number (PIN) has been issued, changes may be made to the information on file. The information that is changing should be completed on the Application as well as boxes 1, 2, 10, 13, 15, 17 and 18. An original signature of the Authorized Official is required. The change request will be denied if the required information is not completed.

Voluntary Termination
Should a provider choose to no longer participate in the section 1011 program, they may terminate their PIN. Sections 1, 2, 10, 13, 15, 17 and 18 must be completed on the application. An original signature of the Authorized Official is required. The termination will not be processed if the required information is not completed.

APPLICATION INSTRUCTIONS

Box 1
List the legal business name that is reported to the Internal Revenue Service (IRS) for tax reporting purposes and also list the physician's name when applicant is a physician as checked in Box 9.

Box 2
Indicate the Doing Business Name if different than **Box 1**.

Box 3
Record the physical address of the facility, ambulance company or physician office.

Box 4
Provide the name and address of the enrollment contact person.

Box 5
Submit the county of the physical address in **Box 3**.

Box 6
Note an e-mail address of the contact person listed in **Box 4**.

Box 7
Provide the state where services will be performed. A separate application is required for each State of Service.

Box 8
List your current Medicare Intermediary or Carrier (if applicable).

APPLICATION DEFINITIONS AND INSTRUCTIONS
Section 1011 Provider Enrollment Application—Form CMS-10115 (Continued)

Box 9
Check the correct box indicating the type of provider you are according to the below defined terms.
Hospital: This term is defined at section 1861(e) of the Social Security Act (42 U.S.C. I395x(e)).
Physician: This term is defined at section 1861(r) of the Social Security Act (42 U.S.C. I395x(r)).

Box 10
Medicare Identification Number is a generic term for any number that uniquely identifies the provider. Hospitals must provide their Medicare Number or CMS Certification Number (CCN) and NPI number; physicians must provide either their UPIN or Provider Transaction Access Number (PTAN), NPI number and SSN; ambulance providers must provide their UPIN or PTAN and their NPI number.

Box 11
HOSPITALS ONLY: Hospitals must select to receive payment for both hospital and physician services or just for hospital services and a portion of on-call payments. Should a hospital elect to receive payment for physician services, Attachment 1 must be completed and the hospital agrees to bill section 1011 for for all physicians employed by or contracted with that hospital and not solely for employed physicians. A hospital electing this option must bill for any and all physician services performed in that hospital, without regard to the legal arrangement with the physician. Hospitals may not submit payment requests for certain physicians while allowing others to bill separately.

Box 12
PHYSICIANS ONLY: Physicians should elect to enroll separately or with a group. Physicians enrolling separately should indicate the hospital name, and NPI for which that physician has privileges. If the physician has privileges at multiple hospitals then Attachment 2 must be completed. Groups enrolling their physicians must complete Attachments 1 and 2 and obtain individual signatures of the physicians in which they are enrolling.

Box 13
List the Tax Identification Number which is the number issued by the Internal Revenue Service (IRS) that is used by the provider to report tax information to the IRS.

Box 14
Furnish the applicable routing and account numbers for banking information and specify whether it is a checking or savings account. Information recorded in this box should also match banking information in the EFT Agreement. The information concerning your financial institution should be available through your organization's treasurer or financial institution. A contact person and telephone number are important for verification purposes. Your financial institution can assist you in providing the correct banking information, including the bank's routing number.

Boxes 15–17:
Provide the name and title of the Authorized Official with an original signature and a phone number. An Authorized Official is an appointed official to whom the provider has granted legal authority to enroll it in section 1011, to make changes and/or updates to the provider's financial information, and to commit the provider to fully abide by the laws and program instructions of section 1011. The authorized official must be the provider's general partner, chairman of the board, chief financial officer, chief executive officer, chief operating officer, president, direct owner of five percent of more of the provider or must hold a position of similar status and authority within the provider's organization such as Director, Administrator, County Commissioner, Chancellor, Chief, Vice President or AVP. **The physician's signature is required on the physician application as the authorized official for individual physician.**

SECTION 1011 PROVIDER ENROLLMENT APPLICATION

ATTACHMENT 1

This attachment is required for hospitals electing to receive section 1011 payment for hospital and physician services and physician groups electing to receive payment for group members (physicians) and must list the names and provider numbers of physicians with hospital privileges. All information is required and a physician signature is required for group applications only.

PHYSICIAN NAME (GROUP ENROLLMENT ONLY)	NPI NUMBER	UPIN OR PTAN	SSN	PHYSICIAN SIGNATURE

SECTION 1011 PROVIDER ENROLLMENT APPLICATION

ATTACHMENT 2

This attachment is required for physicians with privileges at more than one hospital or Physician Group applications.

Physicians with hospital privileges at more than one hospital must list the names, Medicare numbers (CCN) and NPI numbers of the hospitals where they have privileges.

Physician Groups must list the names, Medicare numbers and NPI numbers (CCN) of the hospitals where the group physicians have privileges.

HOSPITAL NAME	MEDICARE NUMBER (CCN)	NPI NUMBER

DEPARTMENT OF HEALTH AND HUMAN SERVICES
CENTERS FOR MEDICARE & MEDICAID SERVICES

FORM APPROVED
OMB NO. 0938-0373

MEDICARE PARTICIPATING PHYSICIAN OR SUPPLIER AGREEMENT

Name(s) and Address of Participant*	National Provider Identifier (NPI)*
_____	_____
_____	
_____	

*List all names and the NPI under which the participant files claims with the Medicare Administrative Contractor (MAC)/carrier with whom this agreement is being filed.

The above named person or organization, called "the participant," hereby enters into an agreement with the Medicare program to accept assignment of the Medicare Part B payment for all services for which the participant is eligible to accept assignment under the Medicare law and regulations and which are furnished while this agreement is in effect.

1. **Meaning of Assignment:** For purposes of this agreement, accepting assignment of the Medicare Part B payment means requesting direct Part B payment from the Medicare program. Under an assignment, the approved charge, determined by the MAC/carrier, shall be the full charge for the service covered under Part B. The participant shall not collect from the beneficiary or other person or organization for covered services more than the applicable deductible and coinsurance.

2. **Effective Date:** If the participant files the agreement with any MAC/carrier during the enrollment period, the agreement becomes effective _____.

3. **Term and Termination of Agreement:** This agreement shall continue in effect through December 31 following the date the agreement becomes effective and shall be renewed automatically for each 12-month period January 1 through December 31 thereafter unless one of the following occurs:

   a. During the enrollment period provided near the end of any calendar year, the participant notifies in writing every MAC/carrier with whom the participant has filed the agreement or a copy of the agreement that the participant wishes to terminate the agreement at the end of the current term. In the event such notification is mailed or delivered during the enrollment period provided near the end of any calendar year, the agreement shall end on December 31 of that year.

   b. The Centers for Medicare & Medicaid Services may find, after notice to and opportunity for a hearing for the participant, that the participant has substantially failed to comply with the agreement. In the event such a finding is made, the Centers for Medicare & Medicaid Services will notify the participant in writing that the agreement will be terminated at a time designated in the notice. Civil and criminal penalties may also be imposed for violation of the agreement.

Signature of participant (or authorized representative of participating organization)	Date
Title (if signer is authorized representative of organization)	Office Phone Number (including area code)

Received by (name of carrier)	Initials of Carrier Official	Effective Date

According to the Paperwork Reduction Act of 1995, no persons are required to respond to a collection of information unless it displays a valid OMB control number. The valid OMB control number for this information collection is 0938-0373. The time required to complete this information collection is estimated to average 15 minutes per response, including the time to review instructions, search existing data resources, gather the data needed and complete and review the information collection. If you have any comments concerning the accuracy of the time estimate(s) or suggestions for improving this form, please write to: CMS, 7500 Security Boulevard, Attn: PRA Reports Clearance Officer, Baltimore, Maryland 21244-1850.

Form CMS-460 (04/10)   1

DEPARTMENT OF HEALTH AND HUMAN SERVICES
CENTERS FOR MEDICARE & MEDICAID SERVICES

INSTRUCTIONS FOR THE MEDICARE PARTICIPATING PHYSICIAN AND SUPPLIER AGREEMENT (CMS-460)

To sign a participation agreement is to agree to accept assignment for all covered services that you provide to Medicare patients.

WHY PARTICIPATE?

If you bill for physicians' professional services, services and supplies provided incident to physicians' professional services, outpatient physical and occupational therapy services, diagnostic tests, or radiology services, your Medicare fee schedule amounts are 5 percent higher if you participate. Also, providers receive direct and timely reimbursement from Medicare.

Regardless of the Medicare Part B services for which you are billing, participants have "one stop" billing for beneficiaries who have Medigap coverage not connected with their employment and who assign both their Medicare and Medigap payments to participants. After we have made payment, Medicare will send the claim on to the Medigap insurer for payment of all coinsurance and deductible amounts due under the Medigap policy. The Medigap insurer must pay the participant directly.

Currently, the large majority of physicians, practitioners and suppliers are billing under Medicare participation agreements.

WHEN THE DECISION TO PARTICIPATE CAN BE MADE:

- Toward the end of each calendar year, all MAC/carriers have an open enrollment period. The open enrollment period generally is from mid-November through December 31. During this period, providers who are currently enrolled in the Medicare Program can change their current participation status beginning the next calendar year on January 1. This is the only time these providers are given the opportunity to change their participation status. These providers should contact their MAC/carrier to learn where to send the agreement, and get the exact dates for the open enrollment period when the agreement will be accepted.

- New physicians, practitioners, and suppliers can sign the participation agreement and become a Medicare participant at the time of their enrollment into the Medicare Program. The participation agreement will become effective on the date of filing; i.e., the date the participant mails (post-mark date) the agreement to the carrier or delivers it to the carrier.

Contact your MAC/carrier to get the exact dates the participation agreement will be accepted, and to learn where to send the agreement.

WHAT TO DO DURING OPEN ENROLLMENT:

If you choose to be a participant:

- Do nothing if you are currently participating, or

- If you are not currently a Medicare participant, complete the blank agreement (CMS-460) and mail it (or a copy) to each carrier to which you submit Part B claims. (On the form show the name(s) and identification number(s) under which you bill.)

If you decide not to participate:

- Do nothing if you are currently not participating, or

- If you are currently a participant, write to each carrier to which you submit claims, advising of your termination effective the first day of the next calendar year. This written notice must be postmarked prior to the end of the current calendar year.

WHAT TO DO IF YOU'RE A NEW PHYSICIAN, PRACTITIONER OR SUPPLIER:

If you choose to be a participant:
- Complete the blank agreement (CMS-460) and submit it with your Medicare enrollment application to your MAC/carrier.
- If you have already enrolled in the Medicare program, you have 90 days from when you are enrolled to decide if you want to participate. If you decide to participate within this 90-day timeframe, complete the CMS-460 and send to your MAC/carrier.

If you decide not to participate:
- Do nothing. All new physicians, practitioners, and suppliers that are newly enrolled are automatically non-participating. You are not considered to be participating unless you submit the CMS-460 form to your MAC/carrier.

We hope you will decide to be a Medicare participant.

Please call the MAC/carrier in your jurisdiction if you have any questions or need further information on participation.

DO NOT SEND YOUR CMS-460 FORM TO CMS, SEND TO YOUR MAC/CARRIER. IF YOU SEND YOUR FORMS TO CMS, IT WILL DELAY PROCESSING OF YOUR CMS-460 FORMS.

To view updates and the latest information about Medicare, or to obtain telephone numbers of the various Medicare Administrative Contractor (MAC)/carrier contacts including the MAC/carrier medical directors, please visit the CMS web site at *http://www.cms.gov/*.

CREDENTIALING APPLICATION
Please complete all sections. Incomplete applications may delay the credentialing process.

PERSONAL IDENTIFICATION DATA

Last Name: _____ First: _____ MI: _____ Degree: _____

Date of
Birth: _____ Social Security #: _____

Please list all other legal names you have used: _____

Applying As: ☐ Primary Care Physician   ☐ Specialist Physician:

    In the specialty of: _____   In the specialty of: _____

    ☐ Hospital-based Physician   ☐ Allied Health Practitioner

    In the specialty of: _____   In the specialty of: _____

Submission of the following information is voluntary. Please be assured that you will not be subjected to any adverse treatment if you do not provide the following:

Gender Classification: ☐ Male   ☐ Female

EEO Classification: ☐ White (not of Hispanic origin)   ☐ Hispanic   ☐ Asian or Pacific Islander

    ☐ African American   ☐ American Indian or Alaskan Native   ☐ Eastern Indian

    ☐ Other:_____

Medicare Number: _____ Medicaid Number: _____ NPI Number: _____

OFFICE / PRACTICE INFORMATION

Primary Location

Your practice is (please check one): ☐ Solo   ☐ Corporation   ☐ Association

Do you offer 24-hour coverage for your patients?   ☐ Yes   ☐ No

If yes, how? _____

Group Practice Name *(if applicable)*: _____

Tax ID Number: _____   Age Limits: _____

		What hours/days are you available to see patients:
Street: _____	Office Hours:	
City: _____	Mon. _____	_____
State: _____ Zip: _____	Tue. _____	_____
County: _____	Wed. _____	_____
Telephone: _____	Thu. _____	_____
Backline Telephone Number *(not for publication)*:	Fri. _____	_____
_____	Sat. _____	_____
Fax: _____	Sun. _____	_____

After Hours Telephone: _____

Office Access: Other languages spoken: _____

☐ Bus   ☐ Other Public Transportation   _____

Is your office Handicap Accessible? ☐ Yes   ☐ No

Credentialing
Contact: _____ Ph: _____ Fax: _____ Email: _____

Office
Manager: _____ Ph: _____ Fax: _____ Email: _____

AvMed requires written notification of address, phone, fax, and Tax ID changes. Notification of Tax ID changes must be submitted with a revised W-9 form as registered with the Internal Revenue Service. Failure to submit notification of changes immediately will result in a delay of claims adjudication.

OFFICE / PRACTICE INFORMATION (cont'd.)

Additional Location #1

☐ Billing only   ☐ Administration only   ☐ Other office where patients are treated

Group Practice Name *(if applicable)*: _____

Tax ID Number: _____

Street: _____

City: _____

State: _____ Zip: _____

County: _____

Telephone: _____

Backline Telephone Number *(not for publication)*:

_____

Fax: _____

After Hours Telephone: _____

Office Hours:

Mon. _____

Tue. _____

Wed. _____

Thu. _____

Fri. _____

Sat. _____

Sun. _____

What hours/days are you available to see patients:

_____

_____

_____

_____

_____

_____

_____

Credentialing
Contact: _____ Ph: _____ Fax: _____ Email: _____

Office
Manager: _____ Ph: _____ Fax: _____ Email: _____

Additional Location #2

☐ Billing only   ☐ Administration only   ☐ Other office where patients are treated

Group Practice Name *(if applicable)*: _____

Tax ID Number: _____

Street: _____

City: _____

State: _____ Zip: _____

County: _____

Telephone: _____

Backline Telephone Number *(not for publication)*:

_____

Fax: _____

After Hours Telephone: _____

Office Hours:

Mon. _____

Tue. _____

Wed. _____

Thu. _____

Fri. _____

Sat. _____

Sun. _____

What hours/days are you available to see patients:

_____

_____

_____

_____

_____

_____

_____

Credentialing
Contact: _____ Ph: _____ Fax: _____ Email: _____

Office
Manager: _____ Ph: _____ Fax: _____ Email: _____

OFFICE / PRACTICE INFORMATION (cont'd.)

Additional Location #3 _(Please attach additional sheet for other locations)_

☐ Billing only   ☐ Administration only   ☐ Other office where patients are treated

Group Practice Name _(if applicable)_: _____

Tax ID Number: _____

Street: _____	Office Hours:
City: _____	Mon. _____
State: _____ Zip: _____	Tue. _____
County: _____	Wed. _____
Telephone: _____	Thu. _____

What hours/days are you available to see patients:

_____

_____

_____

_____

Backline Telephone Number _(not for publication):_   Fri. _____   _____

_____   Sat. _____   _____

Fax: _____   Sun. _____   _____

After Hours Telephone: _____

Credentialing
Contact: _____ Ph: _____ Fax: _____ Email: _____
Office
Manager: _____ Ph: _____ Fax: _____ Email: _____

Please list covering practitioner(s).

Covering practitioners should be participating with AvMed, or be in the process of becoming practitioners in the AvMed Health Plans Network (please attach separate sheet as needed).

1. Name: _____
   Street: _____ City: _____ State: _____ Zip: _____
   Telephone: _____
   Hospital Affiliations _____

2. Name: _____
   Street: _____ City: _____ State: _____ Zip: _____
   Telephone: _____
   Hospital Affiliations _____

3. Name: _____
   Street: _____ City: _____ State: _____ Zip: _____
   Telephone: _____
   Hospital Affiliations _____

OFFICE / PRACTICE INFORMATION (cont'd.)

Do you perform surgery in your office? ☐ Yes ☐ No If 'Yes', please list the types of surgery:

_____

Do you have any allied health professionals providing patient care in your practice (i.e., physician assistant, advanced registered nurse practitioners)?

☐ Yes ☐ No

If yes, do you allow patients to be cared for by allied health professionals when you or your associates are not in the office?

☐ Yes ☐ No

Do you maintain their current credentials? ☐ Yes ☐ No

Do you maintain their current licenses? ☐ Yes ☐ No

Do you maintain their current malpractice information? ☐ Yes ☐ No

Do you recredential them? ☐ Yes ☐ No ☐ annually or ☐ bi-annually?

If you have ARNP's, do you file protocols annually with the Board of Medicine and Nursing? ☐ Yes ☐ No

Please identify all allied health professionals in your practice:

1. Name: _____ Type: _____

Florida Professional License Number: _____ Expiration Date: _____

2. Name: _____ Type: _____

Florida Professional License Number: _____ Expiration Date: _____

3. Name: _____ Type: _____

Florida Professional License Number: _____ Expiration Date: _____

4. Name: _____ Type: _____

Florida Professional License Number: _____ Expiration Date: _____

Does your practice provide laboratory services? ☐ Yes ☐ No

If yes, please describe the type(s) of services provided: _____

_____

Are you in compliance with the Clinical Laboratory Improvement Amendments of 1988 (CLIA)? ☐ Yes ☐ No

If yes, please provide a copy of your Certificate of Waiver or Certificate of Registration.

CLIA Certification number: _____

What outside labs, if any, do you use? _____

Does your practice provide radiology or imaging services? ☐ Yes ☐ No

If yes, please describe the type(s) of services provided: _____

_____

What outside radiology facility do you use? _____

OFFICE / PRACTICE INFORMATION (cont'd.)

Do you perform any other types of procedures in your office utilizing equipment which requires proper instruction and inspection (i.e. pulmonary function tests, etc.)? ☐ Yes ☐ No

If yes, please list the procedures: _____

_____

_____

Do you or a member of your family own, have an investment in, or otherwise have a business interest in any clinical laboratory, diagnostic, or testing center, hospital, surgicenter, or other business dealing with the provision of ancillary health services, equipment or supplies?
☐ Yes ☐ No

If yes, please provide the following information: (*If others, please attach separate sheets.*)

Name of organization: _____ Tax ID #: _____ Telephone _____

Street _____ City: _____ State: _____ Zip: _____

Type of organization: _____ Size of organization: _____ % of business owned: _____

Invested by practitioners or hospitals: _____ Invested by applicant: _____

Type of business interest (i.e. owner, partner, investor). _____

PROFESSIONAL LICENSE

List all current licenses

State: _____ Type: _____

Number: _____ Original Date of Issue: _____

Expiration Date: _____

State: _____ Type: _____

Number: _____ Original Date of Issue: _____

Expiration Date: _____

FEDERAL DEA REGISTRATION

Federal DEA Number: _____ Date Issued: _____

Expiration Date: _____

BOARD CERTIFICATION

1. Are you Board Certified? ☐ Yes ☐ No (If No, please respond to 1b. below)
   1a. List the names of specialty boards by which you are certified.

Specialty board	Date of initial certification	Date of most recent certification	Expiration Date
Specialty board	Date of initial certification	Date of most recent certification	Expiration Date

   1b. **If not certified,** have you applied for the certification examination? ☐ Yes ☐ No

   Have you been accepted to take the certification examination? ☐ Yes ☐ No

   If no, do you intend to apply for the certification examination? ☐ Yes ☐ No

EDUCATION

Schools

Medical/Professional School	Degree	From (MM/YY)	To (MM/YY)

Medical/Professional School	Degree	From (MM/YY)	To (MM/YY)

If foreign medical school graduate, ECFMG #: _____   **Date** _____

Internships *(list every internship begun or completed)*

Institution	Address	Department/Specialty	From (MM/YY)	To (MM/YY)
Institution	Address	Department/Specialty	From (MM/YY)	To (MM/YY)
Institution	Address	Department/Specialty	From (MM/YY)	To (MM/YY)

Residencies *(list every Residency begun or completed)*

Institution	Address	Department/Specialty	From (MM/YY)	To (MM/YY)
Institution	Address	Department/Specialty	From (MM/YY)	To (MM/YY)
Institution	Address	Department/Specialty	From (MM/YY)	To (MM/YY)

Fellowships *(list every Fellowship begun or completed)*

Institution	Address	Department/Specialty	From (MM/YY)	To (MM/YY)
Institution	Address	Department/Specialty	From (MM/YY)	To (MM/YY)
Institution	Address	Department/Specialty	From (MM/YY)	To (MM/YY)

WORK HISTORY

Please provide relevant work history, beginning with current practice.

For all gaps in practice history greater than six months, please explain below.

Relevant experience includes work as a health professional.

Practice/Facility Name:	Location (City and State)	From (Month/Year)	To (Month/Year)
Practice/Facility Name:	Location (City and State)	From (Month/Year)	To (Month/Year)
Practice/Facility Name:	Location (City and State)	From (Month/Year)	To (Month/Year)
Practice/Facility Name:	Location (City and State)	From (Month/Year)	To (Month/Year)
Practice/Facility Name:	Location (City and State)	From (Month/Year)	To (Month/Year)
Practice/Facility Name:	Location (City and State)	From (Month/Year)	To (Month/Year)
Practice/Facility Name:	Location (City and State)	From (Month/Year)	To (Month/Year)
Practice/Facility Name:	Location (City and State)	From (Month/Year)	To (Month/Year)
Practice/Facility Name:	Location (City and State)	From (Month/Year)	To (Month/Year)

GAPS GREATER THAN 6 MONTHS:

From (Month/Year)	To (Month/Year)	Explanation

HOSPITAL AND MEDICAL STAFF ACTIVITIES
(Not applicable for Allied, Hospital-Based, and Non-Admitting Specialty)

List all hospitals where you currently hold privileges (List Primary Admitting first)

Hospital Name	Department	Type of Privileges	Date of Privileges

If you do not have admitting privileges, please indicate who will admit on your behalf.

_____

_____

PROFESSIONAL LIABILITY

Insurance

Identify present carrier. **If none, please submit a signed and dated Financial Responsibility Form****

Carrier Name: _____

Policy #: _____

Policy Period: _____   _____
                            From   To

Levels of Coverage: _____

** To request a blank Financial Responsibility Form, please call (800) 346-0231 x40546

DISCLOSURE QUESTIONS

LICENSURE

1. Has your license to practice in any state ever been relinquished, denied, limited, suspended, or revoked?   ☐Yes* ☐No

2. Have you ever voluntarily relinquished or been asked to surrender your license?   ☐Yes* ☐No

3. Have you ever been suspended, sanctioned, or otherwise restricted from participating in any private, federal, or state health insurance program (e.g., Medicare or Medicaid)?   ☐Yes* ☐No

4. Have you ever been the subject of an investigation by any private, federal, or state agency?   ☐Yes* ☐No

       4a. Are any such investigations pending?   ☐Yes* ☐No

5. Have any disciplinary actions or investigations been initiated against you by any state regulatory agency or medical society?   ☐Yes* ☐No

       5a. Are any such investigations pending?   ☐Yes* ☐No

6. Have you ever been disciplined or given a letter of guidance by any state regulatory agency or medical society?   ☐Yes* ☐No

DEA

1. Has your DEA registration ever been limited, suspended, revoked, restricted, or denied?   ☐Yes* ☐No

2. Have you ever voluntarily relinquished your DEA registration?   ☐Yes* ☐No

BOARD CERTIFICATON

1. Has your board status ever been — on a voluntary or involuntary basis — denied, revoked, suspended, reduced, limited, placed on probation, or relinquished for disciplinary reasons?   ☐Yes* ☐No

PRIVILEGES

1. Has your membership status, clinical privileges, and/or application ever been denied, suspended, reduced, or not renewed at any hospital, managed care organization, or any other institution?   ☐Yes* ☐No

2. Have you ever voluntarily relinquished membership status and/or clinical privileges at any hospital, managed care organization, or any other institution?   ☐Yes* ☐No

3. Have you ever withdrawn your application for appointment, reappointment, or clinical privileges or resigned from the medical staff before a decision was made by a hospital's or healthcare facility's governing board?   ☐Yes* ☐No

4. Have you ever been the subject of disciplinary proceedings or investigations at any hospital, healthcare facility, or managed care organization?   ☐Yes* ☐No

PERSONAL HISTORY

1. Do you have a physical or mental condition that could affect your ability to exercise the privileges requested or would require an accommodation for you to exercise those privileges safely and competently?   ☐Yes* ☐No

2. Do you have any current or prior physical or mental condition(s) that include, but are not limited to, alcohol or drug dependency, participation in aftercare programs for alcohol or drug dependency, medical limitation of activity, workload, etc., and prescribed medications that may affect your clinical judgment or motor skills?   ☐Yes* ☐No

3. Are you currently using any illegal drugs or controlled or dangerous substances?   ☐Yes* ☐No

4. Have you ever been convicted of a crime (other than a minor traffic offense), or do you have any criminal or civil charges pending against you or your practice?   ☐Yes* ☐No

5. Have you ever been named as a defendant in any criminal proceeding or entered a plea for any criminal offense, including but not limited to, domestic violence or driving while under the influence?   ☐Yes* ☐No

6. Have you ever been arrested for or charged with a sexual offense?   ☐Yes* ☐No

7. To your knowledge, has information pertaining to you ever been reported to the National Practitioner Data Bank or the Healthcare Integrity and Protection Data Bank?   ☐Yes* ☐No

*** For any Yes responses to questions on this page, please include a detailed explanation.**

PROFESSIONAL LIABILTY

1. Has your present professional liability insurance carrier excluded any specific area of practice (e.g., obstetrics, surgery) from your coverage? ☐Yes ☐No

    If yes, list the excluded clinical activities: _____

    Provide a full explanation on a separate sheet, including the name of the carrier, the date, and specific information concerning any limitation.

2. Has your professional liability insurance coverage ever been terminated by action of any insurance company? ☐Yes ☐No

    If yes, state when and by what company. _____

4. Have any professional liability claims or suits, including dismissals, ever been filed against you? ☐Yes* ☐No

5. Have any professional liability suits been filed against you that are presently pending? ☐Yes* ☐No

6. Have any judgments or settlements been made against you in professional liability cases? ☐Yes* ☐No

* For any Yes responses to questions 4, 5 or 6 above, please complete the attached
Professional Liability Claims form.

Required Documents

Copies of the following documents are required with this application in order to facilitate the credentialing process. Your application will not be processed without this information.

☐ AvMed Release of Information Form.

☐ Current Malpractice Insurance Face Sheet indicating effective dates and amount of coverage,

   or other means of compliance with state financial responsibility requirements.

☐ CV with Current Work History in month/year format.

☐ GP's only: CME Certificates for the past 2 years

☐ Narratives for positive responses (where indicated)

☐ Professional Liability Claims Form(s) (if applicable)

Affirmation

I represent that information provided in or attached to this application is accurate. I understand that a condition of this application is that any misrepresentation, misstatement, or commission from this application—whether intentional or not—is cause for automatic and immediate rejection of this application and may result in the denial of appointment and clinical privileges. Upon subsequent discovery of such misrepresentation, misstatement, or omission, AvMed Health Plans may immediately terminate my appointment and privileges. I agree to provide AvMed Health Plans with updated information regarding all questions on the application form as new information becomes available. I also agree to provide AvMed Health Plans information that it or one of its authorized representatives may request. Failure to produce any requested information will prevent my application from being processed.

_____   _____   _____
Applicant's signature   *Date*   *Applicant's Name (printed or typed)*

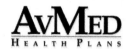

AUTHORIZATION FOR INVESTIGATION AND RELEASE OF INFORMATION

In order for AvMed Health Plan to verify, assess, or update my professional credentials, I:

➤ Authorize AvMed to make inquiries concerning such information about me to my previous employer(s), current employer, educational institutions, State Licensing boards, professional liability insurance carriers, American Medical Association, Federation of state Medical Boards, National Practitioner Data Bank, hospitals, health care facilities, health maintenance organizations, preferred provider organizations, and other professional organizations and/or persons, agencies, organizations, or institutions listed by me as references, and to any other appropriate sources to whom AvMed may be referred by those contacted;

➤ Authorize release of such information and copies of related records and/or documents to AvMed officials;

➤ Release from liability all those who provide information to AvMed in good faith and without malice in response to such inquiries;

➤ Authorize AvMed to disclose to such persons, employers, institutions, boards, or agencies identifying and other information about me sufficient to enable AvMed to make such inquiries.

I understand that:

➤ I have the right to review information obtained by AvMed during the primary verification process;

➤ This information is limited to data that I can obtain from the same primary sources utilized by AvMed (i.e., state licensing boards, National Practitioner Data Bank);

➤ I do not have the right to review information that is peer review protected (i.e., references, recommendations);

➤ Requests for review of information must be in writing, signed by me (original signature required), and submitted to the Credentialing Department;

➤ In the event that I discover erroneous information while reviewing data requested from the Credentialing Department, I will be afforded fifteen (15) calendar days from the receipt of the data in which to advise the Credentialing Department as to the correct information. I will be afforded an additional thirty (30) calendar days to correct the information with the appropriate agency(ies) and advise the Credentialing Department;

➤ If I was denied credentialing or recredentialing based on erroneous information, I will be afforded the right to submit corrected information for reconsideration by the Credentialing Committee no later than sixty (60) calendar days after receipt of the denial notice.

➤ I have the right, upon request, to be informed of the status of my application. Inquiries should be made by phone to AvMed Provider Services Call Center at 800-452-8633.

_____   _____
Signature   Date

_____
Printed Name

PROFESSIONAL LIABILITY CLAIMS

Please list all past or current professional liability claims which have been filed against you or your practice. (Photocopy this page as needed for each claim.)

Date of Occurance: _____   Date Claim Filed: _____

Professional Liability Carrier Involved: _____

Patient Name: _____

Claimant / Plaintiff, if other than patient: _____

Describe your role in the claim: ☐ Primary Defendant   ☐ Co-Defendant

Describe the allegations against you:

_____

_____

Clinical narrative describing your care and treatment of the patient:

_____

_____

_____

_____

_____

_____

_____

Present status of claim: ☐ Closed   ☐ Open

If closed, please indicate the method:

☐ Verdict or judgment for the plaintiff in the amount of $_____
   The portion of the verdict or judgment attributed to me was $_____
   Verdict / Judgment Date _____

☐ Settled out of court for $_____
   The portion of the settlement paid on my behalf was $_____
   Settlement Date _____

☐ Dismissed by the Court (attach a copy of the dismissal)

☐ The claimant/plaintiff voluntarily withdrew the claim (attach documentation)

☐ The claimant/plaintiff voluntarily dismissed me from the lawsuit (attach a copy of the dismissal)

DEPARTMENT OF HEALTH AND HUMAN SERVICES
CENTERS FOR MEDICARE & MEDICAID SERVICES

Form Approved
OMB No. 0938-0581

CLINICAL LABORATORY IMPROVEMENT AMENDMENTS (CLIA)
APPLICATION FOR CERTIFICATION

I. GENERAL INFORMATION

☐ Initial Application   ☐ Survey

☐ Change in Certification Type

☐ Other Changes *(Specify)*

_____

CLIA IDENTIFICATION NUMBER

_____ D _____

(If an initial application leave blank, a number will be assigned)

FACILITY NAME	FEDERAL TAX IDENTIFICATION NUMBER

EMAIL ADDRESS	TELEPHONE NO. *(Include area code)*	FAX NO. *(Include area code)*

FACILITY ADDRESS — *Physical Location of Laboratory (Building, Floor, Suite if applicable.)* Fee Coupon/Certificate will be mailed to this Address unless mailing address is specified

MAILING/BILLING ADDRESS *(If different from street address)*

NUMBER, STREET *(No P.O. Boxes)*	NUMBER, STREET

CITY	STATE	ZIP CODE	CITY	STATE	ZIP CODE

NAME OF DIRECTOR *(Last, First, Middle Initial)*

FOR OFFICE USE ONLY

Date Received _____

II. TYPE OF CERTIFICATE REQUESTED *(Check only one)*

☐ Certificate of Waiver *(Complete Sections I – VI and IX – X)*

☐ Certificate for Provider Performed Microscopy Procedures (PPM) *(Complete Sections I – X)*

☐ Certificate of Compliance *(Complete Sections I – X)*

☐ Certificate of Accreditation (Complete Sections I – X) and indicate which of the following organization(s) your laboratory is accredited by for CLIA purposes, or for which you have applied for accreditation for CLIA purposes

    ☐ The Joint Commission   ☐ AOA   ☐ AABB
    ☐ CAP   ☐ COLA   ☐ ASHI

If you are applying for a Certificate of Accreditation, you must provide evidence of accreditation for your laboratory by an approved accreditation organization as listed above for CLIA purposes or evidence of application for such accreditation within 11 months after receipt of your Certificate of Registration.

NOTE: Laboratory directors performing non-waived testing (including PPM) must meet specific education, training and experience under subpart M of the CLIA requirements. Proof of these requirements for the laboratory director must be submitted with the application.

According to the Paperwork Reduction Act of 1995, no persons are required to respond to a collection of information unless it displays a valid OMB control number. The valid OMB control number for this information collection is 0938-0581. The time required to complete this information collection is estimated to average 30 minutes to 2 hours per response, including the time to review instructions, search existing data resources, gather the data needed, and complete and review the information collection. If you have any comments concerning the accuracy of the time estimate(s) or suggestions for improving this form, please write to: CMS, Attn: PRA Reports Clearance Officer, 7500 Security Boulevard, Baltimore, Maryland 21244-1850.

III. TYPE OF LABORATORY *(Check the one most descriptive of facility type)*

☐ 01 Ambulance	☐ 11 Health Main. Organization	☐ 22 Practitioner Other *(Specify)*
☐ 02 Ambulatory Surgery Center	☐ 12 Home Health Agency	
☐ 03 Ancillary Testing Site in Health Care Facility	☐ 13 Hospice	☐ 23 Prison
☐ 04 Assisted Living Facility	☐ 14 Hospital	☐ 24 Public Health Laboratories
☐ 05 Blood Bank	☐ 15 Independent	☐ 25 Rural Health Clinic
☐ 06 Community Clinic	☐ 16 Industrial	☐ 26 School/Student Health Service
☐ 07 Comp. Outpatient Rehab Facility	☐ 17 Insurance	☐ 27 Skilled Nursing Facility/ Nursing Facility
☐ 08 End Stage Renal Disease Dialysis Facility	☐ 18 Intermediate Care Facility for Mentally Retarded	☐ 28 Tissue Bank/Repositories
☐ 09 Federally Qualified Health Center	☐ 19 Mobile Laboratory	☐ 29 Other *(Specify)*
☐ 10 Health Fair	☐ 20 Pharmacy	
	☐ 21 Physician Office Is this a shared lab? ☐ Yes ☐ No	

IV. HOURS OF LABORATORY TESTING *(List times during which **laboratory testing** is performed in HH:MM format)*

	SUNDAY	MONDAY	TUESDAY	WEDNESDAY	THURSDAY	FRIDAY	SATURDAY
FROM:							
TO:							

(For multiple sites, attach the additional information using the same format.)

V. MULTIPLE SITES *(must meet one of the regulatory exceptions to apply for this provision)*

Are you applying for the multiple site exception?

☐ No. If no, go to section VI.   ☐ Yes. If yes, complete remainder of this section.

Indicate which of the following regulatory exceptions applies to your facility's operation.

1. Is this a laboratory that has temporary testing sites?

   ☐ Yes ☐ No

2. Is this a not-for-profit or Federal, State or local government laboratory engaged in limited (not more than a combination of 15 moderate complexity or waived tests per certificate) public health testing and filing for a single certificate for multiple sites?

   ☐ Yes ☐ No

   If yes, provide the number of sites under the certificate_____ and list name, address and test performed for each site below.

3. Is this a hospital with several laboratories located at contiguous buildings on the same campus within the same physical location or street address and under common direction that is filing for a single certificate for these locations?

   ☐ Yes ☐ No

   If yes, provide the number of sites under this certificate_____ and list name or department, location within hospital and specialty/subspecialty areas performed at each site below.

   If additional space is needed, check here ☐ and attach the additional information using the same format.

NAME AND ADDRESS/LOCATION		TESTS PERFORMED/SPECIALTY/SUBSPECIALTY
NAME OF LABORATORY OR HOSPITAL DEPARTMENT		
ADDRESS/LOCATION *(Number, Street, Location if applicable)*		
CITY, STATE, ZIP CODE	TELEPHONE NO. *(Include area code)*	
NAME OF LABORATORY OR HOSPITAL DEPARTMENT		
ADDRESS/LOCATION *(Number, Street, Location if applicable)*		
CITY, STATE, ZIP CODE	TELEPHONE NO. *(Include area code)*	

In the next three sections, indicate testing performed and annual test volume.

VI. WAIVED TESTING

Identify the waived testing performed. Be as specific as possible. This includes each analyte test system or device used in the laboratory.

    e.g. (Rapid Strep, Acme Home Glucose Meter)

Indicate the estimated **TOTAL ANNUAL TEST** volume for all waived tests performed _____

☐ Check if no waived tests are performed

VII. PPM TESTING

Identify the PPM testing performed. Be as specific as possible.

    e.g. (Potassium Hydroxide (KOH) Preps, Urine Sediment Examinations)

Indicate the estimated TOTAL ANNUAL TEST volume for all PPM tests performed _____

For laboratories applying for certificate of compliance or certificate of accreditation, also include PPM test volume in the "total estimated test volume" in section VIII.

☐ Check if no PPM tests are performed

If additional space is needed, check here ☐ and attach additional information using the same format.

VIII. NON-WAIVED TESTING *(Including PPM testing)*

If you perform testing other than or in addition to waived tests, complete the information below. If applying for one certificate for multiple sites, the total volume should include testing for ALL sites.

Place a check (✓) in the box preceding each specialty/subspecialty in which the laboratory performs testing. Enter the estimated annual test volume for each specialty. Do not include testing not subject to CLIA, waived tests, or tests run for quality control, calculations, quality assurance or proficiency testing when calculating test volume. (For additional guidance on counting test volume, see the information included with the application package.)

If applying for a Certificate of Accreditation, indicate the name of the Accreditation Organization beside the applicable specialty/subspecialty for which you are accredited for CLIA compliance. (The Joint Commission, AOA, AABB, CAP, COLA or ASHI)

SPECIALTY / SUBSPECIALTY	ACCREDITING ORGANIZATION	ANNUAL TEST VOLUME	SPECIALTY / SUBSPECIALTY	ACCREDITING ORGANIZATION	ANNUAL TEST VOLUME
HISTOCOMPATIBILITY			**HEMATOLOGY**		
☐ Transplant			☐ Hematology		
☐ Nontransplant			**IMMUNOHEMATOLOGY**		
MICROBIOLOGY			☐ ABO Group & Rh Group		
☐ Bacteriology			☐ Antibody Detection (transfusion)		
☐ Mycobacteriology			☐ Antibody Detection (nontransfusion)		
☐ Mycology			☐ Antibody Identification		
☐ Parasitology			☐ Compatibility Testing		
☐ Virology			**PATHOLOGY**		
DIAGNOSTIC IMMUNOLOGY			☐ Histopathology		
☐ Syphilis Serology			☐ Oral Pathology		
☐ General Immunology			☐ Cytology		
CHEMISTRY			**RADIOBIOASSAY**		
☐ Routine			☐ Radiobioassay		
☐ Urinalysis			**CLINICAL CYTOGENETICS**		
☐ Endocrinology			☐ Clinical Cytogenetics		
☐ Toxicology			**TOTAL ESTIMATED ANNUAL TEST VOLUME:**		

Form CMS-116 (10/10)

3

IX. TYPE OF CONTROL

VOLUNTARY NONPROFIT

☐ 01 Religious Affiliation

☐ 02 Private Nonprofit

☐ 03 Other Nonprofit

_____
(Specify)

FOR PROFIT

☐ 04 Proprietary

GOVERNMENT

☐ 05 City

☐ 06 County

☐ 07 State

☐ 08 Federal

☐ 09 Other Government

_____
(Specify)

X. DIRECTOR AFFILIATION WITH OTHER LABORATORIES

If the director of this laboratory serves as director for additional laboratories that are separately certified, please complete the following:

CLIA NUMBER	NAME OF LABORATORY

ATTENTION: READ THE FOLLOWING CAREFULLY BEFORE SIGNING APPLICATION

Any person who intentionally violates any requirement of section 353 of the Public Health Service Act as amended or any regulation promulgated thereunder shall be imprisoned for not more than 1 year or fined under title 18, United States Code or both, except that if the conviction is for a second or subsequent violation of such a requirement such person shall be imprisoned for not more than 3 years or fined in accordance with title 18, United States Code or both.

Consent: The applicant hereby agrees that such laboratory identified herein will be operated in accordance with applicable standards found necessary by the Secretary of Health and Human Services to carry out the purposes of section 353 of the Public Health Service Act as amended. The applicant further agrees to permit the Secretary, or any Federal officer or employee duly designated by the Secretary, to inspect the laboratory and its operations and its pertinent records at any reasonable time and to furnish any requested information or materials necessary to determine the laboratory's eligibility or continued eligibility for its certificate or continued compliance with CLIA requirements.

SIGNATURE OF OWNER/DIRECTOR OF LABORATORY *(Sign in ink)*	DATE

THE CLINICAL LABORATORY IMPROVEMENT AMENDMENTS (CLIA) APPLICATION (FORM CMS-116)

INSTRUCTIONS FOR COMPLETION

CLIA requires every facility that tests human specimens for the purpose of providing information for the diagnosis, prevention or treatment of any disease or impairment of, or the assessment of the health of, a human being to meet certain Federal requirements. If your facility performs tests for these purposes, it is considered, under the law, to be a laboratory. CLIA applies even if only one or a few basic tests are performed, and even if you are not charging for testing. In addition the CLIA legislation requires financing of all regulatory costs through fees assessed to affected facilities.

The CLIA application (Form CMS-116) collects information about your laboratory's operation which is necessary to determine the fees to be assessed, to establish baseline data and to fulfill the statutory requirements for CLIA. This information will also provide an overview of your facility's laboratory operation. All information submitted should be based on your facility's laboratory operation as of the date of form completion.

NOTE: WAIVED TESTS ARE NOT EXEMPT FROM CLIA. FACILITIES PERFORMING ONLY THOSE TESTS CATEGORIZED AS WAIVED MUST APPLY FOR A CLIA CERTIFICATE OF WAIVER.

NOTE: Laboratory directors performing non-waived testing (including PPM) must meet specific education, training and experience under subpart M of the CLIA requirements. Proof of these requirements for the laboratory director must be submitted with the application. Information to be submitted with the application include:

- Verification of State Licensure, as applicable

- Documentation of qualifications:
   - Education (copy of Diploma, transcript from accredited institution, CMEs),
   - Credentials, and
   - Laboratory experience.

Individuals who attended foreign schools must have an evaluation of their credentials determining equivalency of their education to education obtained in the United States. Failure to submit this information will delay the processing of your application.

ALL APPLICABLE SECTIONS MUST BE COMPLETED. INCOMPLETE APPLICATIONS CANNOT BE PROCESSED AND WILL BE RETURNED TO THE FACILITY. PRINT LEGIBLY OR TYPE INFORMATION.

I. GENERAL INFORMATION

For an initial applicant, check "initial application". For an initial survey or for a recertification, check "survey". For a request to change the type of certificate, check "Change in certificate type". For all other changes, including change in location, director, etc., check "other changes".

For an initial applicant, the CLIA number should be left blank. The number will be assigned when the application is processed. Be specific when indicating the name of your facility, particularly when it is a component of a larger entity; e.g., respiratory therapy department in XYZ Hospital. For a physician's office, this may be the name of the physician. NOTE: The information provided is what will appear on your certificate.

Facility street address must be the actual physical location where testing is performed, including floor, suite and/or room, if applicable. DO NOT USE A POST OFFICE BOX NUMBER OR A MAIL DROP ADDRESS FOR THE NUMBER AND STREET OF THE ADDRESS. If the laboratory has a separate mailing address, please complete that section of the application.

NOTE: For Office Use Only—Date received is the date the form is received by the state agency or CMS regional office for processing.

II. TYPE OF CERTIFICATE REQUESTED
When completing this section, please remember that a facility holding a:

- **Certificate of Waiver** can only perform tests categorized as waived;*
- **Certificate for Provider Performed Microscopy Procedures** (PPM) can only perform tests categorized as PPM, or tests categorized as PPM and waived tests;*
- **Certificate of Compliance** can perform tests categorized as waived, PPM and moderate and/or high complexity tests provided the applicable CLIA quality standards are met; and
- **Certificate of Accreditation** can perform tests categorized as waived, PPM and moderate and/or high complexity non-waived tests provided the laboratory is currently accredited by an approved accreditation organization.

*A current list of waived and PPMP tests may be obtained from your State agency. Specific test system categorizations can also be found on the Internet at: *http://www.accessdata.fda.gov/scripts/cdrh/cfdocs/cfCLIA/clia.cfm*.

III. TYPE OF LABORATORY
Select your certificate type based on the highest level of test complexity performed by your laboratory. Laboratories performing non-waived tests can choose COA or COC based on the agency you wish to survey your laboratory.

A shared laboratory is when two or more sole practicing physicians collectively pool resources to fund a laboratory's operations. The definition of a shared laboratory may also include two or more physician group practices that share the expenses for the laboratory's operation.

IV. HOURS OF ROUTINE OPERATION
Provide only the times when actual laboratory testing is performed in your facility. Please use the HH:MM format.

V. MULTIPLE SITES
You can only qualify for the multiple site provision (more than one site under one certificate) if you meet one of the CLIA requirements described in 42 CFR 493. Hospice and HHA could qualify for an exception i.e. 493.35(b)(1-3), 493.43(b)(1-3) and 493.55(b)(1-3).

VI. WAIVED TESTING
Indicate the estimated total annual test volume for all waived tests performed. List can be found at: http:www.cms.gov/CLIA/downloads/waivetbl.pdf

VII. PPM TESTING
Indicate the estimated annual test volume for all PPM tests performed. List can be found at: http://www.cms.gov/clia/downloads/ppmp.list.pdf

VIII. NON-WAIVED TESTING *(INCLUDING PPM)*
The total volume in this section includes all non-waived testing, including PPM tests previously counted in section VII. Follow the specific instructions on page 3 of the Form CMS-116 when completing this section. (Note: The Accrediting Organization column should reflect accreditation information for CLIA purposes only; e.g., CAP, etc.).

IX. TYPE OF CONTROL
Select the type of control which most appropriately describes your facility.

X. DIRECTOR OF ADDITIONAL LABORATORIES
List all other facilities for which the director is responsible and that are under different certificate.

Note that for a Certificate of PPM, Certificate of Compliance or Certificate of Accreditation, an individual can only serve as the director for no more than five certificates.

Once the completed Form CMS-116 has been returned to the applicable State agency and it is processed, a fee remittance coupon will be issued. The fee remittance coupon will indicate your CLIA identification number and the amount due for the certificate, and if applicable the compliance (survey) or validation fee. If you are applying for a Certificate of Compliance or Certificate of Accreditation, you will initially pay for and receive a Registration Certificate. A Registration Certificate permits a facility requesting a Certificate of Compliance to perform testing until an onsite inspection is conducted to determine program compliance; or for a facility applying for a Certificate of Accreditation, until verification of accreditation by an approved accreditation organization is received by CMS.

If you need additional information concerning CLIA, or if you have questions about completion of this form, please contact your State agency.

VIII. NON-WAIVED TESTING

TESTS COMMONLY PERFORMED AND THEIR CORRESPONDING LABORATORY SPECIALTIES/SUBSPECIALTIES

HISTOCOMPATIBILITY
HLA Typing (disease associated antigens)

MICROBIOLOGY

Bacteriology
Gram Stain
Culture
Susceptibility
Strep screen
Antigen assays (H.pylori, Chlamydia, etc.)

Mycobacteriology
Acid Fast Smear
Mycobacterial culture
Mycobacterial susceptibility

Mycology
Fungal Culture
DTM
KOH Preps

Parasitology
Direct Preps
Ova and Parasite Preps
Wet Preps

Virology
RSV (Not including waived kits)
HPV assay
Cell culture

DIAGNOSTIC IMMUNOLOGY

Syphilis Serology
RPR
FTA, MHATP

General Immunology
Allergen testing
ANA
Antistreptolysin O
Antigen/Antibody (hepatitis, herpes, rubella, etc.)
Complement (C3, C4)
Immunoglobulin
HIV
Mononucleosis assay
Rheumatoid factor
Tumor marker (AFP, CA 19-9, CA 15-3, CA 125)*

*Tumor markers can alternatively be listed under
Routine Chemistry instead of General Immunology.

HEMATOLOGY
Complete Blood Count (CBC)
WBC count
RBC count
Hemoglobin
Hematocrit (Not including spun micro)
Platelet count
Differential
Activated Clotting Time
Prothrombin time (Not including waived instruments)
Partial thromboplastin time
Fibrinogen
Reticulocyte count
Manual WBC by hemocytometer
Manual platelet by hemocytometer
Manual RBC by hemocytometer
Sperm count

IMMUNOHEMATOLOGY
ABO group
Rh(D) type
Antibody screening
Antibody identification
Compatibility testing

PATHOLOGY
Dermatopathology
Oral Pathology
PAP smear interpretations
Other Cytology tests
Histopathology

RADIOBIOASSAY
Red cell volume
Schilling test

CLINICAL CYTOGENETICS
Fragile X
Buccal smear
Prader-Willi syndrome
FISH studies for: neoplastic disorders, congenital disorders or solid tumors.

CHEMISTRY

Routine Chemistry
Albumin
Ammonia
Alk Phos
ALT/SGPT
AST/SGOT
Amylase
Bilirubin
Blood gas (pH, pO2, pCO2)
BUN
Calcium
Chloride
Cholesterol
Cholesterol, HDL
CK/CK isoenzymes
CO2
Creatinine
Ferritin
Folate
GGT
Glucose (Not fingerstick)
Iron
LDH/LDH isoenzymes
Magnesium
Potassium
Protein, electrophoresis
Protein, total
PSA
Sodium
Triglycerides
Troponin
Uric acid
Vitamin B12

Endocrinology
Cortisol
HCG (serum pregnancy test)
T3
T3 Uptake
T4
T4, free
TSH

Toxicology
Acetaminophen
Blood alcohol
Blood lead (Not waived)
Carbamazepine
Digoxin
Ethosuximide
Gentamicin
Lithium
Phenobarbital
Phenytoin
Primidone
Procainamide
NAPA
Quinidine
Salicylates
Theophylline
Tobramycin
Therapeutic Drug Monitoring

Urinalysis**
Automated Urinalysis (Not including waived instruments)
Microscopic Urinalysis
Urine specific gravity by refractometer
Urine specific gravity by urinometer
Urine protein by sulfosalicylic acid

** Dipstick urinalysis is counted in Section VI. WAIVED TESTING

NOTE: This is not a complete list of tests covered by CLIA. Other non-waived tests and their specialties/subspecialties can be found at **http://www.cms.gov/CLIA/downloads/subject.to.CLIA.pdf** and **http://www.cms.gov/CLIA/downloads/IcCodes.pdf**. You may also call your State agency for further information. State agency contact information can be found at: **http://www.cms.gov/CLIA/downloads/CLIA.SA.pdf.**

GUIDELINES FOR COUNTING TESTS FOR CLIA

- For **histocompatibility**, each HLA typing (including disease associated antigens), HLA antibody screen, or HLA crossmatch is counted as one test.

- For **microbiology**, susceptibility testing is counted as one test per group of antibiotics used to determine sensitivity for one organism. Cultures are counted as one per specimen regardless of the extent of identification, number of organisms isolated and number of tests/procedures required for identification.

- For **general immunology**, testing for allergens should be counted as one test per individual allergen.

- For **hematology**, each **measured** individual analyte of a **complete blood count** or **flow cytometry** test that is ordered **and reported** is counted separately. The **WBC differential** is counted as one test.

- For **immunohematology**, each ABO, Rh, antibody screen, crossmatch or antibody identification is counted as one test.

- For **histopathology**, each block (not slide) is counted as one test. Autopsy services are not included. For those laboratories that perform special stains on histology slides, the test volume is determined by adding the number of special stains performed on slides to the total number of specimen blocks prepared by the laboratory.

- For **cytology**, each slide (not case) is counted as one test for both Pap smears and nongynecologic cytology.

- For **clinical cytogenetics**, the number of tests is determined by the number of specimen types processed on each patient; e.g., a bone marrow and a venous blood specimen received on one patient is counted as two tests.

- For **chemistry**, each analyte in a profile counts as one test.

- For **urinalysis**, microscopic and macroscopia examinations, each count as one test. Macroscopics (dipsticks) are counted as one test regardless of the number of reagent pads on the strip.

- For **all specialties/subspecialities**, do not count calculations (e.g., A/G ratior, MCH, T7, etc.), quality control, quality assurance, or proficiency testing assays.

If you need additional information concerning counting tests for CLIA, please contact your State agency.

Accountable Care Organizations (ACO): A type of healthcare reform in which the third party payer groups providers of different specialties and assigns that group a set of patients. The model ties provider reimbursement to both quality measures and reduction in total healthcare costs by eliminating redundant tests and treatments by coordinating the care of each patient between hospital care and various physician specialists and generalists.

Ad Hoc: A committee or report that is not routine but formed or generated as needed for a specific purpose.

Adjudication: The determination by a third party of its financial obligations after applying the patient's health insurance benefits to a claim.

Adverse Benefit Determination: A determination by a third party that a service for which a claim was received is not payable or that a previously paid service was paid in error and must be refunded.

Age Discrimination in Employment Act (ADEA): An act of Congress passed into federal law in the United States in 1967 making it illegal to discriminate against anyone over the age of 40 years.

Allowed Amount: The amount a third-party payer determines is the full value of a specific service or procedure. Therefore, the total of a patient's responsibility plus the payer's responsibility will not exceed this amount.

Ambulatory Surgery Centers (ASC): A distinct entity with the primary purpose of providing nonemergency surgical procedures that do not usually require overnight hospitalization but are more complex than can routinely be performed in a physician's office setting.

Americans with Disabilities Act of 1990 (ADA): This act was amended in 2008. The law was passed to eliminate discrimination against people with disabilities for the purposes of employment including hiring, promoting, discharging, workers compensation benefits, and job training.

Assets: The total resources of a medical practice including cash, accounts receivables, property, equipment that could be sold for cash, and any other entity which can be legitimately assessed a value.

Assignment of Benefits: The patient signs an agreement whereby the physician will receive any payment for services directly from the patient's insurance company including Medicare.

Authoritarian Leadership: Also known as autocratic leadership, authoritarian leaders provide clear expectations of how, what, and when tasks need to be completed without input from subordinates and within a well-defined position of authority within the company.

Authority: The formal or legitimate authority or power to act on behalf of an organization including the authority to require other employees to act within the limits of the authority figure's scope and within the scope of the employee's job description.

Autocratic Leadership: See authoritarian leadership.

Automatic Fingerprint Identification System (AFIS): A national automated fingerprint identification and criminal history system maintained by the Federal Bureau of Investigation (FBI). AFIS allows search, exchange, and storage capabilities.

Balance Bill: The act of charging a patient (or person financially responsible for the patient) the difference between an insurer's allowed amount and the amount the practice charges for a service.

Balance Sheet: A summary of the financial balances—assets, liabilities, ownership equity as of a given date of a medical practice or any business.

Balanced Score Card (BSC): A strategic performance management framework that allows companies to identify, manage, and measure its strategic objectives from various perspectives.

Behaviorally Anchored Rating Scale: Combines qualitative and quantitative measurement techniques to help managers more accurately evaluate employee performance. These scales take a skill, define it, and then present various levels of performance that are anchored by specific types of behaviors.

Benchmarking: Comparing a practice's performance or work processes against either a national standard representing best practices or an otherwise similar practice that is known to have better performance outcomes especially with regard to quality, timeliness, and cost.

Bottom-Up Budgeting: A participative approach to budgeting in which each unit has input into the budgeting process up through senior management and then the final budget is approved.

Brainstorming: A technique involving a group of people who generate creative ideas in a spontaneous manner in an attempt to solve a problem or make a decision.

Bureaucratic Leadership: Bureaucratic leaders are concerned with ensuring workers follow rules and procedures accurately and consistently.

Business Records Hearsay Exception: Records are considered hearsay (they record what others said and did and are maintained by other than those directly involved in litigation) and are not usually admissible in court. Medical records are the business records of health care and are an exception to the hearsay rule as long as they meet certain criteria such as being maintained in the course of business and recorded at or very near the time of the event by someone who has personal knowledge of the event, that is, a practitioner.

Call Routing or Call Transfer Procedure: A procedure that contains a list of every known type of phone call the office might receive and then describes the action the person receiving the call should take for each type.

Capital Budget: The amount of money projected in addition to the annual operational budget for long-term assets such as large equipment or facilities.

Capitation: A type of managed care that reimburses a physician or group a set amount of money each month for each member of the plan who lists the practice as their primary care physician, regardless of whether that patient received care that month.

Cash Flow Statement: A financial statement that demonstrates how changes in the accounts and income on the balance sheet affect the inflow and outflow of cash.

Center for Information Technology Leadership (CITL): An academic research organization founded in 2002 and focused on assessing the impacts and costs of health information technologies.

Center for Medicare and Medicaid Services (CMS): A division of the Federal Department of Health and Human Services concerned with administering the Medicare and federal portion of Medicaid programs.

Centralization: An organizational theory in which decision making is centralized with top administration based on set policies and communicated down through the organizational structure to the bottom tier.

Certification Commission for Health Care Information Technology (CCHIT): An alliance formed by several professional organizations to: reduce the risk of physicians losing money when they invest in health information technology (HIT), ensure interoperability of electronic health records and other technology, and increase the availability of incentives to accelerate the adoption of interoperable HIT.

Certified Coder Specialist, Physician Based (CCS-P): A credential offered through the American Health Information Management Association designating a professional coder specializing in the coding of physician-based documentation.

Certified Professional Coder (CPC): A credential offered through the American Association of Professional Coders designating a professional coder specializing in the coding of physician-based documentation.

Chain of Command: A system of organization in which authority and decision making flows down from the top through a series of managers in which each manager is generally only accountable to one superior.

Civil Monetary Penalty Act (CMP): An act authorizing the Office of Inspector General to assess and seek civil monetary and other penalties (i.e., exclusion from participation in Medicare) against people who commit health care fraud, violate the antikickback statute, or commit any other abuse of federal health care funds.

Civil Rights Act: Originally passed in 1866 to outlaw certain discriminatory practices for African Americans after the Civil War, it was amended in 1964 to make any type of discrimination against blacks and women illegal. Amended again in 1968 to increase enforcement and include Fair Housing, this law continues to protect minorities from any form of employment discrimination.

Civilian Health and Medical Program of the Department of Veteran Affairs (CHAMPVA): CHAMPVA is a comprehensive health care program in which the Veteran's Administration shares in the cost of health care services and supplies with eligible veterans-those with service related disabilities and certain surviving dependents of deceased eligible veterans.

Claim: A standardized document—CMS 1500 in the case of health care practitioners containing all necessary information and submitted to a third-party payer in order for the practitioner to be reimbursed for eligible services provided to a patient who has health insurance.

Clearinghouse: Practices submit electronic claims to clearinghouses where the claims are scrubbed, formatted, and sent in real time to the appropriate insurance companies in a format acceptable by each insurance company regardless of the software used in the originating medical office.

Clinical Laboratory Improvement Act (CLIA): An act passed in 1988 delineating the conditions a laboratory must meet in order to be certified and therefore to receive any reimbursement under CMS.

CMS 1500: A standardized form originally from the Center for Medicare and Medicaid Services but used to submit claims to most third-party payers so that physician and other eligible practitioners get reimbursed for services covered by the third-party payer.

Coercive Power: One of five recognized forms of power (coercive, reward, legitimate, referent, and expert), coercive power is the power to force someone to do something against their will. It is often physical but may also be psychological or emotional and often uses demonstrations of harm to illustrate what will happen if compliance is not gained.

Coinsurance: A percentage of allowable charges, after any deductible has been satisfied, that the insured must pay. For example, after deductible, a third-party payer may pay 80% of allowed amount and the insured pays the other 20%.

Commercial Health Insurance: A third-party insurance plan that does not receive any funding from the government for administration or payment of benefits.

Computerized Physician Order Entry (CPOE): A process in which a clinician inputs orders for patient care into a computer system that is connected to the appropriate recipient such as a pharmacy, a laboratory or an imaging center. The order is filled or the test is conducted and the results of the test are returned electronically to the clinician.

Communications Services Company: A company that contracts with a medical office to provide various levels of communications support using technology or actual manpower. For example, a communications company is able to remind patients when an appointment is scheduled for the following business day. The services can be very limited or comprehensive.

Consolidated Omnibus Budget Reconciliation Act (COBRA): An act established in 1985 to assist employees who find themselves involuntarily unemployed to continue health care benefits for themselves and their families at the employer's group rates. While the former employee pays the full amount, this option is typically less expensive than the individual or self-insured rate.

Continuing Medical Education (CME): Continuing medical education consists of educational activities which serve to maintain, develop, or increase the knowledge, skills, and performance of a physician and are required for maintenance of credentials.

Continuous Quality Improvement (CQI): A formal method of quality improvement that continuously assesses all aspects of performance and seeks to improve any process, in order of highest impact to lowest impact, so that the practice is continuously improving individual and overall outcomes.

Controlling: One of the traditional functions of management in which the supervisor monitors actual performance against projected performance and determines when corrections need to be made during a certain period of time.

Conventions: Conventions are a tool used in medical coding to alert the coding professional that there is something unique about a code. For example, the code is new this year or the coder has to add another code to the one being considered in a specific sequence, etc.

Coordination of Benefits (COB): A system whereby the order of payment is coordinated among various payers when the patient is covered by more than one third-party payer so that the total combination of multiple payments never exceeds the charges for each service.

Covered Benefit: A term referring to whether a specific third-party payer reimburses for certain services or procedures. For example, one plan may cover an annual physical exam for all of its participants and another may only pay for physicals for children of certain ages.

Covered Entities (CEs): Under HIPAA, any entity defined in the rule as covered must comply with the HIPAA Privacy Rule. Originally, health care payers, health care providers, and medical claims clearinghouses were covered entities but under the Health Care Reform Act of 2009, the list was expanded to include business associates and also to increase the penalties for violation.

CPT Category II Codes: Supplemental tracking codes in the CPT manual that help measure performance compared with national protocols.

Credits: In accounting or bookkeeping, using a double-entry system, there are accounts: assets, expenses, liabilities, owner's equity, and income. Assets plus equity must be equal to liability plus owner's equity plus income. Debits are entries on the left and increase a debit account (e.g., assets and expenses) and decrease a credit account (liabilities, income, and owner's equity). Credits are on the right side and increase a credit account.

Culture of Accountability: A concept that promotes each individual in a medical practice, including each patient, to willingly accept accountability to fulfill their obligations. So, a receptionist is accountable for positive patient communications, providing accurate information to patients and inputting accurate information into the computer system, taking good messages, etc., while a patient is accountable for arriving on time for appointments, meeting all financial obligations in a timely manner, and letting the receptionist know before the actual appointment is scheduled, all of the things that patient would like to discuss with a practitioner so the receptionist can schedule the most appropriate amount of time.

Current Procedural Terminology (CPT): A copyrighted coding system by the American Medical Association that provides a listing of descriptive terms and identifying codes for reporting medical services and procedures performed by physicians and other qualified practitioners.

Debits: In accounting or bookkeeping, using a double-entry system, there are accounts: assets, expenses, liabilities, owner's equity, and income. Assets plus equity must be equal to liability plus owner's equity plus income. Debits are entries on the left and increase a debit account (e.g., assets and expenses) and decrease a credit account (liabilities, income, and owner's equity). Credits are on the right side and increase a credit account.

Decentralization: An organizational structure in which authority to make decisions is delegated downward in an organization rather than centralized with executive management.

Decision Matrix: A graphic tool used to evaluate and prioritize a list of options using weighted criteria determined by the team. For example, a decision matrix can be used to choose an electronic health record vendor or to solve a problem.

Deductible: A predetermined amount for which the patient pays the medical provider(s) the entire cost of treatment (allowed amount if the doctor is participating) up to a specified dollar amount before the third-party payer begins to pay benefits—often a deductible is renewed every year.

Delegate: To ask a subordinate to perform a task for which he or she has the authority to act on the superior's behalf but the superior is still ultimately responsible for the work getting done in a timely and accurate manner.

Departmentalization: A form of organization in which like tasks are grouped together into departments. For example, in a large medical office, laboratory staff may form one department while radiology staff forms another.

Depreciation: The gradual (usually over several years) converting of a capital expense, such as the amount of money spent at one time to purchase a $10,000.00 piece of equipment, into an operational expense (for the annual budget) over the useful life of the asset.

Designated Record Set (DRS): Under the HIPAA Privacy Rule, DRS is any medical record or billing record, including any item or repository containing protected health information, that is used to make decisions about individuals and is collected, maintained, used, or exchanged by or for any covered entity.

Discovery: Part of the pretrial litigation process during which each party requests relevant information and documents from the other side in an attempt to discover facts pertinent to the case and includes depositions, interrogatories, requests for admissions, document production requests, and requests for inspection.

Discrimination: Employment discrimination occurs when an individual receives unequal treatment in an employment situation. In other words, promoting one person over the other based on age discrimination.

Dual Eligibility: A situation in which a patient has both Medicare and Medicaid coverage and no other insurance.

E-Discovery: The collection, preparation, review, and production of electronic documents in litigation discovery. This includes e-mail, attachments, and other data stored on a computer, network, backup, or other storage media.

Electronic Health Records: An electronic record of health-related information on an individual that conforms to nationally recognized interoperability standards and that can be created, managed, and consulted by authorized clinicians and staff across more than on health care organization.

Electronic Medical Record (EMR): An electronic record of health-related information on an individual that can be created, gathered, managed, and consulted by authorized clinicians and staff within one health care organization.

Electronic Patient-Protected Health Information (ePHI): Provision under HIPAA defining any information in electronic format about health status, provision of health care, or payment for health care that can be linked to a specific individual including any part of a patient's medical record or payment history.

Electronic Prescribing: A form of computerized order entry in which the clinician uses a computer to submit an order for a prescription or refill. The order passes through patient safety edits and, once cleared, is pending in the pharmacy computer to fill the order.

Employee Retirement Income Security Act (ERISA): Law enacted in 1974 to protect an employee's pension plan but as employers started to add health insurance as a benefit of employment, health benefits were placed under the protection of this law.

Encoder: Software that facilitates coding medical records by providing sophisticated search tools and logic. Encoders contain updates from coding resources for ICD, CPT, and HCPC codes.

Equal Pay Act (EPA): Law passed in 1974 with the essential purpose of ensuring that women and men receive equal pay for equal work. However, the act protects both genders from wage discrimination based on sex.

Ergonomics: The consideration of the human factors in the design of office equipment and furniture to optimize safety, minimize repetitive stress disorders, and facilitate efficiency.

Established Patient: A patient who has been seen by the same physician or another physician of the same specialty in the same practice within 3 years of a current appointment.

Evaluation and Management: A service performed by a qualified practitioner (e.g., physician) whereby a patient's condition is evaluated by considering patient health history, results of a physical examination, and results of any tests to determine a diagnosis and a plan of managing the diagnosis.

Expert-Based Power: A source of power (the ability to get things done) that is derived from the supervisor having more knowledge than the workers about the work that needs to be accomplished and is therefore an expert in that area gleaning respect from subordinates.

Explanation of Benefits (EOB): A statement from a third-party payer that explains to the patient the result of processing a claim and explains any amount that was not paid for that service.

External Equity: Determining an equitable amount to pay an employee compared to what other similar companies in the same geographic region pay for the equivalent of that employee's job title.

Fair Credit Reporting Act (FCRA): A law that protects the privacy of individuals' consumer credit information, giving them the right to access their credit reports, know when someone has used this information in decision regarding credit, housing, employment, or other benefits, and dispute inaccurate information. With regard to employment, the FCRA places certain restrictions and obligations on employers who wish to access and use information in a potential employee's or current employee's credit report.

Fair Labor Standards Act (FLSA): A federal law that regulates wages and hours. It determines how much workers must be paid, at a minimum, and how many hours they can be required to work.

False Claims Act (FCA): A federal law that imposes penalties, such as fines and imprisonment on persons or companies who defraud any governmental program (e.g., Medicare or Medicaid).

Family and Medical Leave Act (FMLA): A law that provides eligible employees with the right to take up to 12 months of unpaid leave per 12-month period for certain reasons such as to bond with a new child or care for a sick spouse.

Federal Antikickback Statute: A statute that specifies anyone who knowingly and willfully receives or pays anything of value to influence the referral of federal health care program business, including Medicare and Medicaid, can be held accountable for a felony punishable by a fine up to $25,000 per occurrence or imprisonment for up to 5 years or both.

Federal Register: The daily publication of rules, proposed rules, and notices of the federal government.

Fee Schedule: A preset, specific dollar amount that will be charged or reimbursed for each type of service or procedure performed (generally based on individual CPT codes).

Fiscal Year: A 1-year financial cycle that may begin on any day of any month but the first date marks the new financial or budget year for a given practice.

Formal Authority: Formal authority is the power to influence or get things done by position—supervisory authority, for example.

Formulary: A prescription drug formulary is a list of prescription drugs that a given third-party payer will reimburse. Drugs not on that list are only reimbursed on an exception basis.

Gatekeeper: In managed care, a gatekeeper is the primary care physician who must refer patients to specialists or other medical services instead of patients being able to schedule appointments directly with a specialist.

Genetic Information Nondiscrimination Act (GINA): The most recent new civil rights law—GINA prohibits health insurers from using genetic information in decisions about insurance coverage or premiums. With regard to employers, the act prohibits the use of genetic information in employment decisions such as hiring and promotion and requires employers to keep genetic information confidential.

Goals: A goal is a desired outcome or end result of a planned course of action by an individual or a company—usually within a specific frame of time.

Graphic Rating Scales: A method of performance management in which the supervisor lists a number of traits such as job knowledge, reliability, and quality and asks you to rate each employee on a scale ranging from outstanding to unsatisfactory.

Group Model: A HMO managed care model in which the MCO has a contract with a single-multispecialty medical group in each region in which it operates.

Health Information Exchange (HIE): The electronic movement of health-related information among organizations according to nationally recognized standards.

Health Information Organization (HIO): An organization that oversees and governs the exchange of health-related information among organizations according to nationally recognized standards.

Health Insurance Portability and Accountability Act (HIPAA): A law designed to define privacy standards in order to protect the privacy, confidentiality, and security of patient-specific health information.

Health Maintenance Organization (HMO): HMOs are a type of managed care organizations that focus on the maintenance of health in individuals. HMOs encourage healthy lifestyles and early detection of diseases through routine physical exams and screenings. The HMO model is the first managed care model and also the most pure of the managed care philosophy.

HIPAA Privacy Rule: A rule created to put into practice the patient privacy requirements within HIPAA and to protect identifiable patient health information.

HIPAA Security Rules: A rule created to protect ePHI (i.e., PHI that is created, stored, maintained, and communicated by the medical provider electronically).

Immigration Reform and Control Act of 1986 (IRCA): A law containing three major provisions that require employers to verify that all employees are eligible to work in the United States; to keep records of employment verification; and to refrain from discrimination based on citizenship status or national origin.

Incentive Plans: A method of rewarding either individual employees or groups of employees for meeting or exceeding goals, based on paying for performance by awarding extra money or other valuable incentives.

Income Statement: A report of a medical practice's revenue and their expenses, including any applicable taxes. This report will help the practice analyze the cost of providing various services but also is a tool that from the top down shows revenues, total expenses, etc.

Incremental Budgets: A form of budgeting in which an adjustment is made to the previous budget to accommodate known variances such as the cost of health insurance being raised by 5% for all employees.

Indemnity Insurance: Also referred to as traditional or fee-for-service insurance and is considered a non–provider-network (or nonmanaged care) type of coverage.

Individual Practice Association (IPA): A HMO managed care model in which some number of independent physicians form a group that is then able to negotiate with a HMO to offer its members a network of general practitioners and specialists as though they were a network model. The difference is that the IPA is not a "group" for other purposes.

Informal Authority: A source of power (the ability to get things done) derived based on employees looking to a coworker for leadership due to charisma or perceived expertise or some other non–company-sanctioned trait.

Information Security Officer: An identified officer tasked with the development and implementation of the information security policy of the compliance plan for the medical practice.

Insurance or Billing Specialist: A person who is responsible for all of the steps in the revenue cycle that occur from the time a patient is seen by a practitioner until there is a zero balance for that particular encounter.

Internal Equity: Determining that all employees within the same practice are paid within the same range as all other employees with similar job titles, responsibilities, and reporting structure.

International Classification of Diseases (ICD): The official system used to code and classify health conditions, reasons for encounters with health professionals, inpatient hospital procedures for the use of the facility, and other health-related information.

Interoperability: The ability for health information systems, using approved standards, to exchange health care data and information in a meaningful manner between disparate systems and organizations.

Job Analysis: A template that provides a tool for defining the work that is expected to be done by anyone in a specific job title. It forms the basis of the job description.

Job Description: A document that describes each job, by job title, as to what work is performed, the qualifications necessary, the pay grade, and whether or not it is an exempt or nonexempt position, reporting structure, etc.

Legal Health Record (LHR): A medical record that is in full compliance with all rules, regulations, and laws governing how the record is created, updated, maintained, stored, accessed, transmitted to another party, and amended.

Legitimate Power: A source of power (the ability to get things done) which is the perception that the manager has the right to supervise people based on official or legitimate or formal position held by the supervisor.

Line Authority: A position of authority in which at least one person reports to that supervisor. It differs from staff authority because staff authority is a person who has authority to make decisions that affect others but they are not the direct supervisors of those employees.

Long-Term or Strategic Planning: Long-term planning is a function of senior or executive management as to how the practice is going to achieve its mission over a period of time—often 5 years with annual updates,

Magnetic Stripe Security Badge: A type of authentication verification in which a magnetic stripe containing data about the authorized badge owner to ensure the person has legal rights to access PHI. It works like the magnetic stripe on a debit card.

Managed Care Organization (MCO): The concept of managed care is to negotiate discounted rates with providers who treat patients covered by that managed care organization (MCO) and to improve quality of patient care by increasing coverage for preventive medicine and early detection screenings. The providers who agree to specific packages are considered part of that MCO's network.

Management by Objectives: An organization-wide goal-setting method that emphasizes collaboration and buy-in from one level to the next.

Medicaid: A jointly funded health care plan between the federal government and each state that was designed to provide health insurance coverage to people who have limited income and who qualify for coverage.

Medical Necessity: A set of predetermined conditions for which a certain procedure or service is considered to be necessary for health purposes and therefore eligible for reimbursement by a third party. An example is urinalysis. Medicare may pay for this test under certain circumstances but not others.

Medicare: A federal government program administered by the CMS that provides health insurance benefits for people age 65 or older, people under age 65 with certain disabilities, and people of all ages with end-stage renal disease.

Medicare Advantage: Provides an option for Medicare-eligible people to choose a commercial, managed care option for their benefits (Part A, B, and D) instead of traditional Medicare coverage.

Medicare Part A: Designed to provide insurance benefits to help pay for hospital, skilled nursing, and certain other facility charges.

Medicare Part B: Designed to provide medical insurance to help cover doctors' services and outpatient care. It also covers some other medical services that Part A doesn't cover.

Medicare Part C: Part C is also called Medicare Advantage and provides an option for Medicare-eligible people to choose a commercial managed care option for their benefits instead of traditional coverage.

Medicare Part D: Provides coverage for prescription drugs.

Medicare Secondary Payer (MSP): A term used to describe any situation in which a Medicare-eligible person has other coverage that must process benefits as the primary payer and then any balances may be submitted to Medicare for processing.

Medigap: Provides optional supplemental insurance to offset the patient's share of cost for those who have Medicare traditional coverage (not Medicare Advantage), but no other health insurance, including Medicaid.

Medi–Medi: A situation in which the patient has both Medicare and Medicaid coverage.

Merit Pay: A form of individual incentive that differs from bonus payments in that merit pay becomes a part of an employee's base pay. Merit pay is usually in addition to any across-the-board cost of living increases.

Minimum Necessary: A provision under HIPAA that specifies that when using, disclosing, or obtaining from others, protected health information, all effort should be made to only use, disclose, or request the minimum information absolutely needed to satisfy the intention of that use, disclosure, or request.

Modifiers: A two-character suffix added to the end of a CPT or HCPCS code to change or provide more specific information to the basic code description.

Modular: An electronic health record system implementation strategy whereby functional modules, such as e-prescribing, are implemented in a planned manner versus implementing the full EHR at one time.

National Correct Coding Initiative (NCCI): A CMS initiative that includes a policy manual that promotes the accurate coding of claims and is based on input from a diverse group of coding and reimbursement experts. The manual is updated annually.

Nationwide Health Information Network (NHIN): A network that will provide a secure, nationwide, interoperable health information infrastructure that will connect providers, consumers, and others involved in health care. Once in place, it will enable health information to follow the consumer, be available for clinical decision making, and support appropriate use of health care information beyond direct patient care so as to improve health.

National Labor Relations Act (NLRA): A law that regulates what unions and management can and cannot do when interacting with one another and with employees.

National Labor Relations Board (NLRB): The enforcement arm of the NLRA. When a certain jurisdictional standard is reached, the NLRB will enforce the provisions of the act in the event that employees exercise their right to organize.

National Practitioner Data Bank (NPDB): A computerized database of all payments made on behalf of physicians in connection with medical liability settlements or judgments as well as adverse peer-review actions against licenses, clinical privileges, and professional society memberships of physicians and other health care practitioners.

National Uniform Claim Committee (NUCC): A voluntary committee created to develop a standardized data set for use by the non-institutional health care community to transmit claim and encounter information to and from all third-party payers. It is chaired by the American Medical Association (AMA), with the Centers for Medicare and Medicaid Services (CMS) as a critical partner.

Network Model: In a Health Maintenance Organization (HMO), a network model of managed care is a large network of physicians in each geographic area—both single-specialty and multispecialty based on physician practices—who provide services to HMO members and nonmembers but who have a negotiated fee schedule with the HMO for its members.

New Patient: A patient who has not been seen by the same physician or another physician of the same specialty in the same practice within 3 years of a current appointment.

Objectives: A desired result a person or a system envisions, plans, and commits to achieve—a personal or organizational desired end point in some sort of assumed development.

Occupational Safety and Health Act (OSHA): The primary federal law that governs occupational health and safety in the private sector and federal government in the United States.

Office of Civil Rights (OCR): A subagency of the U.S. Department of Education that is primarily focused on protecting civil rights in federally assisted education programs and prohibiting discrimination on the basis of race, color, national origin, sex, handicap, age, or membership in patriotic youth organizations.

Older Workers' Benefit Protection Act (OWBPA): A law that forbids discrimination by employers based on age when providing employee benefits, such as severance, and also ensures that no employee is coerced or pressured into signing legal waivers of rights under the Age Discrimination in Employment Act (ADEA).

ONC-Authorized Testing and Certification Bodies (ONC-ATCBs): Authorized by the Office of the National Coordinator for Health Information Technology, ONC-ATCBs are required to test and certify that certain types of EHR technology (complete EHRs and EHR modules) are compliant with the standards, implementation specifications, and certification criteria adopted by the HHS secretary and meet the definition of certified EHR technology.

Operations Budget: This is the annual budget of an activity and typically contains estimates of the total value of resources required for the performance of the operation as well as estimates of workload in terms of total work units identified by cost accounts.

Organization Chart: A diagram that shows the structure of an organization and the relationships and relative ranks of its parts and positions/jobs.

Organized Health Care Arrangement: An arrangement of covered clinically integrated providers where individuals typically receive care from more than one provider and who present themselves as such and who must have joint utilization review or quality assurance and share financial risk.

Outpatient Code Editor (OCE): It is a software program used by CMS and most claims clearinghouses that identifies errors and inconsistencies on claims that are then electronically returned to the sender to correct before CMS will process the claim for reimbursement.

Paired Comparison Method: A method of analysis where a range of options are compared and the results are tallied to find an overall winner.

Participating Physician: A physician who is contractually bound to a particular program (e.g., one enrolled in the Medicare program) and agrees to accept compensation thereunder.

Participative Leadership: A democratic leadership style that involves and engages team members.

Patient Portals: Health care–related online applications that allow patients to interact and communicate with their health care providers, such as physicians and hospitals.

Pay-for-Performance (P4P) Medical Care: A compensation system whereby providers are rewarded for meeting preestablished quality and efficiency targets for delivery of health care services; opposite of fee-for-services payment model.

Pay-for-Performance Plans (Employee Incentive): Programs where employee compensation is generally given for specific performance results rather than simply for time worked.

Personal Health Records (PHRs): A health record where health data is maintained and controlled by individual users themselves and which conforms to recognized interoperability standards enabling data to be shared at the patient's discretion.

Personal Responsibility and Work Opportunity Reconciliation Act (PRWORA): A reform law that ended welfare as an entitlement program, required recipients to begin working after 2 years of receiving benefits, placed a lifetime limit of 5 years on benefits paid by federal funds, aimed to encourage two-parent families and discourage out-of-wedlock births, and enhanced enforcement of child support.

Physician Credentialing: The process of gathering information and presenting it for review regarding a physician's qualifications for appointment or reappointment to either have privileges at a hospital or to participate with a managed care organization.

Physician Extender: A health care provider who is not a physician but who performs medical activities typically performed by a physician, most commonly a nurse practitioner or physician assistant.

Physician Office Laboratory (POL): A laboratory within the medical practice so that patients or samples don't have to be referred to an outside laboratory for those tests the lab is certified to perform.

Physician Quality Reporting Initiative (PQRI): A 2006 effort at public reporting of health care quality, this program provides incentive payments to physicians who report quality data; however, to date these results are not publicly available for use by consumers.

Plan–Do–Check–Act (PDCA) Cycle: A recurring four-step management process typically used in business; a successive cycle that starts off small to test potential effects on processes, but then gradually leads to larger and more targeted change.

Point-of-Service Plan: A type of managed care health insurance system that combines characteristics of both the HMO and the PPO in which members do not make a choice about which system to use until the point at which the service is being used.

Policies: Definitive courses or methods of action selected from alternatives and in light of given conditions to guide and determine present and future decisions.

Potentially Compensable Event (PCE): An adverse event that occurs in the delivery of health care or services with resulting injury to the patient including any adverse event or outcome, without legal fault, in which the patient experiences any unintended or unexpected negative result.

Power: The ability to get things done regardless of the source of one's power.

Practice Management System (PM): A system (modernly software) that deals with the day-to-day operations of a medical practice allowing for the capture of patient demographics, scheduling of appointments, maintenance of lists of insurance payers, performance of billing tasks, and generation of reports and which is often connected to and overlapping with the electronic health records system.

Preferred Provider Organization (PPO): A managed care organization of medical doctors, hospitals, and other health care providers who have agreed with an insurer or a third-party administrator to provide health care at reduced rates to the insurer's or administrator's clients.

Pregnancy Discrimination Act (PDA): Make illegal discrimination on the basis of pregnancy, childbirth, or related medical conditions constitutes unlawful sex discrimination; women who are pregnant must be treated in the same manner as other applicants or employees with similar abilities or limitations.

Premium: A payment paid by the insured to the insurer, in exchange for the insurer's promise to compensate (indemnify) the insured in the case of a loss to the insured.

Primary Care Physician (PCP): A physician/medical doctor who provides both the first contact for a person with an undiagnosed health concern as well as continuing care of varied medical conditions, not limited by cause, organ system, or diagnosis.

Procedures: In health care, a course of action intended to achieve a result in the care of persons with health problems.

Professional Journal: Publication intended for target marketing to a specific industry or type of trade; examples range from professional magazines to peer-reviewed journals.

Protected Health Information (PHI): Provision under HIPAA defining any information, in any format, about health status, provision of health care, or payment for health care that can be linked to a specific individual including any part of a patient's medical record or payment history.

Provider Enrollment, Chain and Ownership System (PECOS): Supports the Medicare provider and supplier enrollment process by managing, tracking, and validating enrollment data collected in both paper form and electronically via the Internet.

Provider Self-Disclosure Protocol (SDP): Provisions for voluntary disclosure by health care providers of self-discovered evidence of potential fraud to the U.S. Department of Health and Human Services Office of the Inspector General.

Quality Improvement Organizations (QIOs): Private contractor extensions of the federal government that work under the auspices of the U.S. Centers for Medicare and Medicaid Services (CMS) to monitor the appropriateness, effectiveness, and quality of care provided to Medicare beneficiaries.

Ratio: The number of times something occurs divided by the number of times it could have occurred (including the number of times it did occur) multiplied by 100 with the result being the percentage of times the something being measured actually happened.

Reasonable Accommodations: Created under the Americans with Disabilities Act, reasonable accommodations are defined as any modification or adjustment to a job or the work environment that will enable a qualified applicant or employee with a disability to participate in the application process or to perform essential job functions. Reasonable accommodation also includes adjustments to assure that a qualified individual with a disability has rights and privileges in employment equal to those of employees without disabilities.

Recovery Audit Contractors (RACs): Program was created through the Medicare Modernization Act of 2003 (MMA) to identify and recover improper Medicare payments paid to health care providers under fee-for-service Medicare plans (FFS plans).

Red Flags Rule: Policy created by the Federal Trade Commission; sets out how certain businesses and organizations must develop, implement, and administer their identity theft prevention programs.

Reengineering: The analysis and design of workflows and processes within an organization to help rethink or redesign for efficiency.

Regional Extension Centers (RECs): An extension program authorized by the HITECH Act, RECs support and serve health care providers to help them quickly become adept and meaningful users of electronic health records (EHRs).

Regional Health Information Organization (RHIO): A group of organizations within a specific geographical area that share health care–related information electronically according to national standards.

Registered Health Information Administrator (RHIA): Administrators who design and manage medical information systems, ensuring efficient record keeping while meeting state and federal requirements for medical confidentiality.

Registered Health Information Technician (RHIT): Individuals who have been trained and certified by examination to be licensed as a health information technician.

Registration Form: Forms, checklists, and guidelines to meet the management needs of registration department in hospitals and health care providers.

Remittance Advice (RA): A notice of payments and adjustments sent to providers, billers, and suppliers after a claim has been received and processed.

Representative Power: Power democratically delegated by followers to a leader for the purpose of representing followers interests.

Request for Information (RFI): A business process whose purpose is to collect written information about the capabilities of various suppliers, normally following a format that can be used for comparative purposes and often used in combination with the request for proposal (RFP), request for tender (RFT), and request for quotation (RFQ).

Request for Proposal (RFP): A process at the beginning of a project whereby an invitation is presented for suppliers, often through a bidding process, to submit a proposal on a specific commodity or service.

Resource-Based Relative Value Scale (RBRVS): A system used to determine how much money medical providers should be paid used by Medicare in the United States and by nearly all Health Maintenance Organizations (HMOs) utilizing three factors: physician work, practice expense, and malpractice expense.

Revenue Cycle: The process businesses use to describe the financial progression of their accounts receivables from the very beginning, when they first acquire product or deliver a service until they get paid and/or clear the balance owed.

Referent Power: One of five recognized forms of power (coercive, reward, legitimate, referent, and expert), referent-based power is the power derived from another person liking you or wanting to be like you. It is the power of charisma and fame.

Reward-Based Power: One of five recognized forms of power (coercive, reward, legitimate, referent, and expert), reward-based power is the ability to give other people what they want, and hence ask them to do things for you in exchange. Rewards can also be used to punish, such as when they are withheld.

Rules: Laws, bylaws, or regulations adopted to provide guidance for procedure, conduct, or action.

Safe Harbor: Legal provisions that immunize certain payment and business practices that are implicated by the antikickback statute from criminal and civil prosecution under the statute.

Scanlon Plan: A gain-sharing program combining leadership, total workforce education, and widespread employee participation with a reward system linked to group and/or organization performance in which employees share in preestablished cost savings, based upon employee effort.

Secure Messaging: Technology for protecting sensitive data when sent beyond the corporate borders and providing compliance with industry regulations such as HIPAA.

Short-Term Planning Management Strategy: A strategy that takes into account goals and objectives in the near future.

SMART Goals: A mnemonic (specific, measureable, attainable, realistic, timely) used to set objectives in areas such as project management, employee performance management, or personal development.

SOAP Order: A standardized method of documentation of patient symptoms, diagnosis, and care consisting of subjective component, objective component, application or assessment, and plan.

Social Media: The use of Web-based and mobile technologies to turn communication into interactive dialogue creating social interaction.

Society for Human Resource Management (SHRM): A professional human resources association headquartered in Alexandria, Virginia.

Soft Skills: A term relating to a cluster of personality traits, social graces, communication, language, personal habits, friendliness, and optimism (sometimes called an "EQ" or emotional intelligence quotient) that characterize relationships with other people. Soft skills complement hard skills which are the occupational requirements of a job.

Source Document: A document in which data collected for a clinical trial is first recorded.

Span of Control: In business management, refers to the number of subordinates a supervisor has.

Spoliation of Records: The alteration or destruction of medical records.

Staff Authority: Authority to advise, but not to direct, other managers.

Staff Model: A HMO where physicians are employed and all premiums are paid to the HMO and in which covered insurers must select a primary care physician, who has control over referrals to other physicians in or out of the group.

Standards: Models or examples; rules for the measure of quantity, value, extent, or quality.

Stark Law: Regulates physician self-referral for Medicare and Medicaid patients.

Summary Plan Description: A document containing a comprehensive description of a retirement plan that must be filed with the Department of Labor that includes the terms and conditions of participation and which is distributed to all potential participants in advance of enrollment.

Superbill: An itemized form utilized by health care providers for reflecting rendered services; the main data source for creation of a health care claim, which will be submitted to payers (insurances, funds, and programs) for reimbursement.

Sustainable Growth Rate (SGR): The maximum rate at which a company can grow revenue without having to invest new equity capital. For Medicare, SGR pertains to a formula of reimbursement for services that calculates the amount Medicare is able to pay out in benefits based on projected existing and new revenue for the period under consideration and still sustain itself.

SWOT Analysis: A strategic planning method used to evaluate the strengths, weaknesses, opportunities, and threats involved in a project or in a business venture by specifying the objective of the business venture or project and identifying the internal and external factors that are favorable and unfavorable to achieve that objective.

Tax Relief and Health Care Act (TRHCA): Provided key changes to health care savings accounts and modified, extended, and added new provisions regarding tax credits for several different groups.

Team-based Incentive Plans: Compensation plan offering a reward to the entire group for generating positive results.

Telephone Interview: A meeting or consultation between a provider and a patient over the telephone to solicit information regarding treatment, payment, or health care operations.

Top-Down Budgeting: Budgets are created by top management based on organization-wide knowledge of goals and projected revenue and then templates with specific instructions are distributed down to individual department managers from top management to use in developing each department budget.

Total Quality Management (TQM): An integrative philosophy of management for continuously improving the quality of products and processes that contends that the quality of products and processes is the responsibility of everyone who is involved with the creation or consumption of the products or services offered by an organization.

Treatment, Payment, and Operations Information (TPO): Those areas defined in the HIPAA Privacy Rule under which a covered entity is prohibited from using or disclosing protected health information (PHI). The core health care activities of "treatment," "payment," and "health care operations" are defined in the Privacy Rule at 45 CFR 164.501.

Tricare: A health care program of the U.S. Department of Defense Military Health System that provides civilian health benefits for military personnel, military retirees, and their dependents.

Unbundling: There are codes that combine procedures commonly performed together (such as all of the laboratory tests that are typically done to determine a person's overall heart health) into one code. Unbundling is coding each individual code separately instead of using the combination code. Unbundling is not legal or ethical.

Uniformed Services Employment and Reemployment Rights Act (USERRA): A law that establishes, with some exceptions, the cumulative length of time that an individual may be absent from work for military duty and retain reemployment rights to 5 years. USERRA clearly establishes that reemployment protection does not depend on the timing, frequency, duration, or nature of an individual's service as long as the basic eligibility criteria are met.

Unity of Command: Each employee has only one boss. One of the 14 principles of management.

Upcoding: The act of choosing a higher code than warranted by the patient's condition.

Usual, Customary, and Reasonable (UCR): The base amount that third-party payers (including insurance carriers and employers) generally use to determine how much will be paid, on behalf of an enrollee, for services that are reimbursed under a health insurance policy or health plan.

Voice Recognition: A combination of speaker recognition (recognizing who is speaking) and speech recognition (recognizing what is being said). It uses learned aspects of a speaker's voice to determine what is being said. Many electronic medical records (EMRs) applications can be more effective and may be performed more easily when deployed in conjunction with a speech–recognition engine.

Whistle-Blowing: The reporting to the public or someone in authority about alleged dishonest or illegal activities or misconduct occurring in government, public or private organizations, or companies.

Work Simplification: A scientific study of work processes with a view to making that process more efficient and effective by making them more simple and thereby raising productivity and reducing labor, materials, space, time, and energy in the process of producing goods or delivering a services.

Workers' Compensation: A form of insurance that provides wage replacement and medical benefits for employees who are injured in the course of employment. Workers' compensation is administered on a state-by-state basis but is provided in most states by private insurance companies. The federal government has its own workers' compensation program.

INDEX

Note: Page numbers in *italics* denote figures; those followed by a "t" denote tables; those followed by "b" indicate a box